THE WASHINGTON MANUAL™

Gastroenterology Subspecialty Consult

Third Edition

Editor

C. Prakash Gyawali, MD, MRCP
Professor of Medicine
Division of Gastroenterology
Washington University School of Medicine
St. Louis, Missouri

Series Editors

Katherine E. Henderson, MD
Assistant Professor of Clinical Medicine
Department of Medicine
Division of Medical Education
Washington University School of Medicine
Barnes-Jewish Hospital
St. Louis, Missouri

Thomas M. De Fer, MD
Associate Professor of Internal Medicine
Washington University School of Medicine
St. Louis, Missouri

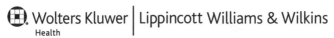

Wolters Kluwer | Lippincott Williams & Wilkins
Health
Philadelphia • Baltimore • New York • London
Buenos Aires • Hong Kong • Sydney • Tokyo

Acquisitions Editor: Sonya Seigafuse
Product Manager: Kerry Barrett
Vendor Manager: Bridgett Dougherty
Marketing Manager: Kimberly Schonberger
Manufacturing Manager: Ben Rivera
Design Coordinator: Stephen Druding
Editorial Coordinator: Katie Sharp
Production Service: Aptara, Inc.

© 2012 by Department of Medicine, Washington University School of Medicine

Printed in China

Library of Congress Cataloging-in-Publication Data
The Washington manual gastroenterology subspecialty consult / editor, C. Prakash Gyawali. — 3rd ed.
   p. ; cm. — (Washington manual subspecialty consult series)
   Includes bibliographical references and index.
   ISBN 978-1-4511-1410-2 (alk. paper) — ISBN 1-4511-1410-9 (alk. paper)
   I. Gyawali, C. Prakash.   II. Series: Washington manual subspecialty consult series.
   [DNLM: 1. Digestive System Diseases—diagnosis—Handbooks.   2. Digestive System Diseases—Therapy—Handbooks. WI 39]
   616.3′3—dc23

                                                                                    2011052164

The Washington Manual™ is an intent-to-use mark belonging to Washington University in St. Louis to which international legal protection applies. The mark is used in this publication by LWW under license from Washington University.

Care has been taken to confirm the accuracy of the information presented and to describe generally accepted practices. However, the authors, editors, and publisher are not responsible for errors or omissions or for any consequences from application of the information in this book and make no warranty, expressed or implied, with respect to the currency, completeness, or accuracy of the contents of the publication. Application of the information in a particular situation remains the professional responsibility of the practitioner.

The authors, editors, and publisher have exerted every effort to ensure that drug selection and dosage set forth in this text are in accordance with current recommendations and practice at the time of publication. However, in view of ongoing research, changes in government regulations, and the constant flow of information relating to drug therapy and drug reactions, the reader is urged to check the package insert for each drug for any change in indications and dosage and for added warnings and precautions. This is particularly important when the recommended agent is a new or infrequently employed drug.

Some drugs and medical devices presented in the publication have Food and Drug Administration (FDA) clearance for limited use in restricted research settings. It is the responsibility of the health care providers to ascertain the FDA status of each drug or device planned for use in their clinical practice.

To purchase additional copies of this book, call our customer service department at (800) 638-3030 or fax orders to (301) 223-2320. International customers should call (301) 223-2300.

Visit Lippincott Williams & Wilkins on the Internet: at LWW.com. Lippincott Williams & Wilkins customer service representatives are available from 8:30 am to 6 pm, EST.

10 9 8 7 6 5 4 3 2 1

CCS0312

Contributing Authors

Anupam Aditi, MD
Resident
Department of Internal Medicine
Washington University School of Medicine
St. Louis, Missouri

Akwi W. Asombang, MD
Fellow
Division of Gastroenterology
Washington University School of Medicine
St. Louis, Missouri

Riad Azar, MD
Associate Professor of Medicine
Division of Gastroenterology
Washington University School of Medicine
St. Louis, Missouri

Elizabeth Blaney, MD
Resident
Department of Internal Medicine
Washington University School of Medicine
St. Louis, Missouri

Benjamin E. Cassell, MD
Resident
Department of Internal Medicine
Washington University School of Medicine
St. Louis, Missouri

Chien-Huan Chen, MD
Assistant Professor of Medicine
Division of Gastroenterology
Washington University School of Medicine
St. Louis, Missouri

Reena V. Chokshi, MD
Fellow
Division of Gastroenterology
Washington University School of Medicine
St. Louis, Missouri

Matthew A. Ciorba, MD
Assistant Professor of Medicine
Division of Gastroenterology
Washington University School of Medicine
St. Louis, Missouri

Jeffrey S. Crippin, MD
Professor of Medicine
Division of Gastroenterology
Washington University School of Medicine
St. Louis, Missouri

Dayna S. Early, MD
Professor of Medicine
Division of Gastroenterology
Washington University School of Medicine
St. Louis, Missouri

Darrell M. Gray, II, MD
Fellow
Division of Gastroenterology
Washington University School of Medicine
St. Louis, Missouri

C. Prakash Gyawali, MD, MRCP
Professor of Medicine
Division of Gastroenterology
Washington University School of Medicine
St. Louis, Missouri

Heba Iskandar, MD
Fellow
Division of Gastroenterology
Washington University School of Medicine
St. Louis, Missouri

John M. Iskander, MD
Fellow
Division of Gastroenterology
Washington University School of Medicine
St. Louis, Missouri

Sreenivasa Jonnalagadda, MD
Professor of Medicine
Division of Gastroenterology
Washington University School of Medicine
St. Louis, Missouri

Thomas A. Kerr, MD
Assistant Professor of Medicine
Division of Gastroenterology
Washington University School of Medicine
St. Louis, Missouri

Kevin M. Korenblat, MD
Associate Professor of Medicine
Division of Gastroenterology
Washington University School of Medicine
St. Louis, Missouri

Gowri Kularatna, MD
Fellow
Division of Gastroenterology
Washington University School of Medicine
St. Louis, Missouri

Mridula V. Kumar, MD
Fellow
Division of Gastroenterology
Washington University School of Medicine
St. Louis, Missouri

Vladimir Kushnir, MD
Fellow
Division of Gastroenterology
Washington University School of Medicine
St. Louis, Missouri

Alexander Lee, MD
Resident
Department of Internal Medicine
Washington University School of Medicine
St. Louis, Missouri

Mauricio Lisker-Melman, MD
Professor of Medicine
Division of Gastroenterology
Washington University School of Medicine
St. Louis, Missouri

Faiz Mirza, MD
Fellow
Division of Gastroenterology
Washington University School of Medicine
St. Louis, Missouri

Daniel Mullady, MD
Associate Professor of Medicine
Division of Gastroenterology
Washington University School of Medicine
St. Louis, Missouri

Amit Patel, MD
Resident
Department of Internal Medicine
Washington University School of Medicine
St. Louis, Missouri

Nishant J. Patel, MD
Resident
Department of Internal Medicine
Washington University School of Medicine
St. Louis, Missouri

Andrew Reinink, MD
Resident
Department of Internal Medicine
Washington University School of Medicine
St. Louis, Missouri

Gregory S. Sayuk, MD
Assistant Professor of Medicine
Division of Gastroenterology
Washington University School of Medicine
St. Louis, Missouri

Jonathan Seccombe, MD
Resident
Department of Internal Medicine
Washington University School of Medicine
St. Louis, Missouri

Anil B. Seetharam, MD
Fellow
Division of Gastroenterology
Washington University School of Medicine
St. Louis, Missouri

Anisa Shaker, MD
Assistant Professor of Medicine
Division of Gastroenterology
Washington University School of Medicine
St. Louis, Missouri

Noura M. Sharabash, MD
Fellow
Division of Gastroenterology
Washington University School of Medicine
St. Louis, Missouri

Jennifer Shroff, MD
Resident
Department of Internal Medicine
Washington University School of Medicine
St. Louis, Missouri

A. Samad Soudagar, MD
Resident
Department of Internal Medicine
Washington University School of Medicine
St. Louis, Missouri

Shelby A. Sullivan, MD
Assistant Professor of Medicine
Division of Gastroenterology
Washington University School of Medicine
St. Louis, Missouri

Hongha (Susan) T. Vu, MD
Fellow
Division of Gastroenterology
Washington University School of Medicine
St. Louis, Missouri

Sachin Wani, MD
Advanced Fellow
Division of Gastroenterology
Washington University School of Medicine
St. Louis, Missouri

Chairman's Note

I t is a pleasure to present the new edition of *The Washington Manual*® Subspecialty Consult Series: Gastroenterology Subspecialty Consult. This pocket-size book continues to be a primary reference for medical students, interns, residents, and other practitioners who need ready access to practical clinical information to diagnose and treat patients with a wide variety of disorders. Medical knowledge continues to increase at an astounding rate, which creates a challenge for physicians to keep up with the biomedical discoveries, genetic and genomic information, and novel therapeutics that can positively impact patient outcomes. *The Washington Manual* Subspecialty Consult Series addresses this challenge by concisely and practically providing current scientific information for clinicians to aid them in the diagnosis, investigation, and treatment of common medical conditions.

I want to personally thank the authors, which include house officers, fellows, and attendings at Washington University School of Medicine and Barnes Jewish Hospital. Their commitment to patient care and education is unsurpassed, and their efforts and skill in compiling this manual are evident in the quality of the final product. In particular, I would like to acknowledge our editor Dr. C. Prakash Gyawali and the series editors Drs. Katherine Henderson and Tom De Fer, who have worked tirelessly to produce another outstanding edition of this manual. I would also like to thank Dr. Melvin Blanchard, Chief of the Division of Medical Education, Department at of Medicine, Washington University School of Medicine, for his advice and guidance. I believe this *Manual* will meet its desired goal of providing practical knowledge that can be directly applied at the bedside and in outpatient settings to improve patient care.

Victoria J. Fraser, MD
Dr. J. William Campbell Professor
Interim Chairman of Medicine
Codirector, Infectious Disease Division
Washington University School of Medicine

Preface

G astroenterology continues to expand as a specialty, with a wealth of new insights on disease pathophysiology, diagnostic tools, and management options. In addition, certain disorders such as eosinophilic esophagitis, autoimmune enteropathy and autoimmune pancreatitis are being increasingly recognized and managed. Genetic testing now has a defined role in many gastrointestinal disorders, including colon cancer, and is actively utilized in clinical gastroenterology. Given these advances, it is clear that there is ongoing need for easy access of concise diagnostic and management direction for the novice and intermediate trainee, a need that this manual fulfills. The unique aspect of this manual is that it is conceived and written by trainees for trainees, with extensive mentoring and editing from academic faculty experts. The manual therefore describes symptoms and disease entities that are encountered most often in clinical units, both ambulatory and inpatient. The manual strives to provide a succinct yet descriptive synopsis of each condition, presenting the reader with disease characteristics, clinical features, investigation, and management.

With the widespread distribution and review of the second edition of the manual, it became evident that certain areas needed additional emphasis. The format of individual diseases and symptoms has been revised to follow specific subheadings to bring uniformity to the manual and to the Subspecialty Consult Series as a whole. The manual has been extensively updated. Two new chapters are included, Liver Transplantation and Genetic Testing in Gastrointestinal Diseases. In addition, the chapter on Nutrition has been revised to reflect Malnutrition. Extended segments have been updated, and in some cases, entire chapters have been rewritten by current Washington University internal medicine residents aspiring to become gastroenterologists and gastroenterology fellows currently enrolled in fellowship training, all under the watchful eyes of faculty experts. The third edition of the manual therefore represents an up-to-date yet concise treatise on current knowledge of common gastrointestinal ailments.

I would like to extend my gratitude to all the trainees and faculty mentors who worked tirelessly to ensure that their chapters were updated and that they conformed to the revised formats. For our trainee authors entering the field of gastroenterology, seeing their contributions in print will hopefully provide them renewed enthusiasm and vigor for continued scholarship and education, and ultimately the opportunity to return the favor by furthering education of future trainees.

—C.P.G.

Contents

PART I. APPROACH TO SPECIFIC SYMPTOMS

PART II. APPROACH TO SPECIFIC DISEASES

Dysphagia

Faiz Mirza

GENERAL PRINCIPLES

- Dysphagia is a common patient complaint that requires prompt evaluation and management.

Definition

- Dysphagia is defined as **difficulty in swallowing or the sensation of an obstruction in the passage of food** (semisolid, solid, and/or liquid) **anywhere from the mouth to the stomach.**[1]
- Dysphagia should be distinguished from the following:
  - **Odynophagia:** pain during swallowing (dysphagia and odynophagia may coexist in the same patient).
  - **Globus:** constant sensation of a lump or fullness in throat without difficulty swallowing.
  - **Aphagia:** inability to swallow, which can result when a food bolus gets impacted in the esophagus, thus blocking passage of any further boluses. Aphagia can also result from pharyngeal muscle paralysis from lower cranial nerve involvement.
  - **Xerostomia:** dryness of the mouth from decreased salivation (from Sjogren's syndrome, radiation to head and neck, medication side effects, etc.), which can cause trouble initiating a swallow because of poor lubrication of the food bolus.

Classification

- Dysphagia can be classified as oropharyngeal or esophageal.[1]
- **Oropharyngeal dysphagia**
  - Arises from disorders that affect the function of the oropharynx, larynx, and upper esophageal sphincter (UES).
  - Typically caused by lesions of the swallowing center, cranial nerves, or oropharyngeal muscles, mucosa, or teeth.[2]
  - Results from defects in oral and pharyngeal phases of swallowing.[3]
  - These disorders cause difficulties with preparing the food for swallowing or with transferring a bolus of food from oral cavity to esophagus.
  - Patients with oropharyngeal dysphagia may report difficulty initiating a swallow, coughing, choking, drooling, or nasal regurgitation. This sensation is typically reported within 1 second of initiating a swallow.[3]
- **Esophageal dysphagia**
  - Arises commonly from structural defects within the body of the esophagus, the lower esophageal sphincter (LES), or gastric cardia.
  - May be caused by diseases of the esophageal smooth muscle, the autonomic nervous system, and/or mucosa of the esophagus.[2]

- ○ Dysphagia is typically reported with solid foods initially.
- ○ Can result from motor abnormalities in lower esophageal sphincter relaxation or the esophageal phase of swallowing. Dysphagia can result from both solids and liquids in neuromuscular disorders.
- ○ Patients may describe the sensation of food sticking in the throat or the chest, retrosternal chest pain, or regurgitation soon after swallowing. The regurgitate may taste similar to food just eaten and not sour or bitter (which implicates retrograde transit from the stomach, as in reflux disease or emesis).
- ○ The sensation of dysphagia may be referred to the sternal notch despite the fact that the point of obstruction may be in the distal esophagus.

Epidemiology

- It is estimated that nearly 16% to 22% of individuals older than 50 years describe symptoms of dysphagia.[3]

Etiology

- Oropharyngeal dysphagia is most commonly caused by neurogenic and myogenic disorders and rarely occurs as a result of oropharyngeal or base-of-skull tumors.
- Esophageal dysphagia is either the result of a structural esophageal (luminal, intramural or extraluminal) lesion or a neuromuscular disorder of esophageal peristalsis. In recent years, eosinophilic esophagitis, an idiopathic eosinophilic inflammatory disease with remodeling of the esophagus, is becoming increasingly recognized as a cause for esophageal dysphagia, particularly in young adults.

Pathophysiology

- **The normal swallowing process can be divided into three phases[4]:**
  - ○ **Oral:** The food bolus is first mechanically prepared by the muscles of the jaw, face, and tongue, and propelled posteriorly and superiorly by the tongue and the palate. This process lasts 1 to 2 seconds.
  - ○ **Pharyngeal:** This phase begins when the bolus passes the anterior tonsillar pillars. The soft palate closes the nasopharynx, and the lips and the jaws remain closed. The larynx elevates and closes the laryngeal valves (epiglottis and vocal cords). This also opens the upper esophageal sphincter, allowing passage of the bolus into the esophagus. The entire process lasts <1 second.
  - ○ **Esophageal:** This phase begins with the entry of the bolus into the esophagus. The upper esophageal sphincter closes, and bolus is propelled efficiently through the esophagus to the stomach. In the upright position, this is facilitated by gravity, with the esophageal muscle contraction stripping the remnants of the bolus through an open lower esophageal sphincter. Secondary esophageal peristalsis may initiate in response to esophageal distension if the primary peristaltic effort is insufficient in propelling the bolus.
- **Dysphagia is caused by a disruption in this process**
  - ○ **Oropharyngeal dysphagia:** occurs when there is a disruption in the oral or pharyngeal phases of swallowing.
  - ○ **Esophageal dysphagia:** occurs when there is a disruption in the esophageal phase of swallowing.

DIAGNOSIS

Clinical Presentation

- **Oropharyngeal**
  - Oropharyngeal dysphagia is **commonly a manifestation of a systemic disorder** (Table 1-1). A careful and directed history specifically intended to include or rule out neurologic, muscular, collagen vascular, and local structural disorders is essential.
  - Patients complain of difficulty initiating a swallow, coughing, choking, drooling, or nasal regurgitation within 1 second of initiating a swallow.
  - Patients have difficulty with swallowing solids and/or liquids.
  - Evidence of neurologic dysfunction in the lower cranial nerves, or of generalized muscle weakness or dystrophy may be evident on physical examination.
- **Esophageal**
  - Esophageal dysphagia is **typically related to an esophageal process, either structural or neuromuscular.**
  - Patients complain of food sticking in the throat or the chest.
  - Symptoms start a few seconds after swallowing.
  - Patients have difficulty swallowing solids at the start, particularly with structural lesions. This can progress to difficulty with liquids. Motor disorders may be associated with dysphagia to both solids and liquids.
  - Regurgitation and chest pain may be associated symptoms.

History
- A carefully taken symptom history can provide clues to the underlying cause of dysphagia.[3]

TABLE 1-1   CAUSES OF OROPHARYNGEAL DYSPHAGIA

Neuromuscular Disorders

Cerebrovascular accident
Parkinson's disease
Amyotrophic lateral sclerosis
Poliomyelitis
Polymyositis
Myasthenia gravis
Brain tumors
Hypothyroidism
Abnormal upper esophageal sphincter relaxation

Structural Lesions

Neoplasm
Inflammation (pharyngitis, radiation)
Plummer-Vinson syndrome
Cervical hyperostosis
Thyromegaly
Lymphadenopathy
Prior oropharyngeal surgery
Zenker's diverticulum

- It is important to determine whether the patient has esophageal or oropharyngeal dysphagia.[3] The following are factors important in making this determination:
  - Duration of symptoms and acuity of onset
  - Whether symptoms are intermittent or progressive
  - The presence or absence of aspiration symptoms, that is, cough or choking episodes while swallowing
  - Symptoms of lower cranial nerve dysfunction, such as regurgitation through the nose, drooling, or food spilling from the corners of the mouth
  - Associated symptoms like heartburn or chest pain
  - Medications the patient takes (including over-the-counter medications). Medications that are commonly prescribed can cause dysphagia in the oropharyngeal or esophageal stages of swallowing. For example, tetracycline, clindamycin, and doxycycline can cause direct esophageal mucosal injury.[5]
  - Other preexisting medical conditions, including atopic disorders and asthma, which may be relevant in eosinophilic esophagitis
  - The patients can be asked to describe where they feel the disturbance is located
  - Food items that typically cause difficulty (specifically, solids, liquids, or both)
  - History of radiation therapy to head and neck
  - The presence of weight loss[1]

Physical Examination

- General examination: evaluate nutritional status (including body weight).
- Complete neurologic examination (attention to resting tremor, cranial nerves, and muscle strength).
- Examine oral cavity, head, and neck.
- If the patient describes easy fatigability, observe the patient while performing a repetitive task (e.g., blinking, counting aloud).[3]
- Observe the patient's gait and balance (one reason for this is to check for Parkinson's disease).
- Examine the skin for thickening or texture changes (especially palms of hands and the soles of feet).[1]
- Evaluate the neck for thyromegaly or other mass.
- Inspect the muscles for wasting and fasciculations and palpate for tenderness to detect an underlying motor neuron disease.[3]

Differential Diagnosis

- **Oropharyngeal dysphagia**
  - Neuromuscular causes are more frequent than structural causes for this type of dysphagia. This is mainly because the nerves that control the muscles in this region have a direct connection to the brain through cranial nerves and can be damaged in accidents or diseases that affect the brain or the cranial nerves.[3]
  - Table 1-1 refers to some of the more frequent causes of oropharyngeal dysphagia.
- **Esophageal dysphagia**
  - Generally, structural causes are a more frequent cause of this type of dysphagia than disorders involving nerves and muscles.
  - A structural disorder will initially cause dysphagia to solid foods but may later include liquids as well. Eosinophilic esophagitis can present with intermittent food bolus impactions.

| TABLE 1-2 | CAUSES OF ESOPHAGEAL DYSPHAGIA |

Structural Causes

Benign stricture
Esophageal cancer
Schatzki ring
Esophageal webs
Foreign bodies
Extrinsic (vascular, cervical osteoarthritis, adenopathy)

Motility Disorders

Achalasia
Scleroderma
Hypertensive lower esophageal sphincter
Diffuse esophageal spasm
Chagas' disease
Nutcracker esophagus

- Patients with a neuromuscular disorder commonly report dysphagia to both solids and liquids from the onset of symptoms.[1]
- Table 1-2 refers to some of the more frequent causes of esophageal dysphagia.

Diagnostic Testing

- **If oropharyngeal dysphagia is suspected:**
  - **A careful neurologic examination is the first step in evaluation.**
  - **Modified barium swallow/videofluoroscopy**[4]: This consists of a radiographic study in which the oral and pharyngeal phases are observed in real time while the patient swallows barium of varying consistencies, such as thin liquids, thick liquids, and barium cookies, or a cracker. This study helps identify abnormalities of the oropharyngeal phases and may direct therapy. Patients may tolerate certain consistencies better than others, and the diet can be modified accordingly.
  - **Laryngoscopy:** If structural lesions are identified, direct laryngoscopy should be performed for further evaluation.
  - **High-resolution manometry:** Newer techniques of esophageal manometry may have value in evaluation of pharyngeal muscle and upper esophageal sphincter function. Recent advances have incorporated tactile sensor technology to high-resolution manometry (3D high-resolution manometry) that may have value in defining sphincter function.
- **If esophageal dysphagia is suspected:**
  - **Upper endoscopy:** This is the most useful initial test, because it allows for direct visualization of the esophagus and permits tissue biopsy and dilation of structural narrowing if found.[6] An upper endoscopy is the test of choice in the evaluation of esophageal dysphagia and should be the first test ordered.
  - **Esophagram (barium swallow):** Alternate test that is useful when subtle strictures or narrowings are suspected or when road mapping of a tight or complicated stricture is desired before endoscopic evaluation. This test can also provide information on the length and degree of narrowing of a structural

lesion.[6] An esophagogram commonly reveals structural esophageal abnormalities such as tumors, webs, and rings, or aids in the detection of subtle abnormalities. Motility disorders, such as achalasia, diffuse esophageal spasm, and scleroderma esophagus, have typical esophagram findings, but esophageal manometry is typically required for a definitive diagnosis.

○ **Esophageal manometry:** This method is considered when no structural or obstructive process is identified on upper endoscopy or barium esophagram in patients presenting with dysphagia.[1] It involves the passage of a thin catheter through the nose, down the esophagus, and past the LES. Pressure measurements are then obtained over the full length of the esophagus, including the UES and the LES, both at rest and during a swallow.[7] High-resolution esophageal manometry involves using a solid state catheter with 36 circumferential sensors 1 cm apart and provides high-fidelity topograms (Clouse plots) of esophageal peristalsis and sphincter function. This has been demonstrated to substantially improve the sensitivity of diagnosis of LES relaxation abnormalities. The addition of stationary impedance to high-resolution manometry and the incorporation of viscous and solid boluses to manometry testing may improve the yield for a motor diagnosis in the evaluation of dysphagia.

TREATMENT

Medications

Medications are **useful only if they can treat the underlying condition causing dysphagia.**

Other Nonpharmacologic Therapies

- **Oropharyngeal dysphagia**
  ○ When possible, treatment should be directed at the underlying disorder.
  ○ However, many patients have irreversible or progressive neurologic diseases, which can lead to worsening oropharyngeal dysphagia.
  ○ **Consultation with a speech therapist** is often helpful in modifying eating behaviors and food consistency.[4]
  ○ Despite these interventions, some patients will still experience oropharyngeal dysphagia placing them at a high risk for aspiration or inadequate caloric intake.
  ○ If significant improvement of oropharyngeal dysphagia is not expected, alternative sources of **nutritional support** should be pursued. Options may include nasogastric feeding tube, or enteral feeding through percutaneous gastrostomy or jejunostomy tubes.
  ○ Excessive drooling or troublesome oropharyngeal secretions can sometimes be suppressed using anticholinergic agents or tricyclic antidepressants.
- **Esophageal dysphagia**
  ○ Management of esophageal dysphagia should be tailored to the underlying disorder (see Chapter 12 for more detail).
  ○ **Endoscopic therapies,** including dilation of strictures and disruption of esophageal rings, can be helpful in the management of structural causes of esophageal dysphagia.
  ○ **Eosinophilic esophagitis can be treated with topical steroids and exclusion diets;** intermittent dilation of dominant strictures may be sometimes necessary.

○ Empiric endoscopic dilation with a large caliber dilator is often performed in patients wherein a definitive etiology for esophageal-type dysphagia is not apparent on routine investigation. This approach may result in symptomatic improvement of varying durations.

○ Obstructing tumors can be treated with dilation or by placement of an endoscopic stent.

○ Some motility disorders are amenable to endoscopic therapy, including botulinum toxin injection into the LES in disorders of LES relaxation.

○ Surgical myotomy and pneumatic dilation are durable options in achalasia.

○ **Gastrostomy tube placement** may be indicated in patients with large, obstructing esophageal tumors that are not amenable to dilation or stent placement.

Lifestyle/Risk Modification

Diet

Treatment of dysphagia can include a change in the patient's diet or the consistency of the diet to aid swallowing. A **modified barium swallow may help identify certain consistencies that can be swallowed** better than others. This is particularly relevant in oropharyngeal dysphagia from neuromuscular disease and in esophageal dysphagia where there is residual dysphagia after treatment.

Activity

A speech–language pathologist can help a patient learn different **exercises and head and neck positions that may help facilitate swallowing.**[3]

SPECIAL CONSIDERATIONS

• **Functional dysphagia:** A disorder that is characterized by a sensation of abnormal bolus transit through the esophagus in the absence of structural lesions, GERD, and histopathology-based esophageal motility disorders. Functional dysphagia includes the sense of solid and/or liquid foods sticking, lodging, or passing through esophagus.[8] This is related to increased perception of esophageal sensation, sometimes triggered by noxious triggers like gastroesophageal reflux disease. In addition to treating associated reflux disease, neuromodulators (e.g., low-dose tricyclic antidepressants) may be of value.

COMPLICATIONS

• The most common complications with dysphagia include **aspiration, pneumonia, and dehydration.**[9] Prolonged dysphagia can lead to weight loss and malnutrition. Aggressive dilation of esophageal strictures can rarely result in esophageal perforation.

REFERRAL

• Treating a patient with dysphagia is often a joint effort of a team of specialists including a gastroenterologist, radiologist, speech–language therapist, neurologist, otolaryngologist, and nutritionist.[3]

OUTCOME/PROGNOSIS

- The improvement of symptoms often depends on the type of dysphagia.
- In the case of strictures, tumors, and cervical webs, surgery, dilation, antineoplastic therapy, or a combination of these treatments may be used.[3] An alternative option, especially with untreatable tumors, is stent placement.
- Certain types of dysphagia such as those caused by acid reflux disease, esophageal infections, and eosinophilic esophagitis may be treated with medical therapy.
- Dysphagia caused by achalasia can be treated with pneumatic balloon dilation, botulinum toxin injection, or myotomy.[6]

REFERENCES

1. Trate DM, Parkman HP, Fisher RS. Dysphagia evaluation, diagnosis, and treatment. *Gastroenterology.* 1996;23:417–432.
2. Schechter GL. Systemic causes of dysphagia in adults. *Otolaryngol Clin North Am.* 1998; 31:525–535.
3. Cook IJ, Kahrilas PJ. AGA technical review on management of oropharyngeal Dysphagia. *Gastroenterology.* 1999;116:455–478.
4. Logemann JA. Swallowing disorders. *Best Pract Res Clin Gastroenterol.* 2007;21:563–573.
5. Spieker MR. Evaluating dysphagia. *Am Fam Physician.* 2000;61:3639–3648.
6. Spechler SJ. AGA technical review on treatment of patients with dysphagia caused by benign disorders of distal esophagus. *Gastroenterology.* 1999;117:233–254.
7. Roman S, Pandolfino J, Mion F. High-resolution manometry: a new gold standard to diagnose esophageal dysmotility? *Gastroenterol Clin Biol.* 2009;33:1061–1067.
8. Galmiche JP, Clouse RE, Balint A, et al. Functional esophageal disorders. *Gastroenterology.* 2006;130:1459–1465.
9. Schindler A, Ginocchio D, Ruoppolo G. What we don't know about dysphagia complications? *Rev Laryngol Otol Rhinol (Bord).* 2008;129:75–80.

Nausea and Vomiting

2

Vladimir Kushnir and C. Prakash Gyawali

GENERAL PRINCIPLES

- Nausea is one of the most common gastrointestinal (GI) symptoms and can be related to a wide variety of GI, systemic, and neurologic disorders.
- Nausea can precede the act of emesis, occur concurrently with emesis, or occur on its own.
- Altered autonomic activity and decreased function of the upper GI tract can accompany severe nausea.

Definitions

- **Nausea** refers to the feeling of an imminent urge to vomit and is usually sensed in the throat or epigastrium. It can be accompanied by transient hypersalivation, lightheadedness or dizziness, and sweating.
- **Vomiting** (or emesis) denotes the forceful ejection of GI contents through the mouth. The act of emesis is a highly coordinated event requiring the integration of both central and peripheral nervous systems.[1]

Epidemiology

- Nausea and vomiting are commonly reported symptoms. Prevalence in the community is estimated at 12%. Nausea and vomiting are frequent reasons for consultation with a gastroenterologist and contribute significantly to hospital costs and physician visits.

Etiology

- Clinically important etiologies of nausea and vomiting are listed in Table 2-1.
- **Medications**
  - **Antiparkinsonian agents** (e.g., l-DOPA, bromocriptine), nicotine, and digoxin produce nausea and vomiting through direct action on receptors in the chemoreceptor trigger zone.
  - **Nonsteroidal anti-inflammatory drugs (NSAIDs) and antibiotics**, such as erythromycin, stimulate peripheral afferent pathways to activate the vomiting center directly.[2]
  - **Opioid analgesics** cause nausea in >25% of patients. Multiple mechanisms have been implicated, including direct stimulation of the chemoreceptor trigger zone, reduced GI motility, or enhanced vestibular sensitivity.
  - **Chemotherapeutic agents** frequently cause nausea and vomiting. Acute vomiting, usually caused by agents such as cisplatin, nitrogen mustard, and dacarbazine, is generally mediated through serotonergic pathways, both centrally and peripherally. Delayed and anticipatory vomiting is serotonin independent.
  - **Cannabis,** when used on a long-term basis, can result in an illness that resembles cyclic vomiting syndrome, termed cannabinoid hyperemesis.

TABLE 2-1	DIFFERENTIAL DIAGNOSIS OF NAUSEA AND VOMITING

Medications

Chemotherapy: cisplatin, dacarbazine, nitrogen mustard

Analgesics

Oral contraceptives

Cardiovascular: digoxin, antiarrhythmics, β-blockers, antihypertensives, calcium channel blockers

Antibiotics: erythromycin, tetracycline, sulfonamides

Sulfasalazine

Azathioprine

Antiparkinsonian agents

Theophylline

Infections

Gastroenteritis

Viral: rotavirus, Norwalk virus, adenovirus, reovirus

Bacterial: *Staphylococcus aureus, Salmonella, Bacillus cereus,* and *Clostridium perfringens* (toxins)

Systemic nongastrointestinal infections

Other Disorders

Pregnancy

Uremia

Diabeti'c ketoacidosis

Addison's disease

Postoperative nausea and vomiting

Cardiac ischemia or infarction

Gastrointestinal and Peritoneal Disorders

Peptic ulcer disease

Appendicitis

Hepatitis

Mesenteric ischemia

Pancreatitis

Cholecystitis

Gastric outlet obstruction

Small bowel obstruction

Gastroparesis

Nonulcer dyspepsia

Central Nervous System Disorders

Increased intracranial pressure: tumor, hemorrhage, pseudotumor cerebri

Migraine

Psychogenic vomiting

Cyclic vomiting syndrome

Anorexia Nervosa

Bulimia nervosa

Labyrinthine disorders

Cannabis-induced autonomic dysregulation and abnormal gastric emptying are thought to be contributing to this process.[3]

- **Infections**
  - **Viral gastroenteritis** is a common cause of acute nausea and vomiting, particularly in the pediatric population. Causative agents include *rotavirus, Norwalk virus, reovirus,* and *adenovirus.*
  - **Bacterial infections** with *Staphylococcus aureus, Salmonella, Bacillus cereus,* and *Clostridium perfringens* are commonly associated with "food poisoning." Enterotoxins act both centrally and peripherally.
  - **Miscellaneous infectious processes,** such as *otitis media, meningitis, urinary tract infections,* and *acute hepatitis,* also commonly produce nausea and vomiting.[2]
- **Endocrine and metabolic disorders**
  - **Pregnancy** is an important cause of nausea and vomiting in women of reproductive age. Nausea and vomiting occurs in ~70% of women during the first trimester. Symptoms typically peak around the ninth week and subside by

the end of the first trimester. Nausea in pregnancy is related to fluctuations in hormone levels, as the symptoms parallel the rise and fall of beta-human chorionic gonadotropin (β-HCG) levels. Hyperemesis gravidarum complicates 1% to 5% of pregnancies, causing intractable vomiting. This condition is serious and can result in significant weight loss and fetal loss.[4]

○ **Uremia, diabetic ketoacidosis,** and **hypercalcemia** are postulated to cause nausea and vomiting through direct action on the area postrema. **Parathyroid, thyroid,** and **adrenal disease** act by disruption of GI motility.

- **Gastrointestinal and peritoneal disorders**
  ○ Nausea can be caused by **gastroesophageal reflux disease** or **peptic ulcer disease.**
  ○ **Functional disorders,** such as *functional nausea and vomiting, chronic idiopathic nausea,* and *cyclic vomiting syndrome,* account for a large proportion of chronic nausea and vomiting. Alterations in motility (e.g., abnormal gastric emptying) may be present but correlate poorly with symptoms.[5]
  ○ **Gastroparesis,** where altered gastric motility leads to a failure or near failure of gastric emptying, is associated with a multitude of systemic disorders, notably diabetes mellitus, systemic lupus erythematosus, scleroderma, and amyloidosis. Upper abdominal fullness, nausea, vomiting (particularly delayed vomiting of food ingested hours or days earlier) and weight loss can be seen.[6]
  ○ **Inflammation of any viscus** can cause nausea and vomiting through activation of afferent pathways. *Pancreatitis, diverticulitis, colitis, appendicitis, cholecystitis,* and *biliary pain* (colic) are common causes. Peritoneal inflammation is usually associated with severe abdominal pain in addition to nausea and vomiting.
  ○ **Mechanical obstruction** at any level in the GI tract can be the cause of nausea and vomiting. Distention of the bowel lumen causes activation of afferent pathways and emesis ensues in an attempt to decrease pressure.
  ○ **Intestinal pseudo-obstruction** usually results from disorders of neuromuscular function in the colon and small bowel. Clinical presentation is similar to that of mechanical bowel obstruction, but no anatomic obstruction is evident on investigation.
- **Central nervous system (CNS) disorders**
  ○ **Increased intracranial pressure** from any cause (malignancy, infection, cerebrovascular accident, hemorrhage) can induce emesis with or without nausea.
  ○ **Vestibular disorders,** including labyrinthitis, cerebellopontine angle tumors, Ménière's disease, and motion sickness, are common causes of nausea and vomiting.[2]

Pathophysiology
- **Initiation of emesis**
  ○ The *vomiting center,* located in the dorsal portion of the lateral reticular formation, serves as the point of integration and initiation of emesis.
  ○ Afferent stimuli are received by the vomiting center from a variety of sources. The vestibular system, particularly the labyrinthine apparatus located in the inner ear, sends afferent signals through the vestibular nucleus and the cerebellum to the vomiting center.[7]
  ○ Peripheral neural pathways from the GI tract play a significant role in the initiation of emesis. Afferent vagal fibers project to the nucleus tractus solitarius and from there to the vomiting center. Serotonergic pathways are also believed to play a large role in peripheral stimulation via 5-hydroxytryptamine (5-HT)-3 receptors located on the afferent vagal nerves.

○ The chemoreceptor trigger zone, located in the area postrema on the floor of the fourth ventricle, is a major mediator of the initiation of emesis. A number of drugs and toxins activate the zone via dopamine D_2, muscarinic M_1, histaminergic H_1, serotonergic 5-HT_3, and vasopressinergic receptors. Several metabolic abnormalities also affect the trigger zone. Once activated, efferent signals are sent on to the vomiting center, where the physical act of emesis is initiated.

- **Mechanisms of emesis**
  ○ Efferent pathways from the vomiting center serve to initiate vomiting. Important pathways include the phrenic nerves to the diaphragm, the spinal nerves to the abdominal musculature, and visceral efferent vagal fibers to the larynx, pharynx, esophagus, and stomach.[7]
  ○ The act of emesis involves a coordinated sequence of events that includes the abdominal wall musculature and smooth muscle of the GI tract. While the lower esophageal sphincter and the gastric body relax, a combination of forceful contractions of the abdominal wall muscles, diaphragm, and gastric smooth muscle causes the expulsion of gastric contents into the esophagus. Reverse peristalsis propels these contents into the mouth, whereas reflex closure of the glottis prevents aspiration and elevation of the soft palate prevents reflux into the nasopharynx.

DIAGNOSIS

In general, a three-step approach is recommended for the evaluation of nausea and vomiting[1]:

1. Assess the degree to which symptoms impair the patient's quality of life and ability to function.
   ○ Patients with refractory symptoms, significant metabolic abnormalities, or evidence of an acute emergency require hospitalization for expedited evaluation and treatment.
2. Investigate and treat the cause of nausea and vomiting.
3. If no cause can be determined, therapy to improve symptoms is initiated.

Clinical Presentation

History
- **Acute vomiting** suggests bowel obstruction, infection, medication-induced cause, or an accumulation of toxins as in uremia or diabetic ketoacidosis.[1]
- **Chronic vomiting,** defined as emesis for ≥1 month, suggests a chronic medical or functional basis for the symptom; rarely, the etiology is psychogenic.
- **Abdominal pain** is commonly associated with nausea and vomiting. This may indicate an inflammatory condition, such as appendicitis or pancreatitis; pain can also occur from violent retching and bruising of abdominal wall musculature.
- **Diarrhea** or **fever** suggests an infectious process.
- **Weight loss** occurs when nutrition is affected in chronic and severe situations; it can also be seen with gastroparesis.
- **Mental status changes** and **headache** indicate meningitis or other CNS abnormalities.

- **Vertigo** and **tinnitus** suggest a labyrinthine process.
- **Timing of vomiting** can offer clues to the etiology of nausea and vomiting:
  - Vomiting that occurs within minutes of a meal can be caused by an obstructive process in the proximal GI tract.
  - Inflammatory conditions generally produce vomiting within approximately 1 hour after meals.
  - Vomiting from gastroparesis can occur several hours after a meal and is typically associated with weight loss.
  - Early morning vomiting often occurs with first-trimester pregnancy and uremia.
  - Neurogenic vomiting is typically projectile and brought on by positions that increase intracranial pressure.
- The **nature of the vomited material** can point to a diagnosis:
  - Vomiting of undigested or partially digested foods suggests gastric retention caused by obstruction or gastroparesis.
  - Blood or the appearance of "coffee grounds" in the emesis indicates an upper GI bleed.
  - Bile rules out the possibility of obstruction proximal to the duodenal papilla.
  - Foul odor can indicate a distal obstruction, coloenteric fistula, or bacterial overgrowth.
  - If the patient reports emesis of food that looks and tastes just like the food they just ate, consider regurgitation of esophageal content instead of emesis, and an obstructive distal esophageal process (e.g., achalasia) needs to be excluded.

Physical Examination

- **Assessment of volume status** should be the initial focus of the physical examination. Orthostatic hypotension and tachycardia indicate hypovolemia and should be corrected immediately with volume resuscitation.[2,8]
- **Examination of the oropharynx** may reveal loss of dental enamel in situations associated with chronic emesis such as bulimia or functional nausea and vomiting. Patients with bulimia may also have callus formation over their knuckles from repetitively inducing vomiting.
- **Abdominal tenderness** suggests an inflammatory condition, and rebound tenderness suggests peritonitis.
- Absence of **bowel sounds** is consistent with ileus, whereas obstruction classically presents with high-pitched, hyperactive bowel sounds.
- **Hepatomegaly** or a tender liver edge may indicate hepatitis.
- **Neurologic examination** can reveal signs of meningitis and other nervous system disorders.

Differential Diagnosis

- Table 2-1 lists the common etiologies of nausea and vomiting.
- Vomiting needs to be distinguished from regurgitation and rumination.
  - **Regurgitation** is the passive retrograde flow of esophageal contents into the mouth, commonly seen in gastroesophageal reflux.
  - **Rumination** is the effortless regurgitation of recently ingested food into the mouth, followed by rechewing and swallowing. In adults, rumination can be seen in association with psychiatric disorders and in individuals with developmental disability.

Diagnostic Testing

Laboratory Testing

- **Basic metabolic panel,** evaluating for electrolyte imbalances, especially hyponatremia elevated blood urea nitrogen and creatinine. This can be seen with uremia and dehydration. Hypokalemia and contraction alkalosis can also occur with prolonged vomiting.
- **Liver chemistries,** which may reveal acute hepatitis or cholestasis.
- Elevated **lipase** and **amylase** levels indicate pancreatitis.
- **Complete blood cell count** may reveal an elevated white blood cell count, suggesting an infectious or inflammatory process. Blood counts show decreased hemoglobin and hematocrit in situations associated with blood loss.
- **Urinalysis** may reveal evidence of urinary tract infection; additionally, ketonuria can be seen in the setting of prolonged fasting or diabetic ketoacidosis.
- Urine or serum β-HCG levels are mandatory in women of reproductive age with acute vomiting to evaluate for pregnancy.

Imaging

- **Plan abdominal radiograph.** Flat and upright plain x-ray films of the abdomen can be obtained, typically termed "obstructive x-ray series." The presence of air–fluid levels and small bowel dilatation indicates ileus or obstruction. Free air under the diaphragm indicates bowel perforation.
- **Computed tomography** of the abdomen may be useful for evaluating hollow viscus for evidence of dilatation and obstruction, evaluating for inflammatory conditions, as well as in looking for structural abnormalities of the liver, the pancreas, and the biliary system.
- An **upper GI x-ray series,** sometimes performed with small bowel follow-through with barium contrast, can further evaluate subtle obstruction and mucosal lesions.
- **Nuclear medicine gastric emptying study** may be useful in cases when gastroparesis or functionally delayed gastric emptying is suspected.
- SmartPill® is an ingestible, wireless capsule that measures pressure, pH, and temperature as it transits the GI tract. The smart pill may be useful in the evaluation of nausea and vomiting when gastroparesis, small bowel, or colonic dysmotility are suspected as the etiology.[9]

Diagnostic Procedures

- **Esophagogastroduodenoscopy (EGD)** allows for direct visualization of the foregut mucosa. An EGD is typically considered if the history points toward a GI etiology for chronic nausea and vomiting; it can also be a key test to exclude mucosal disease when an etiology is not apparent. A number of disorders including reflux esophagitis, peptic ulcer disease, gastric outlet obstruction, and foregut malignancy can be diagnosed during EGD.[2]

TREATMENT

General Principles

- Orthostatic hypotension and sinus tachycardia are signs of hypovolemia (with loss of ~10% of circulating blood volume) and should be corrected immediately with administration of intravenous (IV) fluids.[2]

- Emesis caused by peptic ulcer disease can be treated with acid suppression and eradication of *Helicobacter pylori*.
- Many inflammatory conditions, including appendicitis and cholecystitis, as well as mechanical small bowel or gastric outlet obstruction, require surgical intervention. Antiemetic and promotility agents are useful for symptomatic relief.
- Patients with acute, self-limited nausea and vomiting may only require observation, antiemetics, and hydration.

Antiemetic Medications

- **Antihistamines**
  - *Meclizine* (25 mg PO QID) is used for labyrinthitis, whereas *promethazine* (12.5 to 25 mg PO/IM q6h) is very useful for treating the nausea caused by uremia.
- **Anticholinergics**
  - *Scopolamine* (1.5-mg transdermal patch every 3 days) is used for the nausea of motion sickness.
- **Dopamine receptor antagonists**
  - *Prochlorperazine* (5 to 10 mg PO/IM/IV q6h) and *chlorpromazine* (10 to 50 mg PO/IM q8h) are commonly used in both chronic and acute vomiting. Side effects, which are caused by the action on dopamine receptors throughout the CNS, include drowsiness, insomnia, anxiety, mood changes, confusion, dystonic reactions, tardive dyskinesia, and parkinsonian symptoms.
- **5-HT$_3$ receptor antagonists**
  - Included in the class of 5-HT$_3$ receptor antagonists are *ondansetron* (4 to 8 mg PO/IV q8h) and *granisetron* (1 mg PO q12h), *palonosetron* (0.25 mg PO/IV once a week), which are very useful in nausea caused by chemotherapeutic agents, particularly cisplatin.[10]
- **Miscellaneous agents**
  - *Corticosteroids* and *cannabinoids* exert potent antiemetic effects in patients undergoing chemotherapy. *Aprepitant,* which selectively antagonizes human substance P or neurokinin 1 receptors, is used for the prevention of chemotherapy-related nausea and vomiting.

Prokinetic Medications

- **Metoclopramide** (5 to 20 mg PO QID), which acts on both 5-HT$_4$ and peripheral dopamine receptors, is used for treating nausea. Although it is also used to accelerate gastric emptying in gastroparesis and functional dyspepsia, its promotility action is subject to tachyphylaxis with continued use. Its antiemetic properties, through its central action, may allow suppression of nausea and vomiting despite continued use. Jitteriness, tremors, parkinsonism, and the risk of tardive dyskinesia limit its long-term use. The FDA has recently issued a black box warning related to the risk of irreversible neurologic complications and cardiac arrhythmias associated with the use of metoclopramide.[11]
- **Erythromycin,** a macrolide antibiotic, is a motilin receptor agonist that improves gastric emptying but without significant suppression of nausea. It can be administered intravenously for acute gastric distension to stimulate gastric emptying. Its promotility action is subject to tachyphylaxis and therefore it is not useful for long-term management.
- Cisapride is no longer available in the United States because of its proarrhythmic effects.

- **Domperidone,** also a peripheral dopamine receptor antagonist, is a potent pro-kinetic agent but is not currently available in the United States.
- **Tegaserod,** a 5-HT$_4$ receptor agonist, primarily used in the treatment of irritable bowel syndrome, has modest promotility action in the stomach and can be used to improve gastric emptying. This medication, however, is currently not available for routine use because of its cardiovascular effects.[12]

Complementary and Alternative Therapy

- **Ginger** (*Zingiber officinale*) root extract has been evaluated in the treatment of nausea and vomiting in multiple settings. It appears to act via inhibition of serotonin receptors in the GI tract and in the CNS. It has been most extensively studied and effective in pregnancy-related nausea and vomiting. The typical dose of ginger root extract is 250 mg QID.[13]
- **Acupuncture** has been shown to be an efficacious therapy for acute as well as chronic nausea and vomiting related to a wide variety of etiologies. Acupoint PC6 (Neiguan) has been the most commonly evaluated acupuncture point.[14] Acupressure bands that apply pressure on the ventral aspect of the wrist have also been used in this setting.
- **Hypnosis** has been used for the treatment of functional nausea and vomiting as well as nausea and vomiting related to pregnancy and chemotherapy.[4,15]

SPECIAL CONSIDERATIONS

Refractory Nausea and Vomiting

- Nausea and vomiting are considered refractory if investigation fails to reveal a treatable etiology and if routine measures do not result in symptomatic improvement.
- Two patterns of symptoms are recognized.
  - **Chronic persistent nausea and vomiting,** occurring on a daily or frequent basis. This syndrome is part of the spectrum of functional nausea and vomiting, and it can be effectively treated with neuromodulators, including tricyclic antidepressants, selective serotonin reuptake inhibitors, and to a lesser extent, bupropion and buspirone.[16]
  - **Cyclic vomiting syndrome** (CVS) is a unique disorder characterized by short periods of abdominal pain and violent nausea and vomiting that are separated by symptom-free intervals during which patients are relatively asymptomatic.
  - Current understanding of this condition links it to migraine headaches. The treatment approach is similar to that used for migraine headaches, with both abortive and prophylactic medications.
  - Associated complaints during symptom "attacks" include upper abdominal pain, diarrhea, flushing, and sweating. Some patients report a prodrome lasting several minutes to hours.
  - Abortive therapy could include triptans during the prodromal period and combinations of antiemetic medications, anxiolytics, and narcotic analgesics, in addition to IV hydration, during symptomatic periods.
  - Prophylactic approaches include not only tricyclic antidepressants as first-line medications but also antiepileptic medications such as zonisamide, levetiracetam, or even topiramate.[17]

Treatment of Refractory Nausea and Vomiting

- **Low-dose tricyclic antidepressants,** such as amitriptyline or nortriptyline (10 to 50 mg PO at bedtime), are useful in functional vomiting syndrome and as prophylaxis in CVS.[18]
- **Selective serotonin reuptake inhibitors** (*SSRI*), which are generally used for depression and anxiety disorders, may also block presynaptic serotonin receptors on sensory vagal fibers, helping to control nausea. Use of SSRIs for functional nausea and vomiting is largely based on anecdotal evidence; however, these agents are sometimes better tolerated than tricyclic antidepressants. Their role in CVS has not been established.[19]
- **Bupropion,** an inhibitor of neuronal uptake of norepinephrine and dopamine, is an antidepressant and may additionally help relieve nausea and vomiting. It can be considered if side effects from tricyclic antidepressants (especially anticholinergic effects, sexual side effects, and weight gain) are poorly tolerated.
- **Buspirone** is an anxiolytic drug that binds to serotonin and dopamine receptors. This drug may increase the compliance of the gastric antrum and is useful in functional dyspepsia associated with nausea and vomiting.
- **Sumatriptan** activates $5-HT_1$ receptors and is used as an abortive therapy for migraines. It can be used as part of abortive therapy early during a cyclic vomiting attack, especially during the prodrome.[16]
- **Zonisamide,** an antiepileptic agent, has multiple mechanisms of action, including blockade of voltage-dependent sodium and T-type calcium channels, binding to the γ-aminobutyric acid receptor, and facilitating dopaminergic and serotoninergic neurotransmission. It has been used with some success as a prophylactic agent in the treatment of CVS.[17]
- **Levetiracetam,** another antiepileptic drug with a less well-understood mechanism of action, appears to inhibit bursts of neuronal firing without affecting normal neuronal excitability. It may also be of benefit as prophylactic therapy in CVS.
- **Surgical therapy is considered a last resort** in refractory nausea and vomiting, specifically when significant weight loss results from the symptomatic state or from impaired gastric emptying.
- **Enteral feeding** can be maintained through a *jejunostomy tube,* which can be placed endoscopically, surgically, or with radiologic guidance (depending on local expertise).
- **Gastric stimulator,** a device that delivers electrical stimulation through electrodes implanted into the gastric wall, can be an option for patients with refractory persistent nausea and vomiting. It does not appear to improve gastric emptying and therefore may not benefit advanced gastroparesis wherein impaired gastric emptying leads to weight loss and nutritional issues.[20]

COMPLICATIONS

- Vomiting, particularly when protracted, can lead to a number of life-threatening complications.
  - **Metabolic and electrolyte alterations** can develop rapidly; dehydration with resultant hypotension may lead to syncope and prerenal azotemia. Hypochloremic alkalosis is typically the first electrolyte abnormality to appear due to loss of hydrogen and chloride ions; this is followed by development of

hypokalemia due to renal potassium wasting in response to alkalosis. The resulting metabolic derangement can lead to rhabdomyolysis and cardiac arrhythmias.

○ **Nutritional deficiencies and weight loss** may result in decreased oral intake. Enteral (via jejunostomy or nasojejunal tube) or parenteral nutrition may be needed in both the acute and chronic settings. A more detailed discussion of nutritional issues can be found in Chapter 11.

○ **Dental erosions** may develop in patients with chronic vomiting syndromes as a result of acid- and bile-induced erosion of the dental enamel.

○ **Erosive esophagitis** can develop as a result of protracted vomiting and may range from mild to severe. It is important to distinguish esophagitis that is due to vomiting from that associated with gastroesophageal reflux disease (GERD). On endoscopy, esophagitis related to protracted vomiting extends uniformly up to the proximal esophageal body whereas GERD-related esophagitis is most pronounced in the distal esophagus.

○ **Mallory-Weiss syndrome** can result from forceful and prolonged vomiting episodes and is characterized by longitudinal lacerations of the mucosa near the gastroesophageal junction. These tears can lead to GI bleeding, which is typically self-limited.

○ **Boerhaave's syndrome** refers to free perforation of the esophagus into the mediastinum due to vomiting. It is most often seen in alcoholics and patients with binge-eating disorders. It should be suspected in any patient presenting with severe chest pain and subcutaneous emphysema after an episode of vomiting (Mackler's triad). The diagnosis can be made on the basis of chest computed tomograph or esophagram (with water-soluble contrast). Even with prompt surgical repair, *Boerhaave's syndrome* carries a 25% to 50% mortality rate.[21]

REFERENCES

1. Quigley EM, Hasler WL, Parkman HP. AGA technical review on nausea and vomiting. *Gastroenterology.* 2001;120:263–286.
2. Hasler WL, Chey WD. Nausea and vomiting. *Gastroenterology.* 2003;125:1860–1867.
3. Sullivan S. Cannabinoid hyperemesis. *Can J Gastroenterol.* 2010;24:284–285.
4. Niebyl JR. Clinical practice. Nausea and vomiting in pregnancy. *N Engl J Med.* 2010; 363:1544–1550.
5. Prakash C, Clouse RE. Cyclic vomiting syndrome in adults: clinical features and response to tricyclic antidepressants. *Am J Gastroenterol.* 1999;94:2855–2860.
6. Parkman HP, Yates K, Hasler WL, et al. Clinical features of idiopathic gastroparesis vary with sex, body mass, symptom onset, delay in gastric emptying, and gastroparesis severity. *Gastroenterology.* 2011;140:101–115.
7. Horn CC. Why is the neurobiology of nausea and vomiting so important? *Appetite.* 2008;50:430–434.
8. American Gastroenterological Association medical position statement: nausea and vomiting. *Gastroenterology.* 2001;120:261–263.
9. Sarosiek I, Selover KH, Katz LA, et al. The assessment of regional gut transit times in healthy controls and patients with gastroparesis using wireless motility technology. *Aliment Pharmacol Ther.* 2010;31:313–322.
10. Aapro M. 5-HT(3)-receptor antagonists in the management of nausea and vomiting in cancer and cancer treatment. *Oncology.* 2005;69:97–109.
11. Patanwala AE, Amini R, Hays DP, et al. Antiemetic therapy for nausea and vomiting in the emergency department. *J Emerg Med.* 2010;39:330–336.

12. Degen L, Petrig C, Studer D, et al. Effect of tegaserod on gut transit in male and female subjects. *Neurogastroenterol Motil.* 2005;17:821–826.
13. White B. Ginger: an overview. *Am Fam Physician.* 2007;75:1689–1691.
14. Ouyang H, Chen JD. Review article: therapeutic roles of acupuncture in functional gastrointestinal disorders. *Aliment Pharmacol Ther.* 2004;20:831–841.
15. Chiarioni G, Palsson OS, Whitehead WE. Hypnosis and upper digestive function and disease. *World J Gastroenterol.* 2008;14:6276–6284.
16. Talley NJ. Functional nausea and vomiting. *Aust Fam Physician.* 2007;36:694–697.
17. Clouse RE, Sayuk GS, Lustman PJ, et al. Zonisamide or levetiracetam for adults with cyclic vomiting syndrome: a case series. *Clin Gastroenterol Hepatol.* 2007;5:44–48.
18. Prakash C, Lustman PJ, Freedland KE, et al. Tricyclic antidepressants for functional nausea and vomiting: clinical outcome in 37 patients. *Dig Dis Sci.* 1998;43:1951–1956.
19. Talley NJ. How to manage the difficult-to-treat dyspeptic patient. *Nat Clin Pract Gastroenterol Hepatol.* 2007;4:35–42.
20. McCallum RW, Lin Z, Forster J, et al. Gastric electrical stimulation improves outcomes of patients with gastroparesis for up to 10 years. *Clin Gastroenterol Hepatol.* 2011;9(4): 314–319.e1.
21. Atallah FN, Riu BM, Nguyen LB, et al. Boerhaave's syndrome after postoperative vomiting. *Anesth Analg.* 2004;98:1164–1166, table of contents.

Diarrhea

3

Hongha (Susan) T. Vu

GENERAL PRINCIPLES

Definition

- Diarrhea is defined as increased liquidity/decreased consistency of stools, which may be associated with increased frequency of bowel movements, specifically more than three stools per day.
- The small intestine and colon are highly efficient in reabsorption of water.[1,2]
  - 10 L of intestinal fluid enters the jejunum on a daily basis
  - 1 to 1.5 L of intestinal fluid is passed into the colon
  - 100 mL/day passes out of the colon as stool
- Diarrhea results from the inability or inefficiency of the digestive tract to perform this reabsorptive function.

Classification

- Diarrhea can be classified into acute and chronic, based on the duration of symptoms. **Acute diarrhea** is typically <2 weeks in duration, although some acute diarrheal illnesses may continue to improve over 3 to 4 weeks. Diarrhea lasting longer than 4 weeks can be designated **chronic.**
- Diarrhea can be categorized into several types, based on pathophysiology of the causative process.[1,2]
  - **Osmotic**
    - In this type of diarrhea, large amounts of poorly absorbed solute within the intestinal lumen cause osmotic retention of water in the stool.
    - There are two clinical hallmarks of osmotic diarrhea: (a) the diarrhea ceases with fasting, and (b) the stool osmotic gap is abnormally elevated >125 mOsm/kg.
      - Stool osmotic gap is calculated using the formula: $290 - 2(Na^+ + K^+)$.
      - The body maintains equal fecal and serum osmolality, which is approximately 290 mOsm/kg.
      - The presence of a poorly absorbed substance within the intestinal lumen requires that additional water be retained in the stool to maintain this value, causing an osmotic gap.
      - Osmotic gap <50 mOsm/kg is considered normal.
      - Osmotic gap >125 mOsm/kg is consistent with a pure osmotic diarrhea.
  - **Secretory**
    - Intestinal secretion overcomes the absorptive capability of the small intestine and colon.
    - Secretion of incompletely absorbed electrolytes leads to retention of intraluminal water.

- Because intestinal secretion is a constant process, diarrhea is incessant regardless of fasting state or time of the day.
- Presentation is typically with large amounts of watery diarrhea (1 to 10 L/24 hours).
- The stool osmotic gap is normal.
  - ○ **Inflammatory**
    - Inflammation and ulceration impair the absorptive and digestive functions of normal mucosa.
    - In addition, inflammation itself often elaborates mucus, proteins, fluid, and blood into the bowel lumen, adding to stool volume. Secretory mechanisms may be coexistent.
    - Clinical indicators of inflammatory diarrhea include nocturnal diarrhea and systemic signs, such as fatigue or fever.
  - ○ **Steatorrhea**
    - Any process that affects digestion and absorption of fats, ranging from celiac disease to pancreatic insufficiency, can lead to steatorrhea.
    - In addition, inadequate contact time of bowel contents with the digestive juices and absorptive intestinal mucosa, such as with altered intestinal motility, can also contribute to steatorrhea.
  - ○ **Dysmotility/Functional**
    - Gut dysmotility may cause increased intestinal and colonic transit time as well as decrease contact time with intestinal absorptive mucosa.
    - Functional syndromes such as irritable bowel syndrome (IBS) include a pain component as well as a change in bowel habits.

Epidemiology

- **Acute diarrhea**
  - ○ Worldwide, >2 billion people experience at least one episode of acute diarrhea each year.
  - ○ As a result of poor sanitation and limited access to health care, acute infectious diarrhea remains one of the most common causes of death in developing countries, accounting for >5 million childhood deaths per year.
  - ○ In the United States, nearly 100 million people are affected by acute diarrhea annually. Nearly half of these individuals must limit their activities, 250,000 require hospitalization, and approximately 3000 people die. Most deaths occur in the debilitated and the elderly.[3]
- **Chronic diarrhea**
  - ○ Chronic diarrhea has an estimated prevalence of 3% to 5% in the United States, which may be an underestimation since many patients do not seek medical attention.[1]
  - ○ According to the AGA Burden of Illness study, direct costs of chronic diarrhea is $524 million per year, with $136 million per year for indirect costs.[4]
  - ○ Although it is a major cause of disability, there are limited studies on the economic impact or effect on quality of life that results from chronic diarrhea, diagnostic testing, and treatment.

Etiology

- Etiologies of acute infectious diarrhea[3,5,6] and chronic diarrhea[1,7–10] are listed in Tables 3-1 and 3-2.

TABLE 3-1	CAUSES OF ACUTE INFECTIOUS DIARRHEA

Viruses

Rotavirus
Norwalk virus
Adenovirus
Astrovirus
Hepatitis A

Bacteria

Campylobacter
Salmonella
Shigella
Clostridium difficile
Enterohemorrhagic *E. coli* (EHEC, 0157:H7)
Enterotoxigenic *E. coli* (ETEC)
Enteroinvasive *E. coli* (EIEC)
Vibrio cholerae
Vibrio parahaemolyticus
Yersinia
Listeria
Aeromonas
Plesiomonas

Preformed Toxins

Staphylococcus aureus
Clostridium perfringens
Bacillus cereus

Parasites

Giardia lamblia
Entamoeba histolytica
Cyclospora
Isospora
Cryptosporidium
Strongyloides

Opportunistic

Microsporidia
Mycobacterium avium intracellulare
Cytomegalovirus
Herpes simplex virus

DIAGNOSIS

Clinical Presentation

- **Acute versus chronic**
  - ○ **Acute**
    - ■ Most cases of acute diarrhea are mild and are caused by self-limited processes/infections, lasting <5 days. Symptoms may continue to improve for 2 to 3 weeks after onset in some circumstances.
    - ■ Nearly 90% of cases require no diagnostic evaluation and respond to simple rehydration.
  - ○ **Chronic**
    - ■ Patients may present with symptoms that have been present anywhere from 4 weeks to many years.
    - ■ There are a wide variety of causes (Table 3-2). A careful and detailed history and physical examination, along with judicious use of laboratory tests and investigative procedures, often yield an accurate diagnosis.
    - ■ In contrast to acute diarrhea, chronic diarrhea often has a noninfectious etiology.
- **Noninflammatory versus inflammatory**
  - ○ **Noninflammatory**
    - ■ The presentation typically consists of watery, nonbloody diarrhea associated with periumbilical cramps, bloating, nausea, or vomiting.

TABLE 3-2   CAUSES OF CHRONIC DIARRHEA

Osmotic

Medications: antibiotics, lactulose, antacids, sorbitol, laxative abuse, Mg ingestion

Carbohydrate malabsorption/ disaccharidase deficiencies (i.e., lactose intolerance)

High ingestion of sugar substitutes or fructose

Secretory

Medications: nonosmotic laxatives, stimulants, selective serotonin reuptake inhibitors

Bile salt–induced diarrhea (bacterial breakdown of bile acids stimulates secretion from colonic mucosa): postcholecystectomy or ileal malabsorption

Colitis: inflammatory bowel disease, microscopic colitis, diverticulitis

Bacterial toxins

Neuroendocrine tumors: carcinoid syndrome, insulinoma, Zollinger-Ellison/gastrinoma, VIPoma, medullary carcinoma of the thyroid, somatostatinoma, pheochromocytoma, glucagonoma, mastocytosis

Endocrinopathies: hyperthyroidism, diabetes mellitus, Addison's, hyperparathyroidism

Miscellaneous: villous adenoma (chloride secreting), colon cancer, lymphoma, multiple myeloma, HIV/ AIDS, amyloidosis, vasculitis, cholera, congenital chloridorrhea

Inflammatory

Infection: C. difficile, tuberculosis, Yersinia, cytomegalovirus, herpes simplex virus, amebiasis

Inflammatory bowel disease

Ischemic colitis

Radiation enterocolitis

Eosinophilic enterocolitis

Colon cancer, lymphoma

Steatorrhea

Maldigestion: pancreatic exocrine insufficiency, bile acid deficiency, abetalipoproteinemia

Malabsorption: celiac sprue, tropical sprue, Whipple's disease, short bowel syndrome, small intestinal bacterial overgrowth—bacterial deconjugation of bile acids, mesenteric ischemia, protein-losing enteropathy

Altered intestinal motility: hyperthyroidism, diabetes mellitus, scleroderma, medications (i.e., metoclopramide, erythromycin)

Dysmotility/Functional

Irritable bowel syndrome

Fecal impaction (overflow diarrhea)

Enteric fistula

Systemic disease: diabetes mellitus, hyperthyroidism, Addison's, amyloidosis, scleroderma

---

- This is usually caused by disruption of normal absorption or a secretory process in the small intestine, such as that seen with certain bacterial toxins.
- In most cases, the diarrhea is mild. It may, however, become voluminous, ranging from 10 to 200 mL/kg/24 hours, which can result in dehydration and electrolyte abnormalities.
  ○ **Inflammatory**
    - Inflammatory diarrhea may present with fever, bloody diarrhea, abdominal pain, and tenesmus.

- Infectious agents preferentially involve the colon, leading to a small-volume diarrhea defined as <1 L/day. Because these infectious agents are often invasive, fecal leukocytes can be present.

History

- The following points are elicited when obtaining the **history of diarrhea**[11]:
  - Onset, duration, pattern/frequency
  - Stool characteristics: watery, fatty, or inflammatory (blood or mucus)
  - Systemic symptoms: fever, fatigue
  - Abdominal pain: postprandial?
  - Fecal incontinence
  - Weight loss: suggests decreased intake (volitional to decrease diarrhea?), malabsorption, neoplasm, ischemia
  - Significant weight loss (>10 lb) is more worrisome and often points to nutrient malabsorption.
  - Nocturnal/fasting symptoms
  - Aggravating/mitigating factors: diet, stress, medications
  - Recent exposure to hospitals or antibiotic use
  - Sick contacts/regional outbreak: food-related
- **Past medical and surgical conditions** may be relevant to the history, as follows:
  - Systemic disease: diabetes mellitus, thyroid disease, inflammatory/autoimmune disorder, HIV, immunocompromised state, cancer
  - History indicating factitious symptoms: eating disorder, malingering, secondary gain
  - Previous surgery: gastrectomy, vagotomy, bowel resection, cholecystectomy
  - Previous radiation therapy
- A **family history** of the following conditions may be helpful: inflammatory bowel disease (IBD), celiac sprue, multiple endocrine neoplasia (MEN) syndromes.
- A detailed medication history is obtained, especially inquiring about the use of laxatives, antibiotics, over-the-counter medications.
- A **diet history** may be relevant, especially the following:
  - Recent changes or associated foods
  - Intake of sugar-free substitutes or fructose
  - Exposure to contaminated food or water
    - Time from ingestion: <6 hours suggests a preformed toxin, 8 to 16 hours suggests *Clostridium perfringens* infection, and >16 hours suggests an enteroinvasive viral or bacterial infection.
- **Social history**
  - Alcohol, tobacco, illicit drug use
  - Travel/immigration history
    - Recent travel to endemic areas may suggest traveler's diarrhea, *Giardia* infection, tropical sprue.
    - Recent immigration from a developing country raises the possibility of a parasitic infection.
  - Sexual history

Physical Examination

- Vital signs are obtained to determine if the patient has fever, tachycardia, and hypotension. Orthostatic blood pressure changes may be evident with severe volume depletion from fluid loss.

- General examination takes into account whether the patient is toxic appearing and acutely ill. Cachexia and muscle wasting may indicate a chronic process.
- Volume status is assessed by examining orthostatics, mucous membranes, and skin turgor. A history of oliguria supports volume loss.
- Head and neck examination evaluates the findings of hyperthyroidism (thyroid mass, exophthalmos) and extraintestinal manifestations of IBD (episcleritis, mouth ulcers).
- Flushing, wheezing, and cardiac murmurs can rarely be seen in secretory diarrhea, especially carcinoid syndrome.
- A detailed abdominal examination assesses for tenderness, peritoneal signs, hepatomegaly, masses, and ascites. Surgical scars indicate past surgery. Bowel sounds are evaluated for hyper- and hypomotility.
- Anorectal examination focuses on sphincter tone/contractility, fistulas, fissures, perianal abscess, and blood on the examining finger.
- Other areas examined include the peripheries for edema, arthritis, lymphadenopathy; skin examination for rashes and flushing, and a neurologic examination for neurologic deficits and peripheral neuropathy.

Differential Diagnosis

Clinical patterns can help determine pathophysiologic mechanisms of diarrhea as follows:

- **Watery diarrhea**
  - Osmotic diarrhea decreases with fasting.
  - Secretory diarrhea is voluminous, with no change with fasting. Patients may have nocturnal symptoms.
- **Bloody diarrhea with or without mucus**
  - This suggests inflammatory or infectious etiologies. Patients may also manifest systemic symptoms, fevers, fatigue, abdominal pain, tenesmus, and nocturnal symptoms.
- **Fatty stool**
  - This suggests steatorrhea. Diarrhea typically decreases with fasting and can be foul-smelling. Stool may adhere to the toilet bowl, and the patient may report oil droplets in the toilet water.
- **Functional etiologies**
  - In IBS and other functional disorders, there is a predominance of abdominal pain, lack of nocturnal symptoms, and lack of significant weight loss.

Diagnostic Testing

- **Acute diarrhea.** Testing is indicated in the presence of severe symptoms (hypovolemia, fever, severe abdominal pain, bloody diarrhea) but also in the elderly or immunocompromised individuals and in IBD.[3]
- **Osmotic diarrhea**[1,7–10]
  - Osmotic gap can be checked and is typically >125 mOsm/kg.
  - Stool pH helps assess for carbohydrate malabsorption when it is acidic.
  - Stool magnesium level can assess for excessive intake of magnesium.
- **Secretory diarrhea**
  - Osmotic gap is usually normal (<50 mOsm/kg).
  - Infectious etiologies need to be excluded, as some acute infections can induce a transient secretory pattern.

- ○ Imaging studies and endoscopy can evaluate for structural and inflammatory diseases of the small intestine and colon.
- ○ Specialized tests can be performed to investigate for endocrinopathies and neuroendocrine tumors.
- **Inflammatory diarrhea**
  - ○ Fecal occult blood test (FOBT) and/or fecal leukocytes can be assessed in chronic diarrhea wherein both inflammatory and secretory etiologies are being considered. These tests are consistently positive in bloody diarrhea or where other features suggest an inflammatory etiology. If the history, physical examination, and other testing are convincing for an inflammatory etiology, these tests are redundant and should not be performed.
  - ○ Infectious etiologies need to be excluded, even when IBD is suspected, as infectious superinfection can be seen.
  - ○ Imaging studies and endoscopy are useful to evaluate for structural and/or inflammatory diseases of the small intestine and colon.
- **Steatorrhea**
  - ○ Fecal fat assays are typically abnormal and the osmotic gap is >50 mOsm/kg.
  - ○ Imaging studies and endoscopy are useful for evaluating structural and/or inflammatory diseases of the small intestine and pancreas.
  - ○ Investigation can be performed for evaluating pancreatic exocrine insufficiency.

Laboratories (* = initial tests)
- ***Complete blood cell count with differential.** This may show anemia, leukocytosis (infection), or eosinophila (neoplasm, allergies, parasites, eosinophilic gastroenterocolitis).
- ***Comprehensive metabolic panel.** This evaluates for electrolyte abnormalities, coexistent liver disease, hypoalbuminemia/dysproteinemia (malnutrition, protein-losing enteropathy), or diabetes.
- ***TSH, fT4.** This evaluates for hyperthyroidism, which can rarely cause diarrhea on its own but can potentiate diarrhea from other causes.
- **Stool studies.** The following studies can be performed:
  - ○ Leukocytes, lactoferrin
  - ○ FOBT
  - ○ *Osmolarity, electrolytes (Na, K) to calculate osmotic gap
  - ○ Fat. qualitative/Sudan stain versus 24-, 48-, or 72-hour quantitative collection on a 100 g fat/day diet (<6 g/24 hours is normal, >14 g/24 hours suggests malabsorption/maldigestion, >8% suggests pancreatic insufficiency)
  - ○ *Infectious. bacterial culture, *Clostridium difficile* toxin ×3, O&P ± microscopy ×3, stool wet mount for amebiasis in sexually active male homosexuals or travel to endemic areas
  - ○ pH <5.6 suggests carbohydrate malabsorption (colonic fermentation by bacteria)
  - ○ Mg level
  - ○ Laxative screen
  - ○ α_1-Antitrypsin. This is useful in the assessment of protein-losing enteropathy, when stool α_1-antitrypsin levels are elevated.
  - ○ Chymotrypsin or elastase concentration: These are elevated in the stool in pancreatic insufficiency
- **Urine studies.** The following can be performed:
  - ○ Urinalysis: for protein loss in the urine
  - ○ Laxative screen

- **Secretory diarrhea.** The following can be measured for the assessment of secretory diarrhea: serum levels of VIP, gastrin, calcitonin, pancreatic polypeptide, somatostatin, tryptase, and urinary excretion of 5-hydroxyindoleacetic acid, metanephrines, and histamine, and adrenocorticotropin stimulation test, serum protein electrophoresis, immunoglobulins.
- **Celiac disease.** Testing for celiac disease should be performed early for the evaluation of chronic diarrhea: antitissue transglutaminase antibody, deamidated gliadin peptide, IgA levels (up to 10% of patients will be IgA deficient and have a false-negative result).
- **IBD and immunocompromised patients.** Cytomegalovirus (CMV) DNA polymerase chain reaction and *C. difficile* toxins
- **Rectal swab** in those active in anal intercourse [gonorrhea, *Chlamydia,* herpes simplex virus (HSV)]

Imaging
- The following can be performed to assess for structural/inflammatory disease of the small intestine and pancreas:
  ○ Small bowel follow-through
  ○ CT enterography
  ○ MR enterography
  ○ Dual-phase CT scan of the pancreas
  ○ Abdominal ultrasonography
  ○ Endoscopic ultrasonography

Diagnostic Procedures
- **Endoscopy with biopsies**[12]
  ○ Upper endoscopy with small bowel biopsies (for the evaluation of celiac disease—minimum of four duodenal biopsies, Whipple's disease, protein-losing enteropathy, eosinophilic gastroenteritis, giardiasis, amyloidosis)
  ○ Upper endoscopy with small bowel aspirate [small bowel bacterial overgrowth (SIBO)]
  ○ Flexible sigmoidoscopy or colonoscopy with random biopsies
    ■ Flexible sigmoidoscopy is acceptable in cases of acute diarrhea with suspicion for diffuse colitis, such as graft-versus-host disease, or chronic diarrhea in patients with significant comorbidities or pregnancy.
    ■ Colonoscopy is preferred for evaluation of IBD, microscopic colitis, eosinophilic colitis, amyloidosis, colorectal neoplasia or screening, HIV patients, or in cases with significant blood loss.
- **Endoscopic ultrasonography** (chronic pancreatitis)
- **Breath tests** for specific carbohydrate malabsorption (lactose, sucrose) and SIBO (glucose, lactulose, ^{14}C-xylose, ^{14}C-glycocholate)
- **Secretin test, bentiromide test** to assess for pancreatic exocrine insufficiency

TREATMENT

Medications
Acute Diarrhea
- **Volume status and electrolyte disturbances need to be assessed first.**
  ○ Uncomplicated, mild acute diarrhea is treated with oral fluids containing carbohydrates and electrolytes.

- World Health Organization oral rehydration solution (3.5 g NaCl, 2.9 g trisodium citrate or 2.5 g NaHCO$_3$, 1.5 g KCl, and 20 g glucose or 40 g sucrose per L) is recommended.
  - Pedialyte, Gatorade, and similar sports drinks may also be taken, but the carbohydrate load is greater and the sodium content is lower.
  - In severe diarrhea, intravenous fluids (Lactated Ringer's or 0.9% normal saline) may be necessary to restore volume and to keep up with ongoing losses.
- **Antidiarrheal agents** are safe in mild to moderate diarrhea and may improve patient comfort.
  - Loperamide 4 mg followed by 2 mg after each loose stool up to a maximum daily dose of 16 mg.
  - Diphenoxylate plus atropine (Lomotil) 4 mg QID has combined opioid and anticholinergic effects.
  - Antidiarrheal agents are not recommended in bloody or febrile cases.
- **Traveler's diarrhea.** Bismuth subsalicylate 30 mL QID may reduce symptoms through anti-inflammatory and antibacterial properties.
  - The addition of an antibiotic such as fluoroquinolone or rifaximin 200 to 400 mg PO TID ×3 days may lessen the duration and severity of the illness.
- **Antibiotics.** Empiric treatment with antibiotics is recommended only when invasive bacterial infection is suspected, suggested by high fever, tenesmus, bloody diarrhea, or fecal leukocytes. Use must be weighed against possible risks including antibiotic resistance or other possible complications.[3,5,6]
  - **First line.** Fluoroquinolones ×3 to 7 days (i.e., ciprofloxacin 500 mg BID, norfloxacin 400 mg BID, levofloxacin 400 mg daily)
  - **Alternatives.** Trimethoprim-sulfamethoxazole, azithromycin, or erythromycin (Table 3-3)

TABLE 3-3	TREATMENT OF BACTERIAL DIARRHEA
Campylobacter	Azithromycin 500 mg daily ×3 days
Salmonella	Ciprofloxacin 500 mg BID ×7 days Azithromycin 500 mg daily ×7 days
Shigella	Ciprofloxacin 500 mg BID or 750 mg daily ×3 days Azithromycin 500 mg daily ×3 days
Clostridium difficile	Metronidazole 500 mg TID ×14 days Vancomycin 125 mg PO QID ×14 days in severe/recurrent cases
Enterohemorrhagic *E. coli*	NOT RECOMMENDED
Enterotoxigenic *E. coli*	Ciprofloxacin 500 mg BID or 750 mg daily ×3 days Azithromycin 1000 mg ×1
Enteroinvasive *E. coli*	As for *Shigella*
Vibrio cholerae	Doxycycline 300 mg ×1 Azithromycin 500 mg daily ×3 days
Vibrio parahaemolyticus	As for *Shigella*
Aeromonas	As for *Shigella*
Plesiomonas	As for *Shigella*

- **Giardia/Amebiasis.** Metronidazole 250 to 750 mg TID ×7 to 10 days
- **Cyclospora/Isospora.** Trimethoprim-Sulfamethoxazole DS BID ×7 to 10 days
- Antibiotic treatment is also recommended in **infectious diarrhea caused by sexually transmitted diseases,** such as *Chlamydia* infection, gonorrhea, HSV infection, and syphilis.
- **Enterohemorrhagic** *Escherichia coli* (EHEC) **or** *E. coli* **O157:H7.** Antibiotics are NOT recommended as they have not been shown to hasten recovery or decrease the contagious period. In addition, their use may precipitate the hemolytic–uremic syndrome. Clinical clues to EHEC infection include recent ingestion of raw/undercooked ground meat, bloody diarrhea, abdominal pain, and minimal or lack of fever.

Chronic Diarrhea

- **Volume status, electrolyte disturbances, and vitamin deficiencies** need to be addressed.
  - Uncomplicated, mild diarrhea is treated with oral fluids similar to that in acute diarrhea.
  - In cases of severe diarrhea, intravenous fluids (lactated Ringer's or 0.9% normal saline) may be necessary to restore volume depletion and to keep up with ongoing losses. Rarely, patients may require intravenous fluids long term, administered through a permanent indwelling catheter with the assistance of home health care nursing.
  - Total parenteral nutrition may be required in the hospital or long term at home, requiring an indwelling catheter and home health care nursing.
  - Vitamin deficiencies may occur due to decreased oral intake or malabsorption. Vitamin levels should be monitored and supplemented if deficient, especially the fat-soluble vitamins in those with chronic steatorrhea.
- The **underlying cause needs to be treated** whenever possible.[1,7–10]
  - If there is a reversible cause such as infection, dietary precipitant, medication, or tumors, then chronic diarrhea may potentially be resolved with treatment or by removal of the offending agent.
  - **Microscopic (collagenous/lymphocytic) colitis.** Budesonide 9 mg daily with slow taper. Bismuth subsalicylate, cholestyramine, and mesalamine may also be used. In severe or refractory cases, immunomodulators such as azathioprine or systemic steroids may be required.
  - **Bile acid induced diarrhea.** An empiric trial of cholestyramine (a binding resin) is both diagnostic and therapeutic. Recommended dose is 4 g TID.
  - **Lactose intolerance.** Empiric trial of avoiding dairy products is both diagnostic and therapeutic.
  - **Small bowel bacterial overgrowth.** Clinical response to antibiotics is often rapid; cyclical antibiotics are often necessary unless the predisposing cause for bacterial overgrowth has been addressed.
  - **Pancreatic enzyme replacement.** A therapeutic trial may be beneficial in steatorrhea.
- **Opiate antidiarrheal agents** are safe in mild to moderate diarrhea.
  - **Loperamide** (Imodium) 2 to 4 mg QID or 4 mg followed by 2 mg after each loose stool up to a maximum daily dose of 16 mg.
  - **Diphenoxylate plus atropine** (Lomotil) 4 mg QID has combined opioid and anticholinergic effects.

- ○ Other more potent options include combinations of opiates with antispasmodics, such as tincture of opium (2 to 20 drops QID) with belladonna or hyocyamine.
- ○ Empiric treatment with antidiarrheals without extensive investigation is appropriate for patients without alarm findings such as those with IBS.
- ○ **Psyllium** can be used to increase stool bulk in those with fecal incontinence.
- ○ **Octreotide** (a somatostatin analogue) may be used in secretory diarrhea to decrease the volume of stool.
  - ▪ Octreotide 50 to 250 mcg subcutaneous BID to TID.
  - ▪ Octreotide may also be used in acute postoperative diarrhea, such as with high ostomy output.
    - □ In this scenario, a fluid-filled bowel is often mistaken for postoperative ileus. Clues to this diagnosis are abdominal distention on examination in the presence of significant diarrhea. Cross-sectional imaging reveals a distended, fluid-filled bowel. Symptoms resolve rapidly with decompression by a nasogastric tube and initiation of subcutaneous octreotide.
- **Antibiotics**
  - ○ Empiric treatment can be considered if the patient is at high risk for dehydration or systemic complications, in the setting of a high suspicion of infectious cause, or if there is high prevalence of infectious diarrhea in the community.
  - ○ Metronidazole or fluoroquinolone may be used.

Surgical Management

- Surgery may be indicated to treat the underlying cause, such as with neuroendocrine tumor, severe colitis, or malignancy.

Lifestyle/Risk Modification

Diet

- Malnutrition and vitamin deficiencies may occur due to decreased oral intake or malabsorption.
- Enteral feeds are always recommended when the gut is healthy and functioning, but additional intravenous fluids and total parenteral nutrition may be necessary either temporarily or long term.
- In acute diarrhea, bowel rest or a change to a clear liquid or bland diet that avoids high-fiber foods, fats, milk products, caffeine, and alcohol may improve the patient's symptoms in the short term. Dairy products may not be well tolerated.
- If there is an underlying mucosal cause for malabsorption, such as celiac disease or disaccharidase deficiency, then the diet should be limited to eliminate the offending agent (i.e., gluten or lactose-free diets).
- Vitamin levels should be evaluated and supplemented if deficient. Prophylactic supplementation may be recommended with daily multivitamin, calcium, vitamin D, and B-complex.
- Probiotics are not routinely recommended at this time, given the lack of regulations and consensus on their benefits. However, these agents may be beneficial in chronic diarrhea in the setting of IBS. Anecdotal evidence exists for benefit in other types of chronic diarrhea.

SPECIAL CONSIDERATIONS

- **HIV/AIDS**
  - Patients who are HIV positive with low CD4 counts have high risk of chronic infectious diarrhea. Etiologies include common infectious agents as well as opportunistic infections such as CMV and *Mycobacterium avium intracellulare*. Other causes include intestinal malignancies such as lymphoma and Kaposi sarcoma, AIDS enteropathy, and medication-induced symptoms from HAART treatment such as with nelfinavir and ritonavir. The lack of simple diagnostic tools and directed treatment, however, often relegates these patients to symptomatic therapy.
- **Inflammatory bowel disease**
  - Antimotility agents should be used with caution in patients with severe IBD because of the potential complication of toxic megacolon; patients with bloody diarrhea, high fever, or systemic toxicity should not be given antidiarrheals. Anticholinergic agents are absolutely contraindicated in acute diarrhea because of the rare complication of toxic megacolon.
  - The initial clinical presentation of IBD may be unmasked by acute infectious diarrhea.
  - CMV and *C. difficile* infection should always be ruled out first in IBD patients.
- **Pediatrics**
  - Patients with symptoms suggestive of EHEC/*E. coli* O157:H7 should not be treated with antibiotics, given the risk of precipitating hemolytic-uremic syndrome.
  - Clinical clues to EHEC infection include recent ingestion of raw/undercooked ground meat, bloody diarrhea, and abdominal pain but no or minimal fever.
- **Pregnancy**
  - *Listeria* with or without systemic symptoms should be high in the differential.

COMPLICATIONS

- Dehydration
- Acute renal failure
- Electrolyte abnormalities such as metabolic acidosis, hypokalemia
- Weight loss and wasting
- Malnutrition such as fat-soluble vitamin A, D, E, and K deficiencies with steatorrhea
- Transient acquired mucosal digestive insufficiency such as a secondary lactose malabsorption, following an acute gastroenteritis. This phenomenon often manifests as persistent diarrhea, abdominal cramps, and bloating until normal mucosal enzymatic activity is restored. These symptoms may persist for weeks to months.
- A subset of patients with an acute gastroenteritis develop a chronic postinfectious IBS.

REFERRAL

- Referral to a gastroenterologist/specialist is indicated depending on the following:
  - Severity of disease

○ Diagnosis
○ Need for endoscopy
○ Long-term management (IBD, chronic pancreatitis)

REFERENCES

1. Fine KD, Schiller LR. AGA technical review on the evaluation and management of chronic diarrhea. *Gastroenterology.* 1999;116:1464–1486.
2. Camilleri M. Chronic diarrhea: a review on pathophysiology and management for the clinical gastroenterologist. *Clin Gastroenterol Hepatol.* 2004;2:198–206.
3. DuPont HL. Guidelines on acute infectious diarrhea in adults. The Practice Parameters Committee of the ACG. *Am J Gastroenterol.* 1997;92:1962–1975.
4. American Gastroenterological Association. *The Burden of Gastrointestinal Diseases.* Bethesda, MD: American Gastroenterological Association; 2001:38–40.
5. Pawlowski SW, Warren CA, Guerrant R. Diagnosis and treatment of acute or persistent diarrhea. *Gastroenterology.* 2009;136:1874–1886.
6. Thielman NM, Guerrant RL. Acute infectious diarrhea. *N Engl J Med.* 2004;350:38–47.
7. Schiller LR. Chronic diarrhea. *Gastroenterology.* 2004;127:287–293.
8. Schiller LR. Diarrhea. *Med Clin North Am.* 2000;84:1259–1274.
9. Donowitz M, Kokke FT, Saidi R. Evaluation of patients with chronic diarrhea. *N Engl J Med.* 1995;332:725–729.
10. Headstrom PD, Surawicz CM. Chronic diarrhea. *Clin Gastroenterol Hepatol.* 2005;3:734–737.
11. AGA medical position statement: guidelines for the evaluation and management of chronic diarrhea. *Gastroenterology.* 1999;116:1461–1463.
12. ASGE Standards of Practice Committee, Shen B, Khan K, Ikenberry SO, et al. The role of endoscopy in the management of patients with diarrhea. *Gastrointest Endosc.* 2010;71:887–892.

Constipation

Reena V. Chokshi

GENERAL PRINCIPLES

- Constipation is one of the most common gastrointestinal complaints in the general population. It is associated with decreased work productivity,[1] decreased quality of life,[2] and increased anxiety and depression.[3]
- Constipation encompasses a multitude of disorders and symptoms that affect colonic and anorectal function, and a careful understanding of this heterogeneity is essential for proper patient management.

Definition

- Constipation is a symptomatically defined disorder, characterized by infrequent stools, difficult stool passage, or both.[4] Associated symptoms often include passage of hard stools, straining, unproductive urges, and the sensation of incomplete evacuation.

Classification

- **Primary versus secondary**
  - Secondary constipation occurs as a side effect of various conditions and medications and is important to rule out before embarking on a complex evaluation.
- **Acute versus chronic**
  - A consensus definition has been established to address the varied components of chronic constipation (Table 4-1).

Epidemiology

- Studies estimate the prevalence of chronic constipation between 2% and 27% in North America.[4] It is the primary diagnosis or reason for visit in approximately 2.7 million outpatient and emergency department visits annually and is responsible for another 38,000 inpatient stays.[5]
- More than $1 billion is spent annually on laxatives in the United States.[6]

Etiology

- The potential etiologies of primary constipation can be generally categorized into normal transit constipation, slow transit constipation, pelvic floor dyssynergia, and constipation-predominant irritable bowel syndrome. It is important to note that there is considerable overlap between these categories.[7,8]
  - Patients with **normal transit constipation** have symptoms without evidence of delayed colonic transit.
  - **Slow transit constipation** is an idiopathic entity with delayed transit from the proximal to distal colon.
  - **Pelvic floor dyssynergia** occurs when the puborectalis and anal sphincter muscles fail to relax or paradoxically contract with attempted defecation,

TABLE 4-1	ROME III DIAGNOSTIC CRITERIA FOR FUNCTIONAL CONSTIPATION

At least 3 mo (with symptom onset at least 6 mo prior to diagnosis) of two or more of the following:

- Straining with ≥25% of defecations
- Lumpy or hard stools with ≥25% of defecations
- Sensation of incomplete evacuation with ≥25% of defecations
- Sensation of anorectal obstruction or blockage with ≥25% of defecations
- Manual maneuvers to facilitate ≥25% of defecations
- Fewer than three defecations per week

Loose stools are absent without use of laxatives
Insufficient criteria for the diagnosis of constipation predominant IBS (IBS-C)

Adapted from Longstreth GF, Thompson WG, Chey WD, et al. Functional bowel disorders. *Gastroenterology.* 2006;130:1480–1491.

leading to an inability to defecate at the level of the anorectum; colonic transit to the rectum can be normal in this disorder.

○ **Irritable bowel syndrome** is considered **constipation-predominant** if the patient has <25% loose or watery stools or ≥25% hard or lumpy stools.

Pathophysiology

- Colonic and anorectal function are incompletely understood but are thought to be influenced by various factors, including intrinsic reflexes and autonomic processes, neurotransmitters, diurnal variation, and learned behaviors.[9]

Risk Factors

- Women tend to have more self-reported constipation than men, and the prevalence of constipation increases with age.[9] It has been estimated that 50% of the elderly living in the community suffer from constipation.[10]
- Other risk factors include physical inactivity, malnutrition, restricted diets, polypharmacy, recent abdominal or pelvic surgery, travel, and known comorbid conditions.

DIAGNOSIS

- The workup of the constipated patient requires a thorough history and physical examination. Though not always necessary, a number of diagnostic tests can also be performed to arrive at a diagnosis.

Clinical Presentation

- Patients with constipation present with a wide range of complaints, many of which may create substantial embarrassment for them. A trusting relationship will aid in obtaining a clear and well-defined history.

History

- A well-performed defecation history elicits whether the patient has infrequent stools, hard stools, a sense of incomplete evacuation, straining, need for digital

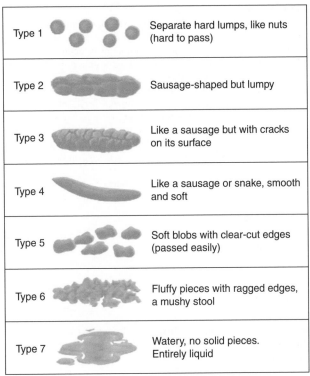

Type 1	Separate hard lumps, like nuts (hard to pass)
Type 2	Sausage-shaped but lumpy
Type 3	Like a sausage but with cracks on its surface
Type 4	Like a sausage or snake, smooth and soft
Type 5	Soft blobs with clear-cut edges (passed easily)
Type 6	Fluffy pieces with ragged edges, a mushy stool
Type 7	Watery, no solid pieces. Entirely liquid

FIGURE 4-1 **Bristol Stool Chart.** (Adapted from Lewis SJ, Heaton KW. Stool form scale as a useful guide to intestinal transit time. *Scand J Gastroenterol.* 1997;32:920–924.)

disimpaction, and associated abdominal pain. Onset and duration of symptoms are also important. For instance, lifelong abdominal discomfort may suggest overlap with irritable bowel syndrome.

- The **Bristol Stool Scale** is the best descriptor of stool form and consistency and can be a very useful tool (Fig. 4-1).
- A complete review of symptoms will help narrow the differential diagnosis. For example, if the patient reports cold intolerance and weight gain, hypothyroidism should be considered. The triad of kidney stones, confusion, and constipation suggests hypercalcemia. Current diuretic use or vomiting may predispose to constipation through hypokalemia and ileus. Esophageal dysmotility associated with constipation can be seen in systemic sclerosis.
- Colon cancer can present with obstructive symptoms, but this is typically a late manifestation; important questions include a history of weight loss, bloody stools, family history of colon cancer, and prior screening colonoscopy.
- A careful medication history should be obtained before embarking on an involved workup of constipation. Numerous medications can be associated with constipation, and simple discontinuation can lead to resolution of symptoms.

Physical Examination

- The physical examination can help identify both gastrointestinal and extraintestinal causes of constipation. For instance, the presence of a thyroid goiter or peripheral neuropathy may suggest an endocrine or neurologic etiology.
- **Abdominal examination** includes inspection for signs of previous surgery; auscultation for the presence and frequency of bowel sounds; and palpation to assess for distention, masses, or retained stool.
- The **perineal and rectal examination** can provide invaluable information. Close inspection helps detect internal hemorrhoids, fissures, or masses. Perineal sensation and the anal wink reflex should also be assessed. Anorectal neuromuscular function can be evaluated on digital examination by checking the sphincter tone both at rest and with squeeze. Gaping of the anal canal on immediate withdrawal of the finger may suggest external anal sphincter denervation. Asking the patient to bear down may reveal rectal prolapse, rectocele, or paradoxical contraction. Significant pain on digital examination can imply a fissure or ulceration.

Differential Diagnosis

- Differential diagnosis is broad and includes myriad conditions and medications as listed in Table 4-2.

Diagnostic Testing

- No single test makes a clear diagnosis, so patients must be assessed thoroughly on an individual basis.

Laboratories

- Initial laboratory tests include **basic chemistry panel with glucose, calcium, thyroid-stimulating hormone,** and **complete blood cell count. Stool should be checked for occult blood.**

TABLE 4-2	DIFFERENTIAL DIAGNOSIS OF CONSTIPATION
Endocrine	Diabetes mellitus, hypothyroidism, hyperparathyroidism, pregnancy, pheochromocytoma
Metabolic	Chronic kidney disease, hypercalcemia, hypokalemia, hypomagnesemia, porphyria, heavy metal poisoning
Neurogenic	Hirschsprung's disease, Chagas' disease, Parkinson's disease, spinal cord injuries or tumors, autonomic neuropathy, intestinal pseudoobstruction, stroke, multiple sclerosis, dementia
Myopathies	Scleroderma, amyloidosis, myotonic dystrophy
Structural	Colon cancer, stricture, external compression, rectocele, fissure, hemorrhoids
Medications	Analgesics, tricyclic antidepressants, anticholinergics, antihistamines, antipsychotics, antiparkinsonian agents, antidiarrheals, antacids, calcium-channel blockers, diuretics, anticonvulsants, cation-containing agents (e.g., iron, bismuth), bile acid resins
Other	Irritable bowel syndrome, anal spasm, rectal prolapse, depression, low-fiber diet, sedentary lifestyle, slow-transit constipation, pelvic floor dysfunction

- More specific testing for endocrinopathies, metabolic disorders, or collagen vascular disorders should be performed only when a high suspicion exists.

Imaging
- **Plain radiographs** can be helpful to investigate possible ileus or obstruction as well as to look for stool retention or megacolon. **Barium radiography** can be performed if plain radiographs are suggestive of megacolon, megarectum, or structural disease with luminal narrowing.
- **Defecography** typically involves placing a small amount of barium into the patient's rectum and then having him or her perform a series of maneuvers. **Dynamic MRI** may be used instead of fluoroscopic techniques to view the pelvis in greater detail. This can prove helpful when previous studies are inconclusive or inconsistent with the clinical scenario.[11]

Diagnostic Procedures
- **Flexible sigmoidoscopy** and **colonoscopy** are typically reserved for new-onset constipation of unclear etiology, especially in the presence of warning signs, such as weight loss, anemia, bloody stools, family history of colon cancer, or hemoccult-positive stools. When seen in patients older than 50 years, these signs should prompt a full workup to rule out colorectal cancer. Other processes that can be detected on colonoscopy, such as hemorrhoids, fissures, and stercoral ulcers, may be the result of long-standing constipation. Melanosis coli, a brownish-black discoloration of the bowel mucosa, is sometimes seen in the presence of chronic anthraquinone laxative use.
- **Colonic transit studies** can be performed to distinguish causes of primary constipation. One type involves ingestion of radio-opaque markers, with plain radiography performed 5 days later. If six or more markers are left scattered throughout the colon, slow transit is suggested. If those markers are confined to the rectosigmoid colon, there may be an element of obstructive defecation. A new, wireless capsule technique, called the Smart Pill, can provide similar information while also assessing transit and pH in the stomach and small bowel.[9]
- **Anorectal manometry** provides an assessment of both pressure activity and sensation of the anorectum and its sphincters. These measures are carefully evaluated during rest, squeeze, and bear down maneuvers. A balloon inflation test measures the patient's symptoms at various pressures. Finally, a balloon expulsion test can be performed to assess the patient's ability to expel a simulated bowel movement within an allotted amount of time, typically within 2 minutes in normal subjects.

TREATMENT

- Initial therapy for chronic constipation involves use of dietary fiber supplementation and laxatives.
- In the event that first-line therapy fails, assessment of colonic and/or anorectal function is appropriate before starting further medications.

Medications

First Line
- **Fiber supplementation** can begin at 10 g/day and increased by approximately 5 g/day each week to a total intake of approximately 25 g/day. It is important to instruct patients to maintain adequate hydration during trials of increased

fiber, as constipation can potentially worsen. Bloating, abdominal distention, and flatulence are side effects seen with fiber supplementation.

- **Osmotic laxatives,** such as lactulose and mixed electrolyte solutions (polyethylene glycol), work by osmotically increasing fluid in the bowel lumen. Adverse effects include electrolyte imbalance, dehydration, and urge incontinence because of the fluid volume delivered to the rectum. Similarly, **saline laxatives** help attract water to the bowel lumen. Examples are magnesium citrate, phosphate, and sulfate. Adverse effects include dehydration, abdominal cramping, and magnesium toxicity (avoid in renal dysfunction).
- **Stimulant laxatives** are the most frequently prescribed laxatives. They work by increasing colonic motility. Anthraquinones additionally increase fluid and electrolyte content in the distal ileum and colon. Examples are senna and bisacodyl. Adverse effects include abdominal cramping, cathartic colon, and melanosis coli (senna, cascara).
- **Emollients** consist of mineral oils and docusate salts. Mineral oil penetrates the stool and softens it, whereas docusate salts lower surface tension of stool, allowing more water through. Adverse effects include malabsorption of fat-soluble vitamins and lipid pneumonia if aspirated.
- **Enemas** use tap water, saline, mineral oil, or sodium phosphate to cause distal colonic distension and reflex evacuation of luminal contents. Adverse effects include mechanical trauma and damage to rectal mucosa with chronic use.

Second Line

- **5-hydroxytryptamine-4 (5-HT$_4$) receptor agonists** have been studied extensively for their prokinetic value. The older drugs in this class, cisapride and tegaserod, have been taken off the market due to potential cardiovascular adverse events. Instead, attention has shifted to newer drugs in this class, such as prucalopride, which has been approved in Europe at a dose of 2 mg/day in adults and 1 mg/day in the elderly.[12]
- **Lubiprostone,** a chloride-channel activator that increases intestinal water secretion, has been approved for use both in constipation predominant IBS (IBS-C) and chronic constipation.[13] Nausea is the most commonly seen adverse effect.
- **Linaclotide** is a guanylate cyclase C activator that leads to intestinal chloride and bicarbonate secretion. Studies are ongoing, and thus far the results have been encouraging.[14]
- **Mu-receptor antagonists** that work in the periphery can be helpful in certain, typically inpatient, situations. Methylnaltrexone, used to treat patients with opioid-related constipation, promotes bowel movements without decreasing the pain-relieving effects of narcotics. Alvimopan has been used successfully in postoperative ileus.[15]

Other Nonpharmacologic Therapies

- **Biofeedback** is a type of behavioral training that has shown benefit in the setting of defecatory disorders, both in improving symptoms and anorectal function.[16] Patients are retrained to relax their pelvic floor muscles and restore normal anorectal synergy during defecation. This method appears to be beneficial primarily in those with outlet dysfunction.[17]
- Other behavioral training includes **ritualization of bowel movement timing.**[9]

Surgical Management

- Surgical intervention can be used in patients with a structural reason for obstructed defecation (e.g., rectocele). It is rarely used in chronic constipation, except in the patient with colonic inertia who has failed prolonged medical therapy.

Lifestyle/Risk Modification

- **Proper fluid intake** and **exercise** could be beneficial in patients with constipation, though there is little evidence to support this.[18]

SPECIAL CONSIDERATIONS

- In the elderly, the etiology of constipation is often multifactorial and can include comorbid illnesses, medications, and decreased mobility.[18] Care should be taken to monitor hydration and electrolytes closely, especially in those with renal disease.
- Constipation is a commonly encountered problem in pregnancy. Oftentimes, patients can be treated with simple reassurance and proper education.[19]

COMPLICATIONS

- Early recognition and management of constipation is important, because chronic constipation can lead to **fecal impaction, pudendal nerve damage, fecal incontinence, rectal prolapse, stercoral ulcers** with perforation or bleeding, **volvulus, hemorrhoids,** or **anal fissures.**
  - These complications tend to occur more frequently in the elderly and nursing home residents. Early recognition of these complications is an effective strategy to reduce morbidity in these patients.
  - Some complications can require surgical management, such as stercoral ulcers with perforation, or anatomic abnormalities that obstruct defecation (e.g., enterocele, rectocele, cystocele). Refractory slow transit constipation or colonic inertia is sometimes managed with total colectomy and ileorectal anastomosis, but pelvic floor dyssynergia is first excluded in these instances.[12,18]
  - Endoscopic therapy of stercoral ulcers may be necessary to achieve hemostasis in the setting of rectal bleeding.
  - Fecal impaction should always be considered in patients with chronic constipation regardless of whether presentation involves constipation or incontinence. Fecal impaction can lead to incontinence by invoking the rectoanal inhibitory reflex, that is, the tendency for the internal anal sphincter to relax in the presence of stool in the rectum. A quick digital rectal examination can often help detect stool in the rectum. However, fecal impaction sometimes occurs higher than the rectum, and absence of stool in the rectum does not exclude the diagnosis. A plain x-ray film of the abdomen may reveal obstructive features and lack of rectal air. Management involves disimpaction, sometimes manually. Oil-based enemas (cottonseed enema, mineral oil enema) may help soften the stool and ease evacuation. Hypaque enemas may provide both diagnosis and therapy of fecal impaction. After disimpaction, an effective oral laxative regimen with or without rectal suppositories or enemas needs to be established.

- Abdominal pain associated with constipation can sometimes lead to unnecessary surgeries, such as appendectomy, hysterectomy, or ovarian cystectomy.

REFERRAL

- Referral to a gastroenterologist may be warranted, especially if specialized studies, such as anorectal manometry, are needed.

REFERENCES

1. Bracco A, Kahler K. Burden of chronic constipation must include estimates of work productivity and activity impairment in addition to traditional healthcare utilization. *Am J Gastroenterol.* 2004;99:S233.
2. Irvine EJ, Ferazzi S, Pare P, et al. Health-related quality of life in functional GI disorders: focus on constipation and resource utilization. *Am J Gastroenterol.* 2002;97:1986–1993.
3. Cheng C, Chan AOO, Hui WM, et al. Coping strategies, illness perception, anxiety and depression of patients with idiopathic constipation: a population-based study. *Aliment Pharmacol Ther.* 2003;18:319–326.
4. American College of Gastroenterology Chronic Constipation Task Force. An evidence-based approach to the management of chronic constipation in North America. *Am J Gastroenterol.* 2005;100(suppl 1):S1–S4.
5. Martin BC, Barghout V, Cerulli A. Direct medical costs of constipation in the United States. *Manag Care Interface.* 2006;19:43–49.
6. Wilbur V, Briscoe T. Constipation, diarrhea, and irritable bowel syndrome. In: Poole Arcangelo V, Peterson AM, eds. *Pharmacotherapeutics for Advanced Practice: A Practical Approach.* 2nd ed. Philadelphia: Lippincott Williams & Wilkins; 2006:386–414.
7. Lembo A, Camilleri M. Chronic constipation. *N Engl J Med.* 2003;349:1360–1368.
8. Cook IJ, Talley NJ, Benninga MA, et al. Chronic constipation: overview and challenges. *Neurogastroenterol Motil.* 2009;21(suppl 2):1–8.
9. Rao SS. Constipation: evaluation and treatment of colonic and anorectal motility disorders. *Gastrointest Endosc Clin N Am.* 2009;19:117–139.
10. Bouras EP, Tangalos EG. Chronic constipation in the elderly. *Gastroenterol Clin North Am.* 2009;38:463–480.
11. Bharucha AE. Constipation. *Best Pract Res Clin Gastroenterol.* 2007;21:709–731.
12. Camilleri M, Bharucha AE. Behavioural and new pharmacological treatments for constipation: getting the balance right. *Gut.* 2010;59:1288–1296.
13. Barish CF, Drossman D, Johanson JF, et al. Efficacy and safety of lubiprostone in patients with chronic constipation. *Dig Dis Sci.* 2010;55:1090–1097.
14. Lembo AJ, Kurtz CB, Macdougall JE, et al. Efficacy of linaclotide for patients with chronic constipation. *Gastroenterology.* 2010;138:886–895.
15. Lembo A. Peripheral opioids for functional GI disease: a reappraisal. *Dig Dis.* 2006;24:91–98.
16. Enck P, Van der Voort IR, Klosterhalfen S. Biofeedback therapy in fecal incontinence and constipation. *Neurogastroenterol Motil.* 2009;21:1133–1141.
17. Chiaroni G, Salandini L, Whitehead WE. Biofeedback benefits only patients with outlet dysfunction, not patients with isolated slow transit constipation. *Gastroenterology.* 2005;129:86–97.
18. Rao SS, Go JT. Update on the management of constipation in the elderly: new treatment options. *Clin Interv Aging.* 2010;5:163–171.
19. Cullen G, O'Donoghue D. Constipation and pregnancy. *Best Pract Res Clin Gastroenterol.* 2007;21:807–818.

Abdominal Pain

5

Akwi W. Asombang

GENERAL PRINCIPLES

- Abdominal pain is one of the most common complaints for which patients visit primary care providers, and one of the most common reasons for gastroenterology consult.[1–3]
- The ability to diagnose and treat abdominal pain accurately and efficiently is of great importance.
- A general understanding of anatomy and physiology is important in formulating a differential diagnosis.
- An orderly approach is essential in the evaluation of abdominal pain, particularly in avoiding unnecessary repetitive testing and potential harmful delays in making the diagnosis.

Classification

- **Parietal pain**
  - The parietal peritoneum lining the abdominal cavity is innervated by somatic nerve fibers.
  - Therefore, the pain caused by irritation of the parietal peritoneum is **usually sharp, well localized, and lateralizes to the site of irritation.**
  - The **most frequent stimulus is inflammation,** often from an inflamed adjacent organ or viscus.
  - Other stimuli that can irritate the parietal peritoneum are blood, gastric acid, or stool.
  - The pain is **constant and worse with motion** of the peritoneum.
  - Pain severity depends on the specific irritating agent and the rate of development.
  - There is open associated reflex muscle spasm of the abdominal muscles referred to as "**involuntary guarding.**"
  - When bowel perforates or when blood collects in the peritoneal cavity, extensive stimulation of the parietal peritoneum results in a board-like **rigid abdomen,** with **diffuse and excruciating pain made worse by even minimal movement.**
- **Visceral pain**
  - Noxious stimuli affecting the abdominal viscera result in the perception of visceral pain.
  - This can result from traction on the peritoneum, distension of a hollow viscus, or muscular contraction, often against an obstructed lumen.
  - The pain fibers innervating the visceral structures are bilateral, so pain is typically perceived in the midline.
  - As opposed to parietal pain, visceral pain is **dull and poorly localized, often remote from the location of the abnormality.**

- ○ The pain is **often intermittent or colicky,** but it can be constant.
- ○ There are often associated autonomic symptoms such as nausea, vomiting, diaphoresis, or pallor.
- **Referred pain**
  - ○ Pain is **felt in areas distant to the diseased organ.**
  - ○ The pain can be well localized and felt in the skin or deeper tissues.
  - ○ Examples include diaphragmatic irritation from a subphrenic hematoma or abscess resulting in shoulder pain, pain in the thigh from a psoas abscess, and radiation of renal colic from loin to groin. Gallbladder and bile duct pain can also be referred to the shoulder or scapular area, particularly on the right side.

Pathophysiology

- Noxious stimuli can result in pain within the abdomen by various mechanisms, and the characteristics of these mechanisms can help in identifying the underlying disease process.[1,3]
- The two principal mechanisms of pain, parietal pain and visceral pain, are discussed below.
- Other mechanisms of pain that may be relevant include ischemia, musculoskeletal pain, referred pain, metabolic derangements, neurogenic pain, and functional pain. A single diseased organ can produce pain through multiple mechanisms.[1–3]

DIAGNOSIS

Clinical Presentation

- A thorough, detailed history and physical examination are keys to efficient evaluation of patients with abdominal pain.
- An accurate diagnosis can be made in most patients only with a meticulous history and physical examination; however, diagnosis can remain elusive regardless of the extensive history and physical examination, in which case consider admission, serial examinations, follow-up calls, or surgical exploration.

History

- This is the **most important part of the evaluation,** thus an organized approach is essential.
- Attempts should be made to identify the pain onset, duration, character, location, severity, exacerbating or alleviating factors, and associated symptoms.[4]
- Other key aspects of the history should include underlying medical conditions, prior surgeries, medications, allergies, family history, travel, contact with animals or sick individuals, and social history including occupation and substance abuse. Some general features regarding these aspects of the history are described here.[4,5]
  - ○ **Onset of pain**
    - ■ It is important to **differentiate acute versus chronic pain.**
    - ■ Severe pain that begins abruptly may indicate an intra-abdominal catastrophe, including ruptured abdominal vasculature, occluded mesenteric vasculature, or perforated viscus. Urgent or immediate surgery may be essential in certain situations for a good patient outcome.
    - ■ Pain that develops rapidly over minutes suggests inflammation or luminal obstruction.
    - ■ Gradual onset over hours may also suggest inflammation.

- Duration
  - Pain caused by irritation of the parietal peritoneum is constant.
  - Obstruction of a hollow viscus typically results in crampy or colicky pain that waxes and wanes.
  - Pain lasting more than 6 months is generally considered as chronic abdominal pain and can remain undiagnosed despite extensive workup.
- Character
  - Parietal pain is usually severe and well localized.
  - Pain associated with visceral noxious stimuli is dull or gnawing and poorly localized.
- Location
  - This is often the most important characteristic in parietal pain. The parietal peritoneum is supplied by somatic nerves, thus pain is perceived in the area where the peritoneum is irritated.
  - Visceral pain is usually midline and poorly localized, but the location may provide useful information regarding the involved organ.
  - Radiation of pain may also help identify the affected organ.
  - Table 5-1 lists the commonly affected organs and perceived areas of pain.
- Severity/Intensity
  - This is very subjective and difficult to measure because it is dependent on the individual patients' point of reference. Other factors influencing severity include past experience of pain, personality traits, or cultural differences.
  - Severe pain suggests ruptured abdominal viscus or vascular structure.
  - Pain that is severe in the setting of a benign examination may suggest mesenteric ischemia.
- Exacerbating and alleviating factors
  - Pain caused by inflammation of the peritoneum is worse with coughing or movement.
  - Patients with renal or intestinal colic may move around in an attempt to get into a comfortable position.
  - Eating exacerbates pain caused by gastric ulcer, chronic mesenteric ischemia, or biliary pain but may alleviate pain caused by duodenal ulcer.
  - The pain associated with pancreatitis is classically relieved by bending forward or curling up in the fetal position.

TABLE 5-1	ORGAN INVOLVEMENT AND PERCEIVED LOCATION OF PAIN
Esophagus	Chest, epigastrium
Stomach	Epigastrium
Small intestine	Periumbilical region
Colon	Lower abdomen
Gallbladder	Right upper quadrant, radiation to scapula, shoulder, back
Liver	Right upper quadrant
Kidney or ureter	Costovertebral angle, flank, radiation to groin
Bladder	Suprapubic region
Aorta	Mid-back region

○ **Associated symptoms**
  ■ Nausea, vomiting, diaphoresis, hematemesis, hematochezia, melena, diarrhea, obstipation, hematuria, and fever may further focus the diagnostic evaluation.

Physical Examination
• As with the history, an organized approach to the physical examination, particularly the abdomen, increases the likelihood of an accurate diagnosis.
• In addition, focusing on key extra-abdominal physical examination findings is crucial because they may provide valuable clues as to the diagnosis.
• An exhaustive review of all the signs is beyond the scope of this chapter; however, several points deserve emphasis.
  ○ **Vital signs**
    ■ Particular attention must be given to frequent hemodynamic monitoring.
    ■ The presence of *tachycardia or orthostatic hypotension* suggests significant volume depletion and should prompt an immediate search for the underlying cause (hemorrhage, vomiting, diarrhea, or third-spacing).
    ■ *Tachycardia* may be the only sign of impending hemodynamic collapse in a patient with vascular catastrophe.
    ■ *Fever* suggests an inflammatory process, often infectious.
    ■ *Tachypnea* is often the earlier sign of sepsis.
  ○ **General appearance**
    ■ Much information can be determined by observing the patients' general appearance.
    ■ This includes an assessment of their overall appearance, respiratory pattern, ability to converse, position in bed, posture, and facial expression. Facial expression should be noted also while palpating the abdomen.
    ■ Patients with peritonitis often lie still, whereas those with renal or intestinal colic writhe in bed.
    ■ Patients with acute inflammatory or vascular disorders frequently appear flushed and systemically toxic.
    ■ Generalized pallor suggests severe anemia, potentially from acute blood loss.
  ○ **Abdominal examination**
    ■ Patients with acute abdominal pain are very apprehensive; hence, it is important to take a gentle, reassuring approach to the abdominal examination.
    ■ The abdomen should be examined with the patients' knees and hips flexed to relax the abdominal muscles.
    ■ First, the abdomen should be visually inspected for surgical scars, distension, bulging flanks, or other obvious abnormalities.
    ■ Next, auscultate for the presence or absence of bowel sounds or bruits.
    ■ Gentle pressure with the stethoscope allows assessment of tenderness without alarming the patient.
    ■ Palpation should begin at the site furthest away from the area of pain and additionally noting any visceral enlargement or masses.
    ■ The presence or absence of guarding, rigidity, or rebound tenderness should be noted, because these may signify peritoneal irritation.
    ■ Peritoneal inflammation is best determined by light percussion on the abdomen, gently shaking the bed or asking the patient to cough.

- Hernial orifices should be inspected and palpated in all instances, and the patient is asked to cough to determine whether an impulse is felt on coughing.
- Digital rectal examinations may have value, not just in anal/rectal palpation and inspecting rectal content on the examining finger but in localizing pain.
- External genitalia should be inspected, particularly the scrotum in males.
- Female patients should have pelvic examinations performed when appropriate.

Differential Diagnosis

- The list of diagnoses that can cause abdominal pain is extensive and includes inflammatory, mechanical, ischemic, metabolic, and neurologic conditions.[5]
- This emphasizes the need for a careful and systematic history and physical examination to narrow the possible diagnoses. Table 5-2 lists some of the common causes of abdominal pain.

Diagnostic Testing

- The differential diagnosis in patients presenting with acute abdominal pain can be determined with a careful history and physical examination; further diagnostic evaluation should be targeted to ruling in or excluding these conditions.[5]

TABLE 5-2 CAUSES OF ABDOMINAL PAIN

Inflammation	Mechanical	Ischemic	Metabolic	Other
Cholecystitis	Small or large bowel obstruction	Mesenteric ischemia	Diabetic ketoacidosis	Thoracic disorders
Pancreatitis	Volvulus	Splenic infarction	Uremia	Herpes zoster
Appendicitis	Biliary obstruction	Testicular torsion	Porphyria	SLE
Diverticulitis	Ureteral stones	Ovarian cyst torsion	Lead poisoning	Musculoskeletal disorders
Hepatitis	Ruptured aortic aneurysm	Incarcerated hernia		Functional abdominal pain
PID	Ruptured ectopic pregnancy			
Peptic ulcer	Intussusception			
Gastroenteritis				
Spontaneous bacterial peritonitis				
Acute colitis				
Pyelonephritis				
Acute cholangitis				

PID, pelvic inflammatory disease; SLE, systemic lupus erythematosus.

- Excessive, undirected testing increases the costs and may cause unnecessary delays in diagnosis and treatment.
- While elaborating all potential tests in the workup of abdominal pain is beyond the scope of this handbook, a few specific tests deserve special mention.

Laboratories

- A **complete blood cell count with differential count** should be ordered in all patients to evaluate for leucocytosis or anemia.
- **Serum electrolytes** (including blood urea nitrogen, creatinine, and glucose) are important to assess fluid status, acid-base status, and renal function.
- **Amylase** and **lipase** are useful in patients with suspected pancreatic disease, but note that these can also be elevated in patients with bowel obstruction or perforation and in patients with renal failure where clearance may be slow.
- **Lactate** levels may be helpful for suspected bowel infarction, but a normal level does not exclude intestinal ischemia.
- **Liver chemistries** should be obtained in patients with upper abdominal pain and those with known liver disease.
- **Coagulation profile** should be checked in those with suspected liver disease.
- All female patients of childbearing age should have pregnancy excluded with a urine or serum beta-human chorionic gonadotrophin (β-**hCG**).

Imaging

- **Standard radiography**
  - ○ Not all patients with acute abdominal pain require plain or upright films of the abdomen.
    - However, if ordered they should include two views of the abdomen: one in supine and one in the upright position.
    - If the patient is unable to sit up, then a lateral decubitus with left side down may identify abnormal gas pattern.
  - ○ Abdominal x-ray films are **useful for diagnosing perforated viscus** (identified as free air under the diaphragm), **ileus or bowel obstruction.**
  - ○ Abdominal films may also demonstrate the calcific changes associated with chronic pancreatitis as well as calcium-containing renal stones.
  - ○ In addition, some features of intestinal inflammation, such as colonic "thumbprinting," may be perceived on abdominal x-ray films.
  - ○ The sensitivity of abdominal radiography in the diagnosis of abdominal pathology in the setting of acute abdominal pain is about 10%; however, they are safe, relatively inexpensive, and can usually be performed quickly and thus should be considered.[6]
- **Ultrasonography**
  - ○ This is the **preferred initial imaging test in biliary tract disease and gallstones.** It is frequently obtained in patients with suspected acute cholecystitis, biliary colic, choledocholithiasis, and cholangitis.
  - ○ Transabdominal ultrasound is also useful for patients with abdominal aortic aneurysms; ectopic pregnancy, tubo-ovarian abscess, and ovarian or testicular torsion.
  - ○ Ultrasonography is safe and can be performed at the bedside in most cases.
- **Computed tomography (CT)**
  - ○ Abdominal CT, especially with rapid spiral scanning techniques, provides a powerful imaging tool.[6]
  - ○ CT allows "three-dimension" imaging of the entire abdomen and pelvis.

○ CT is less operator-dependent than the ultrasound.

○ CT is a sensitive test for identifying bowel obstruction, inflammatory processes (appendicitis, necrotizing pancreatitis, diverticulitis, intra-abdominal abscess), vascular lesion (ruptured aortic aneurysm, portal vein thrombosis), and abdominal or retroperitoneal hemorrhage.

○ Organ-specific protocols require focused helical CT, which requires coordination of oral/IV contrast and image attainment. This is useful to assess perforated viscus or differentiate ischemic, traumatic, or neoplastic lesions of the pancreas or the liver.

○ CT arteriography is another useful tool in assessing the aorta and visceral vasculature.

○ Patient selection for CT imaging is of great importance, as this can be costly and unnecessarily delay diagnosis and treatment especially in patients who require urgent surgery. There is also the risk of nephrotoxicity and anaphylactic reaction that can occur with iodinated contrast dye.

• **Magnetic resonance imaging (MRI)**

○ This is a multiplanar imaging modality using the different intrinsic soft tissue contrast properties to distinguish areas with different degrees of enhancement.[7]

○ MRI can detect subtle lesions that do not conform to organ contours with high sensitivity.

○ MRI is an excellent modality in the evaluation and differentiation of liver and pancreatic lesions.

○ MRI is highly sensitive in evaluating the mesenteric vessels in suspected ischemia.

○ MR cholangiopancreatography (MRCP) has become the noninvasive imaging modality of choice for evaluating abnormalities of the biliary and pancreatic ducts.

○ MR enterography has been used to image the small bowel and colon to detect inflammation, strictures, and fistulae.

○ Advantages over CT:
  ▪ MRI is safer in children and pregnant women because of lack of ionizing radiation.
  ▪ The intravenous contrast medium typically used (gadolinium) is thought to carry less risk of nephrotoxicity.

○ Disadvantages:
  ▪ MRI cannot be used in patients with permanent pacemakers, defibrillators, aneurysm clips, or metallic implants/devices.
  ▪ MRI is not suited for patients with severe claustrophobia because it is performed in a "closed tube"; open MRIs can be considered in such situations.
  ▪ MRI is more costly, time consuming, and requires greater patient cooperation thus making it less desirable in an urgent setting.

Diagnostic Procedures

• **Endoscopy**

○ Endoscopy is useful in evaluation of the esophagus, stomach, small bowel, and colon for ulceration, neoplasia, ischemia, or inflammation. However, bowel integrity has to be intact before performing endoscopy, as air and intestinal content can be pushed into the peritoneal cavity if endoscopy is performed where bowel integrity is compromised by perforation or extensive inflammation. Procedure risk needs to be balanced with potential benefits before performing endoscopy in acute abdominal pain presentations; it remains a very useful test in patients with chronic pain.[7]

- **Peritoneal aspiration or lavage**
  - A peritoneal tap is a useful adjunct for detecting hemoperitoneum from trauma or feculent material from hollow viscus injury/perforation.
  - Peritoneal taps are also performed for evaluation of peritoneal fluid accumulation, particularly in determining portal hypertension as an etiology, and in evaluating for infectious or spontaneous bacterial peritonitis (see also Chapters 10 and 19).
- **Urgent surgical intervention via laparoscopy or exploratory laparotomy** is warranted in patients with intra-abdominal catastrophes such as ruptured abdominal aortic aneurysm or ruptured intra-abdominal organ. Surgical exploration is sometimes performed in severe abdominal pain presentations wherein significant pathology is suspected, especially mesenteric ischemia.

REFERENCES

1. Fauci A, ed. *Harrison's Principles of Internal Medicine.* 16th ed. New York: McGraw-Hill; 2005:1725–1729.
2. Sleisenger MH, Fordtran JS. *Gastrointestinal Disease: Pathophysiology, Diagnosis, Management.* 8th ed. Philadelphia: WB Saunders; 2002:71–82.
3. Yamada T, ed. *Textbook of Gastroenterology.* 4th ed. Philadelphia: Lippincott Williams & Wilkins; 2003:781–801.
4. Wolfe MM. *Therapy of Digestive Disorders.* 2nd ed. Philadelphia: WB Saunders; 2006: 961–968.
5. Flasar MH, Cross R, Goldberg E. Acute abdominal pain. *Prim Care Clin Office Pract.* 2006; 33:659–684.
6. Ahn SH, Mayo-Smith WW, Murphy BL, et al. Acute non-traumatic abdominal pain in adult patients: abdominal radiography compared with CT evaluation. *Radiology.* 2002; 225:159–164.
7. Ginsberg GG, Kochman ML. *Endoscopy and Gastrointestinal Radiology.* 1st ed. Philadelphia: Mosby; 2004:111–133.

Acute Gastrointestinal Bleeding

6

Darrell M. Gray, II

GENERAL PRINCIPLES

- Acute gastrointestinal bleeding (GIB) is a common medical emergency resulting in significant morbidity, mortality, and >300,000 hospitalizations in the United States per year.[1]
- GIB involves a spectrum of clinical presentations based on the cause and site of bleeding. It can occur anywhere in the gastrointestinal (GI) tract from the mouth to the anus.
- This chapter discusses the etiologies, diagnostic strategies, and management of acute GIB.

Classification

- GIB can be subdivided into **upper gastrointestinal bleeding** (UGIB) and **lower gastrointestinal bleeding** (LGIB), based on location of the source in relationship to the ligament of Treitz. UGIB originates proximal and LGIB originates distal to the ligament of Treitz. With the advent of newer investigative modalities targeting the small bowel, LGIB can be further characterized to **small bowel bleeding (middle GIB)** and **colonic bleeding.**

Epidemiology

- Most GIB episodes are self-limited and require only supportive therapy. Despite this, GIB accounts for 16,000 to 20,000 deaths annually.[1]
- The annual incidence of hospitalization for UGIB has declined over recent years; incidence is ~82 per 100,000 population. In contrast, although LGIB is known to have a lower incidence of hospitalization, incidence has been increasing and is estimated to be 44 per 100,000 population.[1]
- It is well established that hospitalization and mortality rates for both UGIB and LGIB increase with age, but recent data also suggest gender differences, with males having higher incidence of UGIB than females, and females being older than males at the time of LGIB occurrence.[2]

Etiology

- **Upper gastrointestinal bleeding**
  - ○ **Erosive/Ulcerative disease**
    - ■ **Peptic ulcer disease.** This includes gastric and duodenal ulcers. Peptic ulcer disease (PUD) is the most common cause of acute UGIB accounting for up to 50% of cases.
      - □ Risk factors include *Helicobacter pylori* infection, nonsteroidal anti-inflammatory drug (NSAID) use, acetylsalicylic acid (ASA) use, and acid hypersecretion as in Zollinger-Ellison syndrome. *Helicobacter pylori* infection and NSAID use are the two most common causes of PUD.

TABLE 6-1	OUTCOME OF BLEEDING ULCERS BASED ON ENDOSCOPIC FINDINGS			
	% (Range)			
Endoscopic Appearance	Prevalence	Rebleeding	Surgery	Mortality
Clean base	42 (19–52)	5 (0–10)	0.5 (0–3)	2 (0–3)
Flat pigmented Spot	20 (0–42)	10 (0–13)	6 (0–10)	3 (0–10)
Adherent clot	17 (0–49)	22 (14–36)	10 (5–12)	7 (0–10)
Visible vessel	17 (4–35)	43 (0–81)	34 (0–56)	11 (0–21)
Active bleeding	18 (4–26)	55 (17–100)	35 (20–69)	11 (0–23)

Adapted from Laine L, Peterson WL. Bleeding peptic ulcer. *N Engl J Med.* 1994;331:717–727.

- □ In patients taking NSAIDs, cofactors such as age (>75 years), concurrent coronary artery disease, previous GIB, and a history of PUD may be independent risk factors for ulcer bleeding.
- □ Predictors for mortality include age >70 years, multiple comorbidities, systolic blood pressure <100 mm Hg, hematemesis on presentation, ulcer rebleeding, and requirement for surgery.
- □ Studies have shown that the endoscopic appearance of ulcers is strongly associated with rebleeding, need for surgery, and mortality (Table 6-1). Despite therapeutic advances, bleeding ulcer–related mortality rate has remained at ~10%.[3–6]
- ■ **Erosive and hemorrhagic gastropathy.** Gastric erosion can be defined as a 3- to 5-mm break in the mucosa that does not penetrate to the muscularis mucosa. This is most commonly the result of medications such as NSAIDs or ASA, which can cause a hemorrhagic gastropathy within 24 hours of administration.
- ■ **Stress ulcers** are distinct from peptic ulcers and occur in the setting of severe medical illness/physiologic stress. The pathophysiology is thought to be related to gastric hypoperfusion as a result of splanchnic vasoconstriction during physiologic stress.[3]
- ■ **Esophagitis.** Causes include gastric reflux, infections (i.e., cytomegalovirus, herpes simplex virus, *Candida albicans* infection), medications/pill-induced (quinidine, tetracycline, alendronate), radiation therapy, and eosinophilic infiltration. This rarely leads to severe bleeding. Common presenting symptoms include heartburn, nausea, epigastric discomfort, and chest pain.[3]
- ○ **Portal hypertension**
  - ■ **Variceal bleeding.** Variceal hemorrhage can originate from esophageal, gastric, and duodenal varices.
    - □ Varices are the result of portosystemic collateral circulation (with a portosystemic gradient >12 mm Hg) in patients with cirrhosis, portal or hepatic vein thrombosis, congenital hepatic fibrosis, and schistosomiasis.
    - □ In the United States, alcoholic cirrhosis is the most common cause of portal hypertension.

- ☐ Esophageal varices account for ~5% to 30% of UGIB cases. The 1-year incidence rate of a first variceal hemorrhage is 5% for large varices and 15% for small varices.
- ☐ Primary risk factors for bleeding from varices include size and wall thickness, presence of endoscopic stigmata such as red signs, severity of liver disease, and portal pressure.
- ☐ The estimated mortality from an episode of variceal bleeding has decreased over the past 2 decades from 30%–50% to ~20%.[7-9]
- **Portal hypertensive gastropathy.** This is characterized by congestion of the gastric mucosa from dilated arterioles and venules mainly in the gastric fundus and cardia. Erythema, petechiae, multiple bleeding areas, vascular ectasias, and congestion are hallmarks. The endoscopic appearance is often described as a mosaic pattern.[10]
- ○ **Vascular malformations**
  - **Vascular ectasias** account for 5% to 10% of UGIB.
    - ☐ Vascular ectasias include isolated arteriovenous malformations and diffuse linear vascular ectasia known as gastric antral vascular ectasia or "watermelon stomach."
    - ☐ Vascular ectasia are formed by a complex tangle of arteries and veins connected by one or more fistulae. The vascular complex is known as the nidus, which is lacking a capillary bed and, therefore, arteries directly drain into veins. The draining veins are known to dilate secondary to high-velocity blood flow and can eventually rupture, resulting in a bleed.
    - ☐ Vascular ectasias have been associated with various medical conditions including chronic renal failure, valvular heart disease, congestive heart failure, hereditary hemorrhagic telangiectasia, and von Willebrand's disease.[11]
  - **Dieulafoy's lesion.** This is an aberrant vessel protruding through the mucosa without an underlying ulcer. This represents <5% of UGIB cases.[11]
- ○ **Traumatic**
  - **Mallory-Weiss tear.** This is classically associated with vomiting or retching and is characterized by mucosal disruption at the gastroesophageal junction. This is responsible for 5% to 15% of all cases of UGIB and is self-limited in the majority of cases with very rare recurrence (0% to 7%).[3] The tear usually heals within a few days; however, continued vomiting and retching can lead to esophageal rupture (Boerhaave's syndrome).
- ○ **Other etiologies**
  - **Foreign body ingestion**
  - **Hemobilia.** This is characterized by bleeding into the duodenum from the biliary tract. It is usually caused by trauma but can be seen in malignant tumors, cholelithiasis, acalculous inflammatory disease, or vascular disorders.
  - **Tumors.** Benign tumors such as GI stromal tumors can bleed when the tumor outgrows its blood supply and ulcerates. Malignant tumors such as esophageal, gastric, and duodenal cancers can also bleed. Bleeding from malignant tumors may not be amenable to endoscopic therapeutic measures or vascular embolization, and surgical resection or radiation therapy may be required.
  - **Aortoenteric fistulas.** These can occur as a late complication after aortic graft surgery and usually involve the third and fourth parts of the duodenum. The fistulas can be difficult to diagnose because visualization of the graft eroding through the intestinal wall is uncommon. The classic "herald bleed" is a small bleed that can occur days to weeks before massive fatal hemorrhage.

TABLE 6-2 SOURCES OF LOWER GASTROINTESTINAL BLEEDING

Source	Frequency, %	Painless Hematochezia	Comments
Diverticulosis	30–65	Yes	Large volume; ~80% stop spontaneously
Angiodysplasia	4–15	Yes	Frequently multifocal; mostly right colon
Hemorrhoids	4–12	Yes	Typically intermittent and small volume
Ischemic colitis	4–11	No	Primarily affects watershed areas of colon
Colitis, other	3–15	No	Includes infection, radiation, and IBD[a]
Neoplasia	2–11	Yes	Rarely causes brisk bleeding
Postpolypectomy	2–7	Yes	Typically occurs within 2 wk
Rectal ulcer	0–8	Yes	Can result in massive hemorrhage
Dieulafoy's lesion, rare		Yes	Usually located in the rectum
Rectal varices, rare		Yes	Commonly linked to chronic liver disease

[a]IBD, inflammatory bowel disease.

Adapted from Strate LL, Naumann CR. The role of colonoscopy and radiological procedures in the management of acute lower intestinal bleeding. *Clin Gastroenterol Hepatol.* 2010;8:333–343.

■ **Hemosuccus pancreaticus.** This is characterized by hemorrhage into the pancreatic duct and occurs primarily in patients with chronic pancreatitis, pseudocyst, pancreatic cancer, aneurysms of the splenic artery, or trauma.[11]
- **Lower gastrointestinal bleeding** (Table 6-2)
  ○ **Diverticular bleeding.** It is the most common cause of major LGIB in the United States, related to the high prevalence of diverticulosis. Diverticula form at sites of weakness in the muscle wall of the colon where arteries penetrate the muscularis layer to reach the mucosa or submucosa.
  ○ **Anorectal disease. Hemorrhoids** and **anal fissures** are common causes of minor intermittent LGIB. The characteristic clinical history of hemorrhoidal bleeding is bright red blood on the toilet tissue or around the stool but not mixed in the stool. Bleeding often occurs with straining or passage of hard stool. A similar history is common in patients with bleeding from anal fissures, with the exception that anal fissures are often painful.
  ○ **Ischemic colitis.** It is typically caused by "low flow states" and small vessel disease rather than large vessel occlusion and most commonly involves the splenic flexure, descending colon, and sigmoid colon. Most cases resolve

spontaneously with observation and medical support. Surgery is reserved for the rare circumstance of clinical deterioration with fever and rising leukocyte count or persistent hemorrhage.

○ **Infectious colitis.** Pathogens such as *Campylobacter jejuni, Shigella* species, invasive *Escherichia coli* or *E. coli* O157:H7, and, rarely, *Clostridium difficile* may cause bloody diarrhea. Cytomegalovirus can cause invasive disease characterized by ulcers that can bleed but limited to immunocompromised states (immunosuppressive of biologic therapy for inflammatory bowel disease, after organ transplant, AIDS, etc.). The degree of blood loss is variable and rarely significant except with anticoagulation or coagulopathy.

○ **Radiation-induced proctopathy and colopathy.** Radiation injury is a chronic or recurrent problem that may follow irradiation immediately or present several years later. Radiation impairs the normal course of repopulation of surface epithelium within the GI tract. The loss of absorptive surface can often lead to malabsorption and diarrhea, but microulcerations can also form. These **microulcerations** can coalesce and form bigger lesions and eventually result in a GI bleed. Alternatively, **telangiectasia** can form in the mucosa, which can also bleed—this mechanism is typically seen as radiation proctopathy after radiation for prostate cancer. Blood loss is rarely massive but can cause iron deficiency or the need for intermittent blood transfusion.

○ **Inflammatory bowel disease.** It usually causes a small to moderate degree of bleeding, although rarely it can be massive. The blood is usually mixed with the stool and is associated with other symptoms of the disease, such as diarrhea, tenesmus, and pain.

○ **Other less common causes**

  ▪ **Meckel's diverticulum.** Meckel's diverticulum is the most frequent congenital anomaly of the intestinal tract, with an incidence of 0.3% to 3.0% in autopsy reports. It develops from incomplete obliteration of the vitelline duct, leaving an ileal diverticulum. Patients present with painless bleeding that may be melenic or bright red. The diagnosis can be made by radiolabeled technetium scanning. Barium filling of the diverticulum may occur, especially with enteroclysis. Surgical excision is the treatment of choice.

  ▪ **Intussusception.** Uncommon in adults, it usually has a leading point, such as a polyp or malignancy. Patients often present with bloody stools mixed with mucus, often described as "currant jelly." The diagnosis may be made by plain abdominal x-ray films and a sausage-shaped mass found during physical examination. Barium enema may be useful for diagnosis; in children, it may be used for therapeutic reduction. Treatment of intussusception in adults is usually surgical.[12–14]

DIAGNOSIS

Clinical Presentation

- The localization of acute GIB should begin with an assessment of the patient's hemodynamic status, and a focused history and physical examination (Table 6-3). However, these measures will not be diagnostic of the source of blood loss and

TABLE 6-3	ASSESSMENT OF ACUTE GASTROINTESTINAL BLEEDING		
Hemodynamics	% Intravascular Volume Loss	Pertinent History	Physical Examination
Normal	<10	Description of bleeding	Vital signs
Orthostatic hypotension	10–20	Duration and frequency	Orthostatic blood pressure
Shock	20–25	Prior bleeding	Stigmata of liver disease
		Comorbidities	Abdominal tenderness
		Medications	Stool color
		Previous surgery	Rectal examination
		Recent polypectomy Prior radiation Associated symptoms	

further investigation, typically including endoscopy and/or radiologic imaging may be required.[15]

Physical Examination
- **Digital rectal examination.** This has been recommended as a part of the initial evaluation in patients with acute LGIB and, in fact, may prove helpful in providing information regarding anorectal pathology prior to any endoscopic intervention. However, a digital examination does not preclude the need for endoscopic evaluation. One study found that 40% of rectal carcinomas diagnosed by proctoscopy were palpable on digital rectal examination.[16]
- **Nasogastric aspiration.** This should be performed if an upper GI source is suspected or if patients have hematochezia with hemodynamic compromise (as UGIB is detected in 10% to 15% of patients presenting with severe hematochezia). A positive gastric aspirate (frank blood, pinkish fluid, or dark "coffee ground" fluid) indicates that bleeding has occurred proximal to the jejunum. A negative aspirate does not rule out an UGIB. In fact, up to 18% of patients with UGIB have a nonbloody aspirate.[17] Hemoccult testing of a clear or nonbloody gastric aspirate does not add to the evaluation, and visual inspection has better value.

Diagnostic Procedures
- **Upper endoscopy.** Esophagogastroduodenoscopy (EGD) is the **preferred method for evaluating patients with UGIB.** Endoscopy allows direct visualization of the mucosa and identification of the bleeding site.
  - Endoscopy within the first 24 hours of presentation is the goal in UGIB, and endoscopy is recommended as soon as the patient is clinically stable when active ongoing bleeding is suspected. Since 10% of severe hematochezia presentations with hemodynamic compromise can be the result of

UGIB, upper endoscopy is indicated as the first step in the evaluation of such presentations.

○ Total cost of hospitalization, length of hospitalization, and need for emergent surgery have all been greatly reduced with early endoscopy, largely because of the therapeutic options available to the endoscopist (i.e., heater probe, argon plasma coagulation, epinephrine injection, band ligation). Definitive diagnosis is made when active bleeding, stigmata of bleeding, or significant lesions are seen.[11]

○ Early endoscopy (i.e., within 24 hours of admission) has not been demonstrated to decrease mortality.

○ It is important that the hemodynamically unstable patient be adequately volume resuscitated and any coagulopathy be corrected before performing upper endoscopy.

○ Morbidity and mortality rates from upper endoscopy have been reported at 1% and 0.1%, respectively.

○ Contraindications for endoscopy include an agitated patient, perforated viscus, and severe cardiopulmonary disease.

- **Colonoscopy.** Colonoscopy is the **most frequently used diagnostic tool for evaluating LGIB.**

  ○ A diagnosis is made in 75% to 100% of patients depending on the definition of the bleeding source, patient selection criteria, and timing of colonoscopy.[18]

  ○ For an optimal procedure, patients should be adequately resuscitated, hemodynamically stable, and free of stool and debris with bowel preparation.

  ○ With regard to timing of colonoscopy, recent data suggest that the use of urgent colonoscopy does not improve clinical outcome or lower hospital costs as compared with routine elective colonoscopy.

  ○ As many as 10% of hematochezia presentations associated with hemodynamic compromise may be due to an upper GI bleeding source. Therefore, under these circumstances, an upper endoscopy may be indicated as the first step in the evaluation of severe hematochezia. It is widely accepted that once an upper GI source has been excluded, the next step in evaluation of a patient with severe hematochezia is generally a colonoscopy, followed by capsule endoscopy to evaluate the small bowel if colonoscopy is unrevealing.

- **Capsule endoscopy.** Although upper endoscopy and colonoscopy are the standard tools utilized to evaluate acute GIB, visualization of the entire small bowel is easily performed with standard endoscopy. Capsule endoscopy **serves a crucial role in the initial evaluation of the small bowel.** In cases when small bowel bleeding is suspected, or when findings on upper endoscopy and colonoscopy are negative, capsule endoscopy can be used for further visualization of the small bowel. The diagnostic yield has been shown to be as high as 92% in carefully selected obscure GIB cases.

- **Tagged red blood cell scan.** The technetium 99m–labeled red blood cell (RBC) scan can be used as a bedside evaluation of active lower GIB. Bleeding must exceed a rate of 0.1 mL/minute to be detected. The procedure is of very low risk; however, the test is positive <50% of the time. One use of this procedure is as a **screening test before angiography.** A patient with a negative tagged RBC scan is unlikely to have a positive angiogram. If the test finding is negative, a colonoscopy is usually warranted for further evaluation of possible bleeding sources in the colon.

- **Angiography.** Angiography offers accurate diagnosis and therapy in the rapidly bleeding patient. Bleeding rates of 0.5 to 1 mL/minute are required to detect extravasation into the bowel from a bleeding site. The overall diagnostic yield from arteriography ranges from 40% to 78%. If a bleeding source is identified, therapeutic modalities, such as infusion of vasopressin or selective embolization, can be used to stop bleeding. Complications of this procedure include contrast allergy, bleeding from arterial puncture, and embolism from dislodged thrombus. Arteriography should be reserved for those patients with massive, ongoing LGIB for which colonoscopy is not feasible, for suspected massive small bowel bleeding, and for UGIB where endoscopy either fails or is unable to localize the source because of rapid bleeding.[19]

- **Other newer modalities. Computerized tomography angiography** is an emerging tool in the evaluation of the actively bleeding patient with suspected small bowel or colonic bleeding. This modality may have utility as the initial test in clinically unstable patients who cannot be sedated for endoscopy, as yields are expected to be higher than with tagged RBC scans.

TREATMENT

- **Resuscitation**
  - **Intravascular volume should be restored initially with either isotonic saline or lactated Ringer's solution.** Two large-bore (≥18-gauge) intravenous (IV) lines should be in place at all times. Centrally inserted, triple lumen catheters are typically placed. Although these may not confer an advantage over peripheral IV lines in terms of rate of fluid administration, they may be easier to place in the setting of vascular collapse or hypotension where peripheral veins are collapsed.
  - **Blood transfusion with packed red blood cells** is the method of choice for volume resuscitation in patients with severe GI hemorrhage. All patients who are admitted for GIB should be typed and crossed, and cross-matched blood should be transfused when possible. In the case of catastrophic bleeding, however, O-negative units should be used without delay. The target hematocrit is 25%, although in patients with coronary disease, a hematocrit of 30% is desirable. In the case of variceal hemorrhage, target transfusion goal is hemoglobin ~8 g/dL, as overtransfusion can lead higher rates of rebleeding and mortality (Table 6-4). Coagulopathy should be corrected with fresh frozen plasma in the unstable patient, but subcutaneous vitamin K (5 to 10 mg) can be used if the patient is hemodynamically stable. Heparin drips and other anticoagulants should be discontinued and protamine used for reversal, if necessary. If the patient is at risk for aspiration, consider endotracheal intubation to protect the airway. It is often required for management of variceal bleeding.

Medications

- **Nonvariceal UGIB**
  - **IV histamine-2 receptor antagonists.** These have not been shown to reduce surgery requirements or mortality rates. These agents are, therefore, **not recommended in the actively bleeding patient.**
  - **Proton pump inhibitors. Proton pump inhibitors** (PPI) have been found to **reduce rates of further bleeding, surgery, and deaths** caused by ulcer complications. The current standard of care is to administer IV PPIs either as intermittent bolus doses or as an infusion for the first 48 to 72 hours. High-dose (double-dose bid) oral PPI therapy is also of value and can be used when IV PPI

is unavailable, or if clinical active bleeding has ceased. It is unclear whether PPI therapy affects mortality despite obvious benefits to morbidity from UGIB.[20]

- **PPIs in prophylaxis of GIB in NSAID and ASA users.** Therapy should be tailored according to risk. American College of Gastrenterology practice guidelines recommend treatment according to risk stratification: low-, moderate-, and high-risk groups. Included in this risk stratification are factors such as age >65, concurrent medications (ASA, high-dose NSAIDs, corticosteroids, or anticoagulants), history of ulcer(s), and *Helicobacter pylori* infection. Low-risk patients, those without risk factors, should not receive prophylactic PPI therapy. Conversely, PPIs are indicated in those patients at moderate (one to two risk factors) and high risk (more than two risk factors or history of ulcer complications) for peptic ulcer(s) and associated complications.[21]

- **PPIs in prophylaxis of GIB in clopidogrel and ASA users.** A recent randomized, double-blinded, placebo-controlled trial found a significant reduction in UGIB in patients on dual therapy with clopidogrel and ASA who were randomized to receive prophylactic omeprazole. Importantly, there was no significant increase in cardiovascular events or mortality with the use of combination clopidogrel and PPI in this study.[22]

- Variceal UGIB
  - Vasoconstrictors. Several vasoconstricting agents are available and are uniformly effective in reducing variceal bleeding rates in the short term (Table 6-4). These agents produce splanchnic vasoconstriction and thus decrease portal blood inflow. Randomized controlled trials comparing different vasoconstrictor agents (vasopressin, somatostatin, terlipressin, octreotide, vapreotide), show no difference in control of hemorrhage and early rebleeding. **Octreotide** has the most favorable side effect profile and is therefore the agent

TABLE 6-4	MANAGEMENT OF ACUTE VARICEAL HEMORRHAGE
Resuscitation	Cautious transfusion of fluid and blood products with goal hemoglobin of ~8 g/dL Ensure airway is protected
Pharmacologic therapy	Octreotide 50 mcg IV bolus followed by continuous infusion 50 mcg/hr (3–5 days)
	Ciprofloxacin 400 mg BID IV or 500 mg BID PO or ceftriaxone 1 g/day IV (3–7 days)
Diagnosis and treatment	Endoscopy (within 12 hr of admission) with endoscopic therapy, preferably ligation
Rescue management	TIPS or shunt therapy in patients with esophageal varices who have failed pharmacologic and endoscopic therapy or in patients with bleeding gastric fundic varices

Adapted from Garcia-Tsao G, Lim J; Members of the Veterans Affairs Hepatitis C Resource Center Program. Management and treatment of patients with cirrhosis and portal hypertension: recommendations from the Department of Veterans Affairs Hepatitis C Resource Center Program and the National Hepatitis C Program. *Am J Gastroenterol.* 2009;104:1802–1829.

of choice in the United States. The recommended dose is 50 mcg IV bolus, followed by continuous infusion of 50 mcg/hour for 3 to 5 days (Table 6-4).
○ **Antibiotic prophylaxis.** It is recommended that all patients with variceal hemorrhage receive antibiotic prophylaxis for 3 to 7 days to prevent development of spontaneous bacterial peritonitis. Regimens typically include ciprofloxacin or ceftriaxone.

Other Nonpharmacologic Therapies

* **Variceal UGIB**
  ○ **Endoscopic variceal ligation,** which involves banding of the base of the varix, is the treatment of choice in acute variceal bleeding. Rubber bands are placed using a device attached through the instrument channel of the upper endoscope, which interrupt blood flow in the variceal column. This mode of therapy is used both for hemostasis in actively bleeding esophageal varices and for prophylaxis of variceal bleeding in patients with large varices. In the latter instance, repeat band ligation is performed every 4 to 8 weeks till all visible varices are obliterated, following which the patient is screened for recurrence every 6 to 12 months. Band ligation is easy to perform and is associated with lower complication rates than sclerotherapy, although rebleeding rates and mortality may not be different.[23]
  ○ **Sclerotherapy.** This involves injection of a variety of sclerosing agents (ethanolamine oleate, sodium tetradecyl sulfate, polidocanol, morrhuate sodium, or ethanol) directly into the varix, achieves hemostasis in >90% of cases. Recurrent bleeding within 10 days occurs in up to 50% of patients, however, and side effects of therapy include fever, ulceration, strictures, perforation, acute respiratory distress syndrome, and sepsis. This form of therapy is currently limited to refractory bleeding, unavailability of endoscopic band ligation, or gastric varices where band ligation cannot be performed.
  ○ **Rescue management of variceal hemorrhage**
    ▪ Balloon tamponade. Balloon tamponade should be restricted to patients with controllable bleeding for whom definitive therapy is planned within 24 hours. Either the Sengstaken-Blakemore tube or the Minnesota tube, both of which have gastric and esophageal balloons, can be used. In contrast, the Linton-Nachlas tube has only a large gastric balloon and can be considered for isolated gastric variceal bleeding. Hemostasis is achieved 70% to 90% of the time. Complications can be severe and include esophageal perforation, aspiration, chest pain, erosion, agitation, and death from asphyxiation from balloon migration with airway occlusion.
    ▪ Transjugular intrahepatic portosystemic shunt. This is reserved for patients with intractable variceal bleeding or if bleeding recurs after two or more unsuccessful endoscopic attempts at treatment of esophageal varices. Transjugular intrahepatic portosystemic shunt (TIPS) creates a direct portosystemic shunt, thereby decreasing pressure within the portal system. Technical success is achieved >90% of the time, but complications include hepatic encephalopathy (in as many as 25% of patients), shunt stenosis, shunt thrombosis, and rebleeding. When TIPS is used in emergency situations, in-hospital mortality is around 10%, and 30-day mortality rate as high as 40%. Contraindications for TIPS include portal vein thrombosis, inferior vena cava obstruction, and polycystic liver disease.

TABLE 6-5	COMMON THERAPIES FOR UPPER GASTROINTESTINAL BLEEDING

Injection Therapy Action

Dilute epinephrine Tamponade, vasospasm, thrombosis
Sclerosants tamponade and thrombosis

Ablative Therapy

Thermocoagulation—heater probe Tissue ablation via direct compressive contact

Electrocoagulation—BICAP, Gold Probe™ Tissue ablation via direct compressive contact

Argon plasma coagulation—noncontact tissue coagulation via argon gas

Mechanical Therapy

Hemoclips	Joins two sides of a vessel to occlude and arrest bleeding
Band ligation	Entrapment of a varix with a rubber band or elastic ring

Adapted from Cappell MS. Therapeutic endoscopy for acute upper gastrointestinal bleeding. *Nat Rev Gastroenterol Hepatol.* 2010;7:214–229.

- **Surgical shunts.** These are rarely used because of the availability of TIPS procedures. Portacaval and distal splenorenal shunts achieve hemostasis 95% of the time but are associated with a high rate of postprocedural encephalopathy; mortality rates of 50% to 80% are reported, largely because of severe underlying liver disease. Surgical shunts are sometimes considered in noncirrhotic portal hypertension and patients with Child's A cirrhosis.[23]
- **Therapeutic upper endoscopy**
  - There are myriad techniques employed to achieve hemostasis and prevent recurrence of UGIB, namely, injection, ablative, and/or mechanical therapy (Table 6-5).[24] Use of a combination of any two of these methods, most commonly injection therapy followed by either ablative or mechanical therapy, has been associated with a dramatic reduction in the risk of ongoing and recurrent bleeding. Studies suggest a risk reduction from 80% to ~15% for an actively bleeding ulcer and from 50% to ~10% for an ulcer with nonbleeding visible vessel.[25,26]
- **Therapeutic colonoscopy**
  - Endoscopic therapy is applied in 10% to 40% of patients undergoing colonoscopy, and immediate hemostasis is achieved in 50% to 100% of these cases.[18]
  - Endoscopic therapy options are similar to those used in upper endoscopy and include thermal coagulation (heater probe, bipolar or multipolar coagulation, argon plasma coagulation), and injection of vasoconstrictors and sclerosants. Placement of metallic hemoclips has also been successful in the treatment of diverticular bleeding.

- **Angiotherapy**
  - When angiographic localization of bleeding is achieved, two modalities of therapy can be instituted directly into the bleeding vessel: vasopressin infusion and embolization. Vasopressin infusion is typically used in bleeding sources in the colon or small bowel, with the intent to induce vasospasm and, consequently, clotting and hemostasis. With superselective cannulation of the bleeding vessel, embolization with coils or gelfoam can be highly successful in both UGIB and LGIB, with low risk of ischemic changes in the affected bowel segment.

Surgical Management

- The role of surgery is as a salvage therapy in the small group of patients in whom bleeding cannot be controlled with endoscopic therapy and/or angiotherapy. In both UGIB and LGIB, surgery should not be postponed excessively in the patient with persistent bleeding and hemodynamic instability because morbidity and mortality increase with delay.
- **Surgery for UGIB.** Surgery is indicated in patients in whom arterial bleeding cannot be controlled during initial endoscopy. However, in patients in whom bleeding recurs after initial endoscopic hemostasis, the management decision is more challenging and the data are conflicting. Some studies support a second endoscopic attempt at hemostasis, whereas others support immediate surgery or angiographic embolization. Surgical series have suggested that high-risk patients (ulcers ≥2 cm located at the lesser curvature or posterior duodenum, shock at presentation, and/or elderly with comorbidities) require aggressive postendoscopic management. Operative mortality following failed endoscopic therapy in some series has been as high as 25%. However, this varies with operator and institution experience in management bleeding peptic ulcers.[27]
- **Surgery for LGIB.** Accurate preoperative localization of LGIB reduces postoperative rebleeding rates. Surgical mortality rates from recent series are 5% to 10%. For the difficult situation of recurrent massive bleeding without demonstration of a bleeding site, a subtotal colectomy may be indicated in patients with a good overall prognosis. When the patient is a high-risk surgical candidate, angiotherapy or a percutaneously or surgically placed portal-hepatic shunt for variceal bleeding can be considered as alternatives.[13,14]

SPECIAL CONSIDERATIONS

- **Prokinetics in UGIB**
  - A recent meta-analysis showed that **IV erythromycin or metoclopramide** immediately before EGD significantly reduces the need for a repeat EGD. These agents promote gastric emptying and thus administration can improve visualization by evacuation of stomach contents (blood, clot, fluid).[28]

REFERENCES

1. Zhao Y, Encinosa W. Hospitalizations for gastrointestinal bleeding in 1998 and 2006: HCUP statistical brief #65. http://www.hcup-es.ahrq.gov/reports/statbriefs/sb65.pdf. Accessed December 10, 2010.
2. Lanas A, Garcia-Rodriguez LA, Polo-Tomas M, et al. Time trends and impact of upper and lower gastrointestinal bleeding and perforation in clinical practice. *Am J Gastroenterol.* 2009;104:1633–1641.

3. Laine L. Upper gastrointestinal bleeding. *ASGE Clin Update.* 2007;14:1–4.
4. Barkun A. Systematic review of the symptom burden, quality of life impairment and costs associated with peptic ulcer disease. *Am J Med.* 2010;123:358–366.
5. Chui PWY, Ny EKW, Cheung FK, et al. Predicting mortality in patients with bleeding peptic ulcer after therapeutic endoscopy. *Clin Gastroenterol Hepatol.* 2009;7:311–316.
6. Laine L, Peterson WL. Bleeding peptic ulcer. *N Engl J Med.* 1994;331:717–727.
7. Garcia-Tsao G, Bosch J. Management of varices and variceal hemorrhage in cirrhosis. *N Engl J Med.* 2010;362:823–832.
8. Chalasani N, Kahi C, Francois F, et al. Improved patient survival after acute variceal bleeding: a multicenter, cohort study. *Am J Gastroenterol.* 2003;98:653–659.
9. D'Amico G, Pagliaro L, Bosch J. Pharmacologic treatment of portal hypertension: an evidence-based approach. *Semin Liver Dis.* 1999;19:475–505.
10. Perini RF, Camara PRS, Ferraz JGP. Pathogenesis of portal hypertensive gastropathy: translating basic research into clinical practice. *Nat Clin Pract Gastroenterol Hepatol.* 2009;6:150–158.
11. Esrailian E, Gralnek I. Nonvariceal upper gastrointestinal bleeding: epidemiology and diagnosis. *Gastroenterol Clin North Am.* 2005;34:589–605.
12. Strate LL. Lower GI bleeding: epidemiology and diagnosis. *Gastroenterol Clin North Am.* 2005;34:643–664.
13. Green BT, Rockey DC. Lower gastrointestinal bleeding-management. *Gastroenterol Clin North Am.* 2005;34:665–678.
14. Davila RE, Rajan E, Adler DG, et al. ASGE guideline: the role of endoscopy in the patient with lower-GI bleeding. *Gastrointest Endosc.* 2005;62:656–660.
15. Rockey DC. Gastrointestinal bleeding. *Gastroenterol Clin North Am.* 2005;34:581–588.
16. Bindewald H. Indikationen und treffsicherheit der rektoskopie. *MMW Much Med Wochenschr.* 1976;118:1271–1272.
17. Ahmad A, Bruno JM, Boynton R, et al. Nasogastric aspirates frequently lead to erroneous results and delay of therapy in patients with suspected UGI bleeding. *Gastrointest Endosc.* 2004;59:163.
18. Strate LL, Naumann CR. The role of colonoscopy and radiological procedures in the management of acute lower intestinal bleeding. *Clin Gastroenterol Hepatol.* 2010;8:333–343.
19. Laine L, Shah A. Randomized trial of urgent vs. elective colonoscopy in patients hospitalized with lower GI bleeding. *Am J Gastroenterol.* 2010;105:2636–2641.
20. Leontiadis GI, Sharma VK, Howden CW. WITHDRAWN: proton pump inhibitor treatment for acute peptic ulcer bleeding. *Cochrane Database Syst Rev.* 2010;12(5):CD002094.
21. Lanza FL, Chan FKL, Quigley EMM, et al. Guidelines for prevention of NSAID-related ulcer complications. *Am J Gastroenterol.* 2009;104:728–738.
22. Bhatt DL, Cryer BL, Contant CF, et al. Clopidogrel with or without omeprazole in coronary artery disease. *N Engl J Med.* 2010;363:1909–1917.
23. Garcia-Tsao G, Lim J. Members of the Veterans Affairs Hepatitis C Resource Center Program. Management and treatment of patients with cirrhosis and portal hypertension: recommendations from the Department of Veterans Affairs Hepatitis C Resource Center Program and the National Hepatitis C Program. *Am J Gastroenterol.* 2009;104:1802–1829.
24. Cappell MS. Therapeutic endoscopy for acute upper gastrointestinal bleeding. *Nat Rev Gastroenterol Hepatol.* 2010;7:214–229.
25. Laine L. Multipolar electrocoagulation in the treatment of active upper gastrointestinal tract hemorrhage: a prospective controlled trial. *N Engl J Med.* 1987;316:1613–1617.
26. Laine L. Multipolar electrocoagulation in the treatment of peptic ulcers with nonbleeding visible vessels: a prospective, controlled trial. *Ann Intern Med.* 1989;110:510–514.
27. Cheung FKY, Lau JYW. Management of massive peptic ulcer bleeding. *Gastroenterol Clin North Am.* 2009;38:231–243.
28. Barkun AN, Bardou M, Martel M, et al. Prokinetics in acute upper GI bleeding: a meta-analysis. *Gastrointest Endosc.* 2010;72:1138–1145.

Occult and Obscure Gastrointestinal Bleeding

7

John M. Iskander

GENERAL PRINCIPLES

- Occult and obscure gastrointestinal (GI) bleeding ranks among the most common reasons for referral to a gastroenterologist. These can often present significant diagnostic and therapeutic challenges, causing much frustration to both patients and their physicians.[1–4]
- In this chapter, the causes, diagnostic approaches, and treatment options for both occult and obscure GI bleeding are discussed.

Definition

- **Occult bleeding** is defined as either a positive fecal occult blood test (FOBT) or iron-deficiency anemia (IDA) without other evidence of visible blood in the stool. GI bleeding is the most common cause of IDA, especially in men and postmenopausal women.[1,2,5]
- **Obscure bleeding** refers to GI bleeding that persists or recurs, with no identifiable origin after initial endoscopic evaluation. It can present in both the obscure-occult or obscure-overt forms depending on the presence of visible blood.[1,2]

DIAGNOSIS

Occult Bleeding

An extensive list of disorders can cause occult GI bleeding, with or without IDA. Table 7-1 lists the common causes of occult blood loss.

Clinical Presentation
Although, by definition, no known symptoms exist for occult GI bleed, the association with new abdominal symptoms, changes in bowel movements, dietary alterations, or constitutional symptoms remains important.

History
In particular, careful attention must be paid to **medication history,** especially over-the-counter nonsteroidal anti-inflammatory drugs (NSAIDs). Symptoms such as fatigue, exertional dyspnea, tachycardia, and pica suggest possible IDA.[6]

Physical Examination
Physical findings of IDA are rare in developed countries but may include brittle nails with longitudinal furrows or spooning (koilonychia), glossitis, cheilitis, and atrophic rhinitis. The Patterson-Kelly or Plummer-Vinson syndrome of postcricoid esophageal webs and IDA may occur. A GI source must be assumed in the evaluation of IDA, in the absence of menorrhagia, gross hematuria, or other obvious etiologies.

TABLE 7-1 SOURCES OF OCCULT GASTROINTESTINAL BLEEDING	
Source	Incidence, %
Colorectal	25
Colorectal cancer	7
Polyps	9
Angiodysplasia	4
Colitis	1
Upper gastrointestinal tract	41
Duodenal ulcer	5
Gastric ulcer	5
Esophagitis	11
Gastritis	8
Angiodysplasia	4
Gastric cancer	2
Celiac disease	1
No source found	41

Diagnostic Criteria

- **Fecal occult blood tests**
  - Although useful for initial screening, a positive FOBT does not always indicate true disease. False-positive results can occur because of diet, medications, or trauma while obtaining a sample. In fact, physiologic bleeding of up to 1.5 mL/day can occur in healthy patients. The four basic types of FOBT are as follows[2,7]:
    - **Guaiac (hemoccult) test** is widely available, simple, and inexpensive, and thus most commonly used. It is a qualitative test and provides little quantitative information. A colorless compound obtained from tree bark that turns blue with peroxidase-like substances, such as heme and hydrogen peroxide, guaiac detects free heme or heme bound to its apoprotein (e.g., globin, myoglobin, and certain cytochromes). Heme degradation products that may form with more proximal (upper GI) bleeding are not detected. Because guaiac reacts with any peroxidase substance, the test can give false-positive results with red meats or blood-containing foods, as well as plant peroxidases such as that found in radish. Iron, however, does not cause false-positive results. Vitamin C can cause a false-negative result.
    - The **radiochromium-labeled erythrocyte test** remains the accepted gold standard for quantifying GI blood loss. It has limited clinical utility, however, because of cost, complexity, and requirement of ≥3 days of stool collection.
    - **Immunochemical tests** use antibodies against human hemoglobin. They do not react with free heme and thus, require no dietary restrictions before the test. Some of these tests may also provide quantitative information. Because these antibodies interact with the globin chain, they are only useful for colorectal bleeding, because globin from gastric bleeding is degraded.
    - **Heme porphyrin assay (HemoQuant)** is a quantitative fluorometric assay of both heme and its degradation products. Although it has the advantage of detecting proximal bleeds, it is a complex test that requires confirmation in a reference laboratory.

Diagnostic Testing and Procedures

Endoscopic evaluation remains the primary means of investigation in occult GI bleeding, because it allows direct visualization of the mucosa, tissue sampling, and therapeutic intervention.[2,8]

- Both **colonoscopy** and **esophagogastroduodenoscopy** **(EGD)** can be performed during the same endoscopic session for a complete evaluation to eliminate the need for repeat sedation.
  - Colonoscopy is typically performed first, especially in patients older than 50 years, because current colon cancer screening guidelines recommend evaluation of the colon after positive FOBT in this group of patients.
  - Current data support proceeding with EGD after a negative colonoscopy result, because the upper GI tract has been shown to be a significant source for occult bleeding.
    - Often, endoscopy is required after an abnormal radiographic study. Therefore, it is preferable to perform endoscopy as the initial test whenever possible.
- Because most cases of occult bleeding with no clear source do not evolve into obscure bleeding, **further testing beyond initial endoscopy is generally not indicated even if no cause is identified.** In these cases, the patients should receive iron supplementation and be closely monitored for a response. If IDA is profound at the outset, if it persists despite oral iron supplementation, if bleeding recurs, or if FOBT remains positive, further evaluation should proceed according to the obscure bleeding algorithm (see Obscure Bleeding section).

Obscure Bleeding

Obscure bleeding can present as both overt and occult bleeding and can originate from one or more lesions anywhere in the GI tract. As a result, the list of disorders that can cause obscure bleeding is exhaustive, encompassing those of both overt and occult bleeding.[4,9] Table 7-2 lists the causes of obscure gastrointestinal bleeding.

Clinical Presentation

Patients presenting with obscure bleeding have symptoms similar to those of acute overt and occult bleeding. Careful history and physical examination may help delineate the possible source of the bleeding.[2,4,8]

Diagnostic Testing and Procedures

Repeat EGD and colonoscopy remain the initial step in the evaluation of obscure bleeding. Previous studies have shown that repeat EGD and colonoscopy can identify initially missed lesions in 35% to 75% of patients. If repeat endoscopic studies give negative results, several other diagnostic modalities exist to help determine the source of bleeding.[1,2,7,10]

- **Enteroscopy** allows direct visual examination of portions of the small bowel, using a longer endoscope. Different methods of enteroscopy exist, including push enteroscopy and deep enteroscopy.
  - **Push enteroscopy** involves advancing a longer endoscope manually into the small bowel. During repeat endoscopic evaluations of obscure bleeding, EGD is generally replaced by enteroscopy for a more thorough evaluation of the proximal gut. This technique allows visualization of up to 50 cm of the small bowel beyond the ligament of Treitz.

TABLE 7-2 SOURCES OF OBSCURE GASTROINTESTINAL BLEEDING

Colorectal	Neoplasia
Colitis	Ischemia
Ulcerative colitis	HIV-related causes
Crohn's colitis	Bacterial infection
Ischemic colitis	Celiac disease
Infectious colitis	**Upper gut**
Angiodysplasia	Peptic ulcer disease
Diverticulosis	Esophagitis
Neoplasia	Angiodysplasia
Radiation proctopathy	Gastric antral vascular ectasia
Rectal ulcer	Dieulafoy's lesion
Endometriosis	Lymphoma
Amyloidosis	Neoplasia
Lymphoma	Hemobilia
Small bowel	Hemosuccus pancreaticus
Andiodysplasia	Sarcoidosis
Crohn's disease	Aortoenteric fistula
Meckel's diverticulum	Metastatic cancer

○ **Deep enteroscopy** can be performed by a variety of techniques including **single-balloon enteroscopy (SBE)** and **double-balloon enteroscopy (DBE)**.[11] Both these techniques utilize a modified enteroscope with one or two balloons attached toward the distal end. Although similar, the systems vary with regard to whether a balloon is attached only to the overtube (SBE) or also to the tip of the enteroscope (DBE). The balloon system serves as an anchor by gripping on to the intestinal wall to allow further advancement of the endoscope. Alternatively, **spiral enteroscopy** can be used for an antegrade investigation of the small bowel by using an overtube with a soft raised helix at its distal end. The spiral enteroscope usually requires two operators for advancement by pleating the small bowel over the instrument.[7] By utilizing both the oral (antegrade) and anal (retrograde) approaches, SBE or DBE may allow evaluation of the entire small bowel. In addition to its expanded diagnostic capacity, deep enteroscopy also contains intervention capabilities, including hemostasis, biopsy, polypectomy, and dilation.[3,11] Furthermore, lesions identified on endoscopy that are not amenable to conventional endoscopic therapies can be marked using mucosal tattoos or hemoclips near the bleeding source. This may be useful for future localization of the site during interventional radiology or exploratory surgery.

• **Capsule endoscopy** was introduced almost a decade ago and has become the standard in recent years for the examination of the small bowel in obscure GI bleeding. Capsule endoscopy involves ingestion of a capsule containing a small camera that sends images to a recorder worn on the patient's belt. Images are transmitted at a rate of two pictures per second.[9,10,12,13] Relying on normal intestinal peristalsis for the advancement of the capsule, this test is virtually pain free and noninvasive. It is limited, however, by the inability to either perform biopsy or intervene; studies can also be incomplete if the cecum is not traversed within the battery life of the capsule (typically 8 hours). Without air insufflation, rinsing, or control of direction, parts of the mucosal surface may not be visualized, as the capsule gets pushed along by peristalsis. Capsule entrapment or retention, particularly in patients with stricture or diverticula, remains the major risk, which occurs in <1% of cases. If within reach, retained capsules can be retrieved using an enteroscope; if beyond the reach of endoscopic instruments, surgery may be necessary.[9,10]

- **Small bowel series** and **enteroclysis** use oral contrast to identify mucosal lesions in the GI tract radiographically. With a low sensitivity, they are generally reserved either for cases in which more invasive testing cannot be performed or for ruling out endoluminal narrowing before capsule endoscopy.

- **Technetium 99m–labeled erythrocyte scans** can help identify the origin of obscure bleeding when other modalities fail to reveal a source. The test, however, must be performed during episodes of active bleeding at a rate exceeding 0.1 to 0.4 mL/minute. Results of the scan should be confirmed by an alternative test, such as angiography, because of significant false localization rate. Radionuclide imaging using **technetium 99m pertechnetate** (Meckel's scan) can be used to localize Meckel's diverticulum, one of the causes of obscure GI bleeding. This compound is taken up by heterotrophic gastric mucosa within the Meckel's diverticulum and can be localized on a radionuclide scan.

- **Angiography** usually follows a tagged erythrocyte scan and allows visualization of bleeding of at least 0.5 mL/minute and additionally may offer therapeutic interventions such as vasopressin infusion and embolization. Highly vascular lesions such as angiodysplasia and neoplasms can sometimes be identified during angiography by demonstrating typical vascular patterns, even if active bleeding is not manifest. Caution is advised, and pretreatment might be needed in patients with suspected contrast allergy or renal insufficiency. Both **computed tomography and magnetic resonance angiography** are techniques that use dye to highlight vasculature.[14] These techniques can also be useful to localize acute bleeding.

- **Intraoperative enteroscopy** may allow better and more complete visualization of the entire small bowel. It is usually reserved for transfusion-dependent bleeding without a source despite extensive diagnostic evaluation. This is also used to precisely localize bleeding lesions at surgery after initial diagnosis with capsule endoscopy or other diagnostic modalities. The risks of continued bleeding should also be carefully evaluated and must outweigh the surgical risks of laparotomy.[15]

TREATMENT

Treatment of obscure bleeding should be directed at the primary disorder leading to the bleeding.[8,9] The treatment modalities generally fall into four main categories:

- **Endoscopic therapy**
  - The basis for endoscopic therapy of obscure bleeding is accurate localization and identification of the bleeding source. A second-look endoscopy (i.e., repeat upper endoscopy and colonoscopy) or a second-opinion endoscopy may have value in obscure GI bleeding. When this is performed, the upper endoscopy is typically replaced by push enteroscopy to allow inspection of

the proximal small bowel. Some of the reports that use this approach show sources of bleeding in as many as two-thirds of patients. If no source is identified, further testing typically hinges on video capsule endoscopy and deep enteroscopic techniques in stable patients and on radiologic techniques in unstable or rapidly bleeding patients.

○ Endoscopic techniques utilized include epinephrine injection, thermal therapy with a heater probe, bipolar cautery, argon plasma coagulation, endoscopic mucosal resection, and band ligation depending on the lesion identified. See Chapter 6 for further details on these techniques.

- Angiographic therapy
  ○ Infusion of vasopressin into the bleeding vessel can induce spasm and allow hemostasis. This is possible when the bleeding lesion is identified on angiography. Alternatively, gelfoam or coils can be used to embolize and occlude the bleeding vessel. The risk of ischemic changes in the affected bowel segment is greatly reduced with superselective catheterization of bleeding vessels.

- Pharmacologic therapy
  ○ Depending on the lesion identified, simple measures may include acid suppression, avoidance of NSAIDs or aspirin, and optimization of INR or prothrombin time in patients on warfarin or heparin therapy. Misoprostol can sometimes be used for mucosal protection in patients requiring aspirin or NSAID therapy—there is limited evidence that misoprostol may provide mucosal protection extending into the small bowel, whereas proton pump inhibitors provide benefit that is limited to the gastroduodenum under similar circumstances.[9]

  ○ When numerous angiodysplasia are noted, ablation of each of these lesions may not be feasible. In such instances, the initial approach is to replete iron, either orally or parenterally, and to maintain a stable blood count with intermittent transfusions. When this approach fails, pharmacologic therapy with combination of estrogen-progesterone (birth control pills), danazol, amino caproic acid, tranexamic acid, octreotide and thalidomide have been anecdotally used with varying success.[2,9]

- Surgery
  ○ Depending on the lesion identified, surgical resection may sometimes be necessary, especially with stromal tumors and other neoplastic lesions. Rapid bleeding localized to a limited bowel segment may require laparotomy and **intraoperative enteroscopy** for precise localization; some of these procedures are followed by resection of the segment with the bleeding lesion.

If all evaluations give negative results, nonspecific therapy, including iron supplementation, correction of coagulopathy or platelet disorders, or intermittent transfusion, should be continued.

REFERENCES

1. Concha R, Amaro R, Barkin JS. Obscure gastrointestinal bleeding: diagnostic and therapeutic approach. *J Clin Gastroenterol.* 2007;41(3):242–251.
2. Zuckerman G, Prakash C, Askin M, et al. AGA medical position statement: evaluation and management of occult and obscure gastrointestinal bleeding. *Gastroenterology.* 2000;118: 197–200.
3. Bresci G. Occult and obscure gastrointestinal bleeding: causes and diagnostic approach in 2009. *World J Gastrointest Endosc.* 2009;1:3–6.

4. Raju GS, Gerson L, Das A, et al. American Gastroenterological Association (AGA) Institute medical position on obscure gastrointestinal bleeding. *Gastroenterology.* 2007;133:1694–1696.
5. Richter JM. Occult gastrointestinal bleeding. *Gastroenterol Clin North Am.* 1994;23:53–66.
6. Rockey DC, Cello JP. Evaluation of the gastrointestinal tract in patients with iron deficiency anemia. *N Engl J Med.* 1993;329:1691–1695.
7. Rockey DC, Koch J, Cello JP, et al. Relative frequency of upper gastrointestinal and colonic lesions in patients with positive fecal occult blood tests. *N Engl J Med.* 1998;339:153–159.
8. ASGE Standards of Practice Committee; Fisher L, Lee KM, et al. The role of endoscopy in the management of obscure GI bleeding. *Gastrointest Endosc.* 2010;72(3):471–479.
9. Pasha AF, Hara AK, Leighton JA. Diagnostic evaluation and management of obscure gastrointestinal bleeding: a changing paradigm. *Gastroenterol Hepatol (NY).* 2009;5(12):839–850.
10. Adler DG, Knipshield M, Gostoud C. A prospective comparison of capsule endoscopy and push enteroscopy in patients with GI bleeding of obscure origin. *Gastrointest Endosc.* 2004;59:492–498.
11. Gerson LB, Flodin JT, Miyabayashi K. Balloon-assisted enteroscopy: technology and troubleshooting. *Gastrointest Endosc.* 2008;68:1158.
12. Fireman Z. Capsule endoscopy: future horizons. *World J Gastrointest Endosc.* 2010;2(9):305–307.
13. Leighton JA. The role of endoscopic imaging of the small bowel in clinical practice. *Am J Gastroenterol.* 2011;106(1):27–36.
14. Huprich JE. Multiphase CT enterography in obscure GI bleeding. *Abdom Imaging.* 2009;34(3):303–309.
15. Somsouk M, Gralnek IM, Inadomi JM. Managements of obscure occult gastrointestinal bleeding: a cost-minimization analysis. *Clin Gastroenterol Hepatol.* 2008;6:661–670.

Jaundice

8

Noura M. Sharabash

GENERAL PRINCIPLES

- Jaundice is a common condition encountered in both inpatient and outpatient settings, with a broad spectrum of causes, ranging from benign to life-threatening. An in-depth understanding of the presentation and pathophysiology of jaundice is essential for appropriate investigation and accurate diagnosis.

Definition

- Jaundice is defined as a yellow discoloration of skin, sclera, and mucous membranes caused by accumulation of bilirubin, a by-product of heme metabolism.
  - The upper limit of normal for total serum bilirubin is 1.0 to 1.5 mg/dL, of which conjugated bilirubin constitutes <0.3 mg/dL.[1] Hyperbilirubinemia (total serum bilirubin >1.5 mg/dL) may be present without overt jaundice, but it nevertheless represents an abnormal condition.
  - Jaundice typically becomes apparent when the serum total bilirubin concentration reaches 2.5 to 3.0 mg/dL. Increased bilirubin levels may be caused by a defect at any site along the bilirubin metabolic pathway, from increased bilirubin production, decreased bilirubin clearance, or a combination of factors.[1]

Classification

- There are two approaches to the classification of jaundice. The first is according to the location of the defect in the bilirubin pathway (prehepatic, intrahepatic, or posthepatic). The second is classification by the predominant type of bilirubin that is found in the blood (unconjugated vs. conjugated).
- Jaundice can be classified as prehepatic, intrahepatic, or posthepatic.
  - *Prehepatic* jaundice may be due to overproduction of bilirubin.
  - *Intrahepatic* jaundice can be caused by abnormalities in bilirubin transport, conjugation, or excretion.
  - *Posthepatic* jaundice is due to biliary obstruction.
- Jaundice can also be classified as primarily unconjugated bilirubin, conjugated bilirubin, or both.[2]
  - *Unconjugated bilirubin* is mostly water-insoluble and reversibly binds to albumin in the blood. Unconjugated hyperbilirubinemia may be due to bilirubin overproduction, impaired uptake, decreased storage, or abnormal bilirubin conjugation.
  - *Conjugated bilirubin* is conjugated with glucuronic acid, becomes water-soluble, and is subsequently excreted in the stool and urine. The half-life of conjugated bilirubin bound to albumin is approximately 17 days, thus explaining the slow recovery from jaundice even after resolution of the

illness. Conjugated hyperbilirubinemia may be due to decreased bilirubin excretion, hepatocyte dysfunction, or biliary obstruction.

○ *Combination hyperbilirubinemia* can also be seen in hepatocellular disease, biliary obstruction, and decreased canalicular excretion.

Etiology

- *Unconjugated hyperbilirubinemia*
  ○ **Bilirubin overproduction**
    - *Hemolysis* and *ineffective erythropoiesis* are seen with sickle-cell anemia, thalassemia, G6PD deficiency, pyruvate kinase deficiency, malaria, ABO blood group mismatch, and lead toxicity. Bilirubin is usually <3 to 5 mg/dL, and overt jaundice is uncommon in the absence of severe hemolysis or concomitant liver disease. Hemolysis can be evaluated with measurement of lactate dehydrogenase (LDH), haptoglobin, reticulocyte count, and a peripheral smear.
    - Resorption of *large hematomas* results in bilirubin overproduction and subsequent unconjugated hyperbilirubinemia.
  ○ **Impaired hepatic bilirubin uptake**
    - *Decreased hepatic blood flow* can result in impaired hepatic bilirubin uptake and is caused by cirrhosis, portocaval shunts, or congestive heart failure.
    - *Drugs* that can cause impaired bilirubin uptake include rifampin, probenecid, sulfonamides, aspirin, nonsteroidal anti-inflammatory drugs, and contrast dye.
  ○ **Impaired conjugation of bilirubin**
    - Inherited uridine diphosphate glucuronyl transferase (UGT) deficiencies include Gilbert's syndrome and Crigler-Najjar syndrome. *Gilbert's syndrome* affects 3% to 10% of the population (predominantly men) and presents with intermittent jaundice often precipitated by illness, stress, fatigue, or fasting. It is the most common cause of unconjugated hyperbilirubinemia and is benign with no deleterious long-term consequences. *Crigler-Najjar* syndrome is less common and can be of two types: Type I with complete deficiency of UGT 1A1 and type II with partial inactivation of the enzyme.
    - **Neonatal jaundice** can be due to physiologic jaundice due to an initial relatively low activity of UGT and is usually seen between 5 and 14 days in full-term infants. On the other hand, breast milk jaundice is seen later in life and is due to an inhibitor of UGT activity in breast milk. Unconjugated hyperbilirubinemia in newborns can also be caused by ABO incompatibility, G6PD deficiency, hypothyroidism, and so forth. Newborns with severe elevations of unconjugated bilirubin are often treated to prevent kernicterus, which manifests as hypotonia, lethargy, and seizures.
- **Conjugated hyperbilirubinemia**
  ○ **Intrahepatic cholestasis**
    - *Hepatitis* including alcoholic hepatitis, hepatitis B, hepatitis C, Epstein-Barr virus, and cytomegalovirus can present with cholestatic hepatitis.
    - *Primary biliary cirrhosis* is an autoimmune disorder commonly seen in middle-aged women.
    - *Primary sclerosing cholangitis (PSC)* is a chronic liver disease with scarring of the bile ducts ("beads on a string") and is commonly associated with inflammatory bowel disease.

- *Postoperative cholestasis* may have many causes including hemolysis, ischemia, anesthetics, and so forth.
- *Total parenteral nutrition (TPN)* can cause intrahepatic as well as extrahepatic cholestasis.[3]
- *Cholestasis of pregnancy* may be due to morbid pregnancy-related conditions such as HELLP syndrome (hemolysis, elevated liver enzymes, and low platelet count) and acute fatty liver of pregnancy or the more common, but benign, intrahepatic cholestasis of pregnancy (the cause of 30% to 50% of jaundice in pregnancy).
- *Infiltrative disorders:* granulomatous disease (sarcoidosis, lymphoma, mycobacterial infection, Wegener's granulomatosis), amyloidosis, and malignancy (paraneoplastic syndrome: renal cell carcinoma).
- *Infections* such as bacterial, sepsis, fungal, or parasitic.
- *Vascular* causes such as hepatic vein thrombosis (Budd-Chiari syndrome) or shock liver.
- *Stem cell transplant-related* such as sinusoidal obstruction syndrome (venoocclusive disease), graft-versus-host disease, or chemotherapy-induced hepatitis.
- *Drugs* that cause a predominantly cholestatic picture (elevated alkaline phosphatase [AP] and total bilirubin) include anabolic steroids, oral contraceptives, estrogens, amoxicillin–clavulanic acid, chlorpromazine, clopidogrel, erythromycin, irbesartan, mirtazapine, phenothiazines, terbinafine, and tricyclics.
  - Extrahepatic cholestasis
    - *Choledocholithiasis* which is the presence of gallstones in the common bile duct (CBD).
    - *Primary sclerosing cholangitis* can also have dominant extrahepatic biliary strictures.
    - *AIDS cholangiopathy* has an appearance similar to PSC, presents with elevated AP, and is caused by opportunistic infections of the biliary tree.
    - *Malignancy* such as hepatocellular carcinoma (manifest as intraluminal with tumor thrombus or fragments, extraluminal tumor, or hemobilia), cholangiocarcinoma, pancreatic cancer, and ampullary tumors.[4]
    - *Pancreatitis* (acute, chronic, or autoimmune) can be associated with cholestasis.
    - *Mirizzi syndrome* caused by gallstones compressing the common hepatic duct.
    - *Postsurgical* strictures may cause obstruction resulting in extrahepatic cholestasis.
    - *Choledochal cystic disorders* including Caroli's disease and choledochal cysts.
    - *Vascular enlargement* from aneurysms or portal cavernoma.
  - **Congenital and familial causes of cholestasis:** Rotor syndrome; Dubin-Johnson syndrome; progressive familial intrahepatic cholestasis: PIFC-1 (Byler disease), PIFC-2 (BSEP mutation), and PIFC-3 (MDR-3 mutation); benign recurrent intrahepatic cholestasis (BRIC).
- **Mixed conjugated and unconjugated hyperbilirubinemia**
  - A mixed pattern of hyperbilirubinemia may be seen in hepatocellular disorders. A combination of unconjugated hyperbilirubinemia and parenchymal liver disease can also result in a mixed pattern of hyperbilirubinemia.
  - **Hepatocellular disorders:** Viral hepatitis, alcoholic liver disease, Wilson's disease, Reye's syndrome, hemochromatosis, autoimmune hepatitis, α_1-antitrypsin

deficiency, celiac sprue, nonalcoholic steatohepatitis, pregnancy related (acute fatty liver of pregnancy and preeclampsia).

○ **Drugs:** Acetaminophen, amiodarone, clindamycin, colchicine, ketoconazole, niacin, nonsteroidal anti-inflammatory drug, salicylates, calcium channel blockers.[5]

Pathophysiology

• Bilirubin is the end product of degradation of the heme moiety of hemoproteins, including hemoglobin (Fig. 8-1).

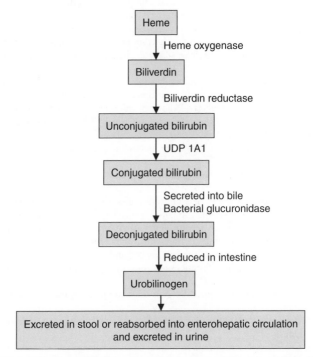

FIGURE 8-1 Bilirubin metabolism. Heme oxygenase catalyzes the rate-limiting step within the reticuloendothelial system. Unconjugated bilirubin is transported bound primarily to albumin, at which point it is taken up by the hepatocyte and undergoes glucuronidation by uridine diphosphate glucuronyl transferase (UGT-1A1). It is then secreted in the water-soluble conjugated form into the canaliculi (70% to 90% diglucuronide and 5% to 25% monoglucuronide). Within the intestine, it is deconjugated and reduced by bacterial β-glucuronide to urobilinogen, which is either excreted in stool or reabsorbed into the enterohepatic circulation. A defect at or before glucuronidation results in primarily unconjugated hyperbilirubinemia, whereas problems after this step cause conjugated hyperbilirubinemia.

○ Hemoglobin from senescent red blood cells accounts for 80% to 90% of the daily bilirubin production, with the remainder coming from ineffective erythropoiesis and degradation of heme-containing proteins (cytochrome P450, peroxidase, and catalase).

○ Normal daily bilirubin production averages 4 mg/kg of body weight (~300 mg). The reticuloendothelial system has the capacity to metabolize up to 1500 mg daily, so hemolysis rarely causes jaundice by itself, unless this ceiling is exceeded or the hemolysis is associated with liver disease.

• Unconjugated or indirect hyperbilirubinemia is present when >80% to 85% of the total bilirubin is unconjugated. Defects proximal to, and including, the conjugation step result in primarily unconjugated hyperbilirubinemia. Defects after the glucuronidation step within the hepatocyte result in primarily conjugated hyperbilirubinemia. Conjugated or direct hyperbilirubinemia is present when >30% of the total bilirubin is in the conjugated form.

DIAGNOSIS

• The history, physical examination, and initial laboratory evaluation should be directed at answering the following questions:
○ Is the process acute or chronic?
○ Is the hyperbilirubinemia unconjugated, conjugated, or mixed?
○ If there is unconjugated hyperbilirubinemia, is it caused by increased production, decreased uptake, or impaired conjugation?
○ If there is conjugated hyperbilirubinemia, is it caused by intrahepatic or extrahepatic cholestasis?

Clinical Presentation

History

• A detailed history is important for developing a differential diagnosis and identifying the cause of the patient's jaundice. Factors that can provide clues to the diagnosis include the following[6]:

○ **Age:** Patients younger than 30 years are more likely to have acute parenchymal disease, including acute viral hepatitis, biliary tract disease, alcoholic liver disease, and autoimmune hepatitis, whereas those older than 65 years are more likely to have gallstones, malignancy, or drug-induced hepatotoxicity in the setting of polypharmacy. Autoimmune disease can have a second peak in the elderly.

○ **Gender:** In male patients, consider alcohol, pancreatic cancer, hepatocellular carcinoma, and hemochromatosis. In female patients, gallstones, primary biliary cirrhosis, and autoimmune hepatitis are more common.

○ **Acute versus chronic** jaundice can be differentiated by a thorough history, physical examination, and laboratory tests. Xanthelasma, spider angioma, presence of ascites, and hepatosplenomegaly are indicative of a chronic process. Similarly, hypoalbuminemia, thrombocytopenia, and prolonged prothrombin time (PT) are mostly seen in the setting of chronic jaundice.[6] Fever, chills, right upper quadrant abdominal pain, leukocytosis, and hypotension are not only indicative of an acute cause but suggest ascending cholangitis and require urgent intervention. Asterixis, confusion, or stupor could represent fulminant hepatic failure and require immediate therapy.

○ Patients with **viral hepatitis** often give a history of a viral prodrome, including anorexia, malaise, and myalgias. Infectious sexual exposures, intravenous drug use, and prior blood transfusions also support a diagnosis of viral hepatitis. Essential are a careful travel history and human immunodeficiency virus status, as well as alcohol and drug history, including over-the-counter and herbal remedies, because a multitude of drugs can cause jaundice by diverse mechanisms, including hemolysis, hepatocellular damage, and cholestasis.

○ **Pruritus** suggests a longer duration of disease and can be seen in both intrahepatic cholestasis and biliary obstruction. Increased urine urobilinogen may represent increased bilirubin production and subsequent enterohepatic circulation or decreased hepatic clearance of urobilinogen and, therefore, does not distinguish between hemolysis and liver disease. In the presence of cholestasis, however, conjugated bilirubin is filtered in the urine. Bilirubin in the urine is a definitive indicator of conjugated hyperbilirubinemia. Abdominal pain with radiation to the back can suggest pancreatic disease, whereas a right upper quadrant aching pain is frequently seen in patients with viral hepatitis.

Physical Examination
- The physical examination can reveal evidence of chronic liver disease and may also provide evidence of less common forms of liver disease.
  ○ **Chronic liver disease** is manifested by muscle wasting, cachexia, palmar erythema, Dupuytren contracture, parotid enlargement, leuconychia, gynecomastia, and testicular atrophy.[6]
  ○ **Cirrhosis** is suggested by the findings of spider angiomata, palmar erythema, and caput medusae (or dilated veins).
  ○ **Liver size and consistency** should also be evaluated. A shrunken and nodular liver would suggest cirrhosis, whereas a palpable mass can be indicative of a malignancy or an abscess. An enlarged liver with a span of >15 cm may be seen in nonalcoholic fatty liver disease, infiltrative disease, or congestive hepatopathy.
  ○ **Ascites** is typically seen in advanced cirrhosis but may also be seen with severe viral and alcoholic hepatitis.
  ○ **Asterixis** is indicative of end-stage liver disease and hepatic failure.
  ○ Other useful findings include hyperpigmentation (**hemochromatosis**), xanthomas (**primary biliary cirrhosis**), and Kayser-Fleisher rings (**Wilson's disease**).

Diagnostic Testing

Laboratories
- Essential initial laboratory tests should include levels of direct and indirect bilirubin, transaminases (aspartate aminotransferase and alanine aminotransferase), AP, total protein, albumin, and PT. If available, results of prior liver biochemical test are essential to evaluate the trend of changes.
- If laboratory results are consistent with **unconjugated hyperbilirubinemia,** a hemolysis workup should be initiated (reticulocyte count, lactate dehydrogenase, haptoglobin, Coomb's test, and peripheral smear). In the absence of hemolysis, most asymptomatic healthy patients with isolated unconjugated hyperbilirubinemia have Gilbert's disease and require no further evaluation.[1]
- If laboratory results demonstrate **conjugated hyperbilirubinemia** or are indeterminate, then additional workup is required.

○ Patients with transaminases elevated out of proportion to the AP most likely have a hepatocellular disorder. Levels of transaminases <300 IU/mL are seen in alcoholic hepatitis, drug-induced injury, and chronic liver disease and obstruction. Levels >1000 IU/mL are indicative of acute hepatitis, drug-induced hepatotoxicity (acetaminophen toxicity), and shock liver.

○ If AP is elevated (usually more than three times upper limit of normal) out of proportion to the transaminases, this suggests intrahepatic cholestasis or extrahepatic obstruction. An increased γ-glutamyl transferase (GGT), 5′-nucleotidase, or leucine aminopeptidase confirms the hepatic origin of an elevated AP.

○ Disproportionate elevation of AP compared with bilirubin could be seen in partial biliary obstruction or in early intrahepatic cholestasis (primary biliary cirrhosis and PSC). High levels of AP and bilirubin may, however, indicate presence of a CBD stone.

○ High levels of GGT could be seen in many other medical conditions other than biliary disease, including congestive heart failure, alcohol intake, pancreatitis, chronic lung disease, renal failure, and diabetes, and as a result of use of many drugs.

• The presence of **low albumin** or **prolonged PT** suggests chronic liver disease with impaired synthetic function.

○ In cirrhotic patients, high levels of globulins and low albumin levels are frequently seen.

○ Prolonged PT may, however, also be seen in obstructive jaundice. Of note, parenteral administration of vitamin K corrects the coagulopathy in patients with obstructive jaundice but not hepatocellular disease.

○ Testing for urinary bilirubin or urobilinogen may be of some use, because clinical jaundice may lag behind bilirubinuria.

○ High cholesterol levels are seen in patients with cholestasis.

• If the initial evaluation does not reveal an obvious etiology (alcohol, drugs, infections), then **specific biochemical studies** should be ordered, including viral hepatitis serologies, antinuclear antibody, antimitochondrial antibody, antismooth muscle antibody, serum quantitative immunoglobulins, iron studies, ceruloplasmin, and α_1-antitrypsin levels.

○ If the cause still remains unclear, then liver biopsy should be considered. Figure 8-2 is helpful in planning the evaluation of the patient with jaundice.

• The evaluation of **conjugated hyperbilirubinemia** requires careful selection of the appropriate imaging procedure, because many of these studies are expensive or invasive.

○ If the initial evaluation suggests a possible vascular cause (Budd-Chiari syndrome or shock liver), then ultrasound with Doppler should be the initial study to evaluate patency of the hepatic and portal veins and hepatic artery.

○ Increased transaminases should prompt a search for hepatocellular disorders.

○ If the history and examination cause concern for malignancy, then an abdominal computed tomographic scan and α-fetoprotein levels should be ordered, followed by ultrasound- or computed tomography (CT)-guided liver biopsy, if appropriate.

• Patients with **increased AP** should be evaluated for causes of cholestatic jaundice.

○ Ultrasound should be the initial study to evaluate for evidence of biliary ductal dilatation. Abdominal CT can also be used to evaluate for ductal dilatation, but it has specific limitations.

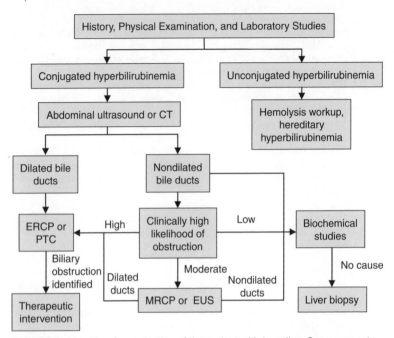

FIGURE 8-2 Algorithm for evaluation of the patient with jaundice. See comments in text regarding selection of appropriate imaging study when given a choice in the algorithm. ERCP, endoscopic retrograde cholangiopancreatography; EUS, endoscopic ultrasound; MRCP, magnetic resonance cholangiopancreatography; PTC, percutaneous transhepatic cholangiography.

○ If ductal dilatation is present, or if the suspicion for obstruction remains high despite a normal study finding, then endoscopic retrograde cholangiopancreatography (ERCP) or percutaneous transhepatic cholangiography (PTC) should be performed. Of note, patients who have had prior cholecystectomy normally have a dilated CBD.

○ If ductal dilatation is not seen and the suspicion for obstruction is low, then biochemical studies should be ordered as above to look for parenchymal disease.

○ Again, liver biopsy should be considered if no etiology can be identified.

Imaging

- **Ultrasound**
  ○ Ultrasound is the best initial study for detection of biliary obstruction as evidenced by ductal dilatation. It has a sensitivity of 77% and specificity of 83% to 95% for identification of bile duct dilation. Its advantages are portability, noninvasiveness, and relatively low cost. Disadvantages include operator-dependent nature and decreased image quality in obese patients or in those with overlying bowel gas and poor visualization of distal ducts in 30% to 50% of patients.

- Nondilated ducts, especially in the setting of acute or intermittent obstructions, cannot definitively rule out biliary obstruction, however. Therefore, additional studies are required if a high suspicion of obstruction remains.
- Ultrasound can also identify hepatic parenchymal lesions, gallbladder disease, cholelithiasis, and choledocholithiasis.

- *Abdominal CT*
  - Abdominal CT is a first-line study for evaluation of hepatic parenchymal lesions; it is also an alternative to ultrasound for identifying biliary obstruction. Its advantages are a less operator-dependent nature and improved images in obese patients. Limitations include higher cost, lack of portability, inability to detect noncalcified gallstones, and requirement of radiocontrast dye.

- *Magnetic resonance imaging*
  - Magnetic resonance imaging is a useful test for assessing liver parenchyma, specifically focal and malignant lesions. It is also sensitive in assessment of liver fat and iron. Magnetic resonance cholangiopancreatography is a special technique used to visualize the biliary tract. Advantages include its noninvasive nature and ability to accurately identify various liver lesions. Unlike ERCP, it does not have therapeutic capabilities.

- *Hepatic iminodiacetic acid (HIDA) scan*
  - The test of choice, if acute cholecystitis with cystic duct obstruction or biliary leakage is suspected, is a HIDA scan. False-negative results should be expected, however, in the setting of TPN use or with fasting serum bilirubin concentrations >5 mg/dL.

Diagnostic Procedures

- *Endoscopic retrograde cholangiopancreatography*
  - ERCP provides direct visualization of the biliary and pancreatic ducts and identifies the site of obstruction in >90% of patients. Advantages include high accuracy in locating the site of obstruction, as well as the ability to perform therapeutic interventions (sphincterotomy, stone extraction, stent placement, cytology, and brushing and direct visualization using SpyGlass). Disadvantages include expense, invasiveness, difficulty after certain surgeries (Roux-en-Y), and morbidity. Complications of perforation, bleeding, cholangitis, and pancreatitis are uncommon but can be serious (2% to 3% overall morbidity rate).

- *Endoscopic ultrasound*
  - Endoscopic ultrasound can detect small CBD stones with similar accuracy to ERCP and no risk of post-ERCP pancreatitis. It can detect small (<3 cm) pancreatic tumors that are usually not discovered by CT scans. Bile duct stones cannot be removed by endoscopic ultrasound, which is a major disadvantage to ERCP.

- *Percutaneous transhepatic cholangiography*
  - PTC is also an excellent test for evaluating biliary obstruction, with accuracy similar to ERCP (up to 90% to 100%) in identifying the site of biliary obstruction if the ducts are dilated. Advantages include lower cost and therapeutic capabilities (decompression of biliary system).
  - This test is less accurate than ERCP, however, if there are nondilated ducts, and several passes into the liver may be required to access the biliary tree. Aside from limited usefulness with nondilated ducts, other problems include inability to perform the test in the presence of coagulopathy (PT >16 seconds

and platelets <50,000) and ascites, as well as complication risks (bleeding, arteriovenous fistulas, sepsis, pneumothorax, peritonitis). The decision of whether to perform ERCP or PTC should be based partially on local expertise of the gastroenterologists and radiologists.

- *Liver biopsy*
  - If imaging studies are inconclusive and a hepatocellular process is suspected, a liver biopsy may be useful. It is an invasive procedure, however, and a complication rate of 0.1% to 3% is expected. Complications include pain, hemobilia, hemoperitoneum, arteriovenous fistula, pneumothorax, or hemothorax. Ultrasound guidance may decrease some of the risks. In patients with thrombocytopenia, coagulopathy, and ascites, a transjugular approach is recommended.

TREATMENT

- **Management of jaundice should be directed at the underlying cause.** These management options are discussed in detail elsewhere in this handbook.
  - Watchful waiting can be appropriate for acute viral hepatitis, where recovery is expected in most instances. Hepatitis B and C have chronic phases that require monitoring and management with interferon and/or antiviral agents as described in Chapter 19. Liver transplant may be an option for end-stage liver disease with decompensation.
  - Discontinuation of offending medications or toxins is recommended for drug- or toxin-induced jaundice. Specific treatment with *N*-acetyl cysteine is available for acetaminophen-induced liver damage but is effective only in early disease course.
  - Management of chronic autoimmune liver diseases causing jaundice may include use of corticosteroids, immune modulators, and liver transplantation. See Chapter 19 for further details.
  - The goal of treating a patient with bile duct obstruction is to drain the bile to decrease the risk of complications and to provide symptom relief. In patients with choledocholithiasis, a laparoscopic cholecystectomy with CBD exploration using intraoperative or postoperative ERCP is recommended. In many cases of CBD stones, an ERCP with sphincterotomy and stone extraction would be the appropriate therapeutic procedure. In old or frail patients who cannot undergo surgery, externally inserted drains into the gallbladder or main hepatic ducts would be suggested to overcome malignant strictures or for temporary relief of symptoms.

SPECIAL CONSIDERATIONS

- **Pregnancy**
  - In pregnant patients, jaundice could be caused by disorders that are unique to pregnancy or coincident with, or exacerbated by, pregnancy (hepatitis E, herpes simplex, Budd-Chiari syndrome, choledocholithiasis).
  - Low serum albumin level and high AP (up to two to four times normal from placenta), fibrinogen, transferrin, and cholesterol levels can be considered part of expected pregnancy-related changes. Levels of transaminases, bilirubin, and GGT do not change with pregnancy, however, and abnormal levels need to be further investigated.[7]

○ Liver diseases associated with pregnancy occur at special time points.[8]

- **Hyperemesis gravidarum** may cause mild elevations of AP, bilirubin, and transaminases during the first trimester.

- **Intrahepatic cholestasis of pregnancy** normally presents with intense itching in the third trimester (up to 100 times increase in total serum bile acids).

- In **Dubin-Johnson syndrome** exacerbated by pregnancy, jaundice develops in the second or third trimester.

- Chronic hepatitis, autoimmune disease, Wilson's disease, and primary biliary cirrhosis may be exacerbated during pregnancy as well. Gallstone disease can occur at anytime.

- **Acute fatty liver of pregnancy** (with marked elevations of transaminases), **preeclampsia** or **eclampsia,** and **HELLP** (hemolysis, elevated liver enzymes, and low platelet count) syndrome could present with jaundice, usually late in the pregnancy. When jaundice occurs late in the course of these hepatocellular diseases, it indicates severe hepatic dysfunction.

- **Critically ill patients**
  ○ Jaundice is commonly seen in patients in the intensive care unit, where it is usually nonobstructive and multifactorial.[9] Bilirubin overproduction caused by hemolysis of transfused blood (10% of red blood cells in a transfused unit are hemolyzed within 24 hours), drug-induced hemolysis, and prosthetic valves are most common explanation of this finding. Hepatocellular dysfunction secondary to ischemia (shock liver), right-sided heart failure, anesthetic agents, sepsis with multisystem organ failure, viral hepatitis, and TPN should also be considered in the differential diagnosis of nonobstructive jaundice.[10]
  ○ Obstructive jaundice seen in critically ill patients is usually due to choledocholithiasis, cholangitis, cholangiocarcinoma, pancreatic duct stricture, or pancreatic head mass. Acalculous cholecystitis causes jaundice, especially after vascular surgeries, trauma, and burns. Injuries of the biliary tract are commonly seen in patients who have recently undergone cholecystectomy or other upper abdominal surgeries.[11]

- **Liver transplantation**
  ○ Biliary strictures are a major source of morbidity after liver transplantation. The incidence has been reported as 5% to 15% after deceased donor liver transplant and 28% to 32% after living donor right lobe transplant. Strictures can often be managed endoscopically with a success rate of 70% to 100% for anastomotic strictures and 50% to 75% for nonanastomotic strictures.[12]
  ○ Cholestasis after liver transplantation can be related to early or late complications (using an approximate cutoff of a 6-month period) or can be mild with no clinical significance.[13] Early complications include acute rejection, ischemia-reperfusion injury (cold and rewarming ischemia), primary graft nonfunction, acute rejection, bacterial or viral infections, and drug-induced cholestasis. Late complications are predominantly related to chronic rejection and recurrence of the original disease.[14]

COMPLICATIONS

- Complications of jaundice will depend on the primary cause and severity of the jaundice.

○ **Kernicterus** caused by deposition of bilirubin in the brain can result in irreversible motor and cortical impairment. This is seen in infants when levels of total bilirubin are >20 mg/dL.

○ **Mechanical obstruction of the extrahepatic ducts** can predispose to life-threatening complications, including cholangitis, secondary biliary cirrhosis, and hepatic abscess formation.

○ **Other long-term complications** include hepatic osteodystrophy, malabsorption of fat and fat-soluble vitamins, and pruritus.

ADDITIONAL RESOURCES

AGA technical review on the evaluation of liver chemistry tests. http://www.gastrojournal.org/article/S0016-5085(02)00241-X/fulltext

American Association for the Study of Liver Diseases (AASLD) Practice Guidelines. http://www.aasld.org/practiceguidelines/Pages/default.aspx

MELD score calculator of survival probability of a patient with end-stage liver disease. http://www.mayoclinic.org/meld/mayomodel6.html

REFERENCES

1. Feldman M, Friedman LS, Brandt LJ. *Sleisenger and Fordtran's Gastrointestinal and Liver Disease.* 9th ed. Philadelphia: Saunders Elsevier; 2010.
2. Green RM, Flamm S. AGA technical review on the evaluation of liver chemistry tests. *Gastroenterology.* 2002;123:1367–1384.
3. Yamada T, Alpers DH, Kalloo AN, et al. *Textbook of Gastroenterology.* 5th ed. Hoboken: Wiley-Blackwell; 2008.
4. Qin LX, Tang ZY. Hepatocellular carcinoma with obstructive jaundice: diagnosis, treatment and prognosis. *World J Gastroenterol.* 2003;9:385–391.
5. Navarro VJ, Senior JR. Drug-related hepatotoxicity. *N Engl J Med.* 2006;354:731–739.
6. Schiff ER, Sorrell MF, Maddrey WC. *Schiff's Diseases of the Liver.* 10th ed. Philadelphia: Lippincott William & Wilkins; 2007.
7. Jamjute P, Ahmad A, Ghosh T, et al. Liver function test and pregnancy. *J Matern Fetal Neonatal Med.* 2009;22:274–283.
8. Knox TA, Olans LB. Liver disease in pregnancy. *N Engl J Med.* 1996;335:569–576.
9. Bansal V, Schuchert VD. Jaundice in the intensive care unit. *Surg Clin North Am.* 2006; 86:1495–1502.
10. Fuchs M, Sanyal AJ. Sepsis and cholestasis. *Clin Liver Dis.* 2008;12:151–172.
11. Faust TW, Reddy KR. Postoperative jaundice. *Clin Liver Dis.* 2004;8:151–166.
12. Sharma S, Gurakar A, Jabbour N. Biliary strictures following liver transplantation: past, present and preventive strategies. *Liver Transpl.* 2008;14:759–769.
13. Ben-Ari Z, Pappo O, Mor E. Intrahepatic cholestasis after liver transplantation. *Liver Transpl.* 2003;9:1005–1018.
14. Corbani A, Burroughs AK. Intrahepatic cholestasis after liver transplantation. *Clin Liver Dis.* 2008;12:111–129.

Abnormal Liver Chemistries

9

Noura M. Sharabash

GENERAL PRINCIPLES

- The evaluation of a patient with suspected hepatic or biliary disease can be aided by the measurement of various serum markers of liver function or injury. A thorough understanding of these markers of hepatic disease is essential for proper interpretation and accurate diagnosis. Whereas a single laboratory value rarely leads to a diagnosis in patients with hepatic disease, the pattern of liver enzyme abnormalities together with a thorough history and physical examination can help direct additional workup to arrive at a diagnosis.

Definition

- Abnormal liver chemistries are commonly referred to as "liver function tests" although they do not necessarily measure the function of the liver. Furthermore, they can be abnormal in patients with healthy livers and normal in patients with advanced liver disease. The most common liver chemistries can be classified as serum enzymes, excretory products, and measures of synthetic liver function.
- **Serum enzymes and excretory products**
  - **Aminotransferases**
    - Aspartate aminotransferase (**AST**, previously called SGOT) and alanine aminotransferase (**ALT**, previously called SGPT) are sensitive markers of hepatocellular injury or necrosis. Injury to hepatocytes results in translocation of these enzymes across the disrupted membranes and a subsequent rise in serum levels. ALT is a more specific indicator of liver injury because it is found primarily in the liver, whereas AST can be found in liver, cardiac and skeletal muscles, kidney, brain, pancreas, leukocytes, erythrocytes, and other organs.[1]
    - The **degree and pattern of elevation** of aminotransferases can offer clues to the etiology. Small to moderate elevations in the aminotransferases can be seen in almost any liver disease, including chronic viral hepatitis, alcohol abuse, autoimmune hepatitis, nonalcoholic fatty liver disease, biliary obstruction, hemochromatosis, Wilson's disease, α_1-antitrypsin deficiency, and as a side effect of various medications (Table 9-1). Whereas marked elevations in AST and ALT (often >1000 U/L) are seen primarily in acute viral, toxin-induced, or ischemic hepatitis, these can also be encountered with acute Budd-Chiari syndrome, fulminant Wilson's disease, autoimmune hepatitis, or acute bile duct obstruction (Table 9-2).[2]
    - The **ratio of AST and ALT** can also aid in focusing the differential diagnosis (Table 9-3). An AST:ALT ratio of ≥2 with an AST <300 U/L is highly suggestive of alcohol-induced injury, whereas a ratio of <1 is usually seen in patients with acute or chronic viral hepatitis, nonalcoholic steatohepatitis

TABLE 9-1	DRUGS COMMONLY ASSOCIATED WITH ELEVATED LIVER ENZYMES
Antiarrhythmics	Amiodarone
Analgesics	Acetaminophen, nonsteroidal anti-inflammatory drugs
Antibiotics	Synthetic penicillins, ciprofloxacin, nitrofurantoin, ketoconazole, fluconazole, isoniazid, erythromycin
Antihypertensives	Methyldopa, captopril, enalapril
Antiepileptics	Phenytoin, carbamazepine
Drugs of abuse	Anabolic steroids, cocaine, 3,4-methylelenedioxy-methamphetamine ("ecstasy")
Herbal substances	Ephedra, Jin bu huan, Senna, chaparral
HMG CoA inhibitors	Atorvastatin, pravastatin, lovastatin, simvastatin
Sulfonylureas	Glipizide
Toxins	Chloroform, phencyclidine, toluene-containing glues, trichloroethylene

TABLE 9-2	CAUSES OF HEPATOCELLULAR INJURY PATTERN OF LIVER CHEMISTRIES*

Viral hepatitis
Hepatitis A, B, C, D, E, and other viruses (cytomegalovirus, Epstein-Barr virus, herpes simplex virus, varicella zoster virus)

Drugs and toxins
Alcoholic liver disease, medications, herbals, and drugs of abuse

Metabolic syndrome
Nonalcoholic fatty liver disease and nonalcoholic steatohepatitis

Autoimmune
Autoimmune hepatitis, thyroid disorders, celiac disease

Vascular
Budd-Chiari syndrome, ischemia and shock liver (hypotension), congestive hepatopathy, veno-occlusive disease

Hereditary
Hemochromatosis, Wilson's disease, α_1-antitrypsin deficiency

Pregnancy associated
Acute fatty liver of pregnancy, preeclampsia, eclampsia, HELLP syndrome

HELLP, hemolysis, elevated liver enzymes, and low platelet count.

*Predominately elevated AST and ALT with or without mild to moderate elevations of alkaline phosphatase and bilirubin.

(NASH), or extrahepatic biliary obstruction. In cases of isolated elevations of AST, a nonhepatic source should be considered (e.g., acute rhabdomyolysis). In acute muscle injury, the AST:ALT ratio may initially be ≥3 but quickly declines to 1 because of the shorter half-life of AST.

○ **Alkaline phosphatase**
  ■ Alkaline phosphatase (AP) is an enzyme found in the bile canalicular membranes. Elevated AP levels arise from two main sources—liver and bone—but the enzyme is also found in other tissues, including placenta, intestines, and kidneys. Marked elevations in AP are typically seen in cholestatic

---

TABLE 9-3 SCREENING FOR ALT AND AST ELEVATIONS

Less than five times the upper limit, screen for:

1. **Alcohol abuse:** Elevation of AST > ALT, especially a ratio of >2:1 (AST rarely exceeds 300) with a twofold elevation of GGT.
2. **Hepatotoxic medications** or herbal supplements identified by history.
3. **Hepatitis B:** Screening tests include hepatitis B surface antigen and antibody, hepatitis B core antibody.
4. **Hepatitis C:** Screen with hepatitis C antibody. Confirm with viral load (hepatitis C RNA by PCR).
5. **Hereditary hemochromatosis:** Serum iron and TIBC to calculate iron saturation (serum iron/TIBC), if saturation is >45%, check ferritin; a ferritin level >400 in men and >300 in women supports the diagnosis. Liver biopsy to assess severity of liver injury and genetic testing should follow.
6. **NASH:** More common in women, associated with obesity and diabetes mellitus type 2. Ratio of AST:ALT usually <1. Obtain imaging studies (ultrasound/CT/MRI).
7. Rarer nonhepatic etiologies include celiac disease, muscle disorders (e.g., rhabdomyolysis or polymyositis), thyroid disorders, adrenal insufficiency, and anorexia nervosa.

AST and ALT elevations >15 times the upper limit, screen for:

1. **Drug-induced hepatotoxicity:** Acetaminophen overdose is the most common cause of drug-induced fulminant hepatic failure.
2. **Acute viral hepatitis** (A-E, Herpes simplex)
3. **Ischemic hepatitis**
4. **Autoimmune hepatitis:** More common in young women. Screen with SPEP (80% of patients have hypergammaglobulinemia) followed by antinuclear (ANA) and antismooth muscle Ab (SMA). Liver biopsy is required to confirm the diagnosis.
5. **Wilson's disease:** Serum ceruloplasmin, ophthalmologic examination for Kayser-Fleischer rings, occasionally a 24-hour urine for copper excretion
6. **Acute bile duct obstruction:** Screen with an ultrasound, CT, MRCP initially. ERCP can be therapeutic.
7. **Acute Budd-Chiari syndrome:** Screen with an abdominal ultrasound with Dopplers.

ALT, alanine aminotransferase; AST, aspartate aminotransferase; GGT, gamma-glutamyl transpeptidase; NASH, nonalcoholic steatohepatitis; SPEP, serum protein electrophoresis; TIBC, total iron binding capacity.

TABLE 9-4	CAUSES OF A CHOLESTATIC INJURY PATTERN OF LIVER CHEMISTRIES*
Malignancy (intrahepatic or extrahepatic)	Rotor's or Dubin-Johnson syndrome
Choledocholithiasis	Biliary stricture
Primary biliary cirrhosis	Sepsis
Primary sclerosing cholangitis	Medications

*Predominately elevated alkaline phosphatase and bilirubin with or without mild to moderate elevations of AST and ALT.

syndromes (e.g., biliary obstruction, primary biliary cirrhosis, primary sclerosing cholangitis, and drug-induced cholestasis, Table 9-4). Moderate elevations in AP are seen with infiltrative processes (sarcoidosis, other granulomatous diseases, Table 9-5), liver metastasis, and other forms of liver disease. Elevations in AP can be confirmed as hepatic in origin by measuring AP isoenzymes, γ-glutamyltransferase (GGT), or 5′-nucleotidase.

○ γ-Glutamyltransferase
  ■ GGT is found in bile duct epithelial cells, hepatocytes, and other tissues, including kidney, pancreas, and intestine. Elevations in GGT can be seen in a number of disorders such as diabetes, pancreatitis, and obesity, as well as with the use of phenytoin, warfarin, barbiturates, and other drugs that induce microsomal enzymes. GGT has two main uses in the evaluation of hepatobiliary disease. An elevated level can confirm a hepatobiliary origin of elevated AP. In addition, GGT has been shown to be elevated in persons who consume alcohol on a regular basis and is sometimes used to monitor alcohol use or abuse in patients receiving treatment. However, its low specificity and low positive predictive value limit the clinical use of GGT for the screening of alcohol abuse.[3]

○ Bilirubin
  ■ Bilirubin is a degradation product of heme metabolism and is composed of conjugated (direct) and unconjugated (indirect) fractions. **Unconjugated hyperbilirubinemia** results from excessive production, reduced hepatic

TABLE 9-5	CAUSES OF AN INFILTRATIVE INJURY PATTERN OF LIVER CHEMISTRIES*
Metastatic cancer	Tuberculosis
Lymphoma	Sarcoidosis
Leukemia	Histoplasmosis
Primary hepatic tumors	Medications

*Predominately elevated alkaline phosphatase with near normal AST, ALT, and bilirubin.

uptake, or impaired conjugation of bilirubin. **Conjugated hyperbilirubinemia** occurs as a result of impaired intrahepatic secretion of bilirubin or extrahepatic biliary obstruction. Both forms of hyperbilirubinemia manifest clinically as jaundice. Usually a serum bilirubin concentration of >3 mg/dL is required for clinical detection of jaundice. A complete discussion of the pathophysiology and differential diagnosis of jaundice can be found in Chapter 8.

- **Measures of synthetic function**
  - ○ Hepatic synthetic function is **commonly evaluated with prothrombin time (PT) and albumin.** Abnormalities in these markers of synthetic function are seen with severe liver disease and should result in urgent evaluation and treatment of the cause of the abnormality. Acute liver disease is discussed in more detail in Chapter 18. Chronic liver disease and cirrhosis are discussed in Chapters 19 and 20.
  - ○ **Clotting factors**
    - ■ Many of the proteins involved in hemostasis, including the coagulation factors, are synthesized in the liver. Normal activity of clotting factors II, VII, IX, and X depends on normal hepatic synthetic function, as well as the presence of vitamin K. As a result, two forms of hepatobiliary dysfunction can lead to coagulopathy manifested by prolongation of PT. First, significant hepatocellular injury or necrosis can impair hepatic synthetic function of clotting factors and leads to PT prolongation. Second, cholestatic syndromes may also prolong PT by interfering with intestinal absorption of vitamin K via impaired lipid absorption. This form should respond to parenteral administration of vitamin K, whereas coagulopathy purely from impaired hepatic synthesis will not.
  - ○ **Albumin**
    - ■ Serum albumin concentration, which is often decreased in chronic liver disease, reflects decreased synthesis. Other disease states as well as plasma volume expansion can also decrease albumin concentration. Levels may be normal in acute liver disease because of a half-life of approximately 20 days. The shorter half-life of prealbumin (1.9 days) makes it a sensitive marker of liver function in patients with acute acetaminophen overdose.

DIAGNOSIS

- A series of laboratory tests alone rarely leads to a diagnosis in a patient suspected of having hepatobiliary disease. Instead, the clinical context must be considered and tests carefully chosen; disease-specific laboratory tests and other appropriate studies are necessary to arrive at a diagnosis.

Clinical Presentation

History

- A thorough and accurate history is essential in the approach to a patient with abnormal liver chemistries; it should include the following:
  - ○ Duration and extent of abnormal liver chemistries.
  - ○ Symptoms of liver disease (e.g., weight loss, anorexia, fever, nausea, vomiting, abdominal pain, pruritus, and jaundice).

○ Medical and surgical history, including details of other medical illnesses, such as cardiac disease, inflammatory bowel disease, diabetes, arthritis, thyroid diseases, and so forth.

○ Risk factors for the metabolic syndrome including a detailed history of weight gain/loss, cholesterol levels, diabetes, and so forth.

○ Pregnancy can predispose to intrahepatic cholestasis of pregnancy, pre-eclampsia/eclampsia, and acute fatty liver of pregnancy. Isolated AP elevation in the third trimester can be from a placental source of the enzyme.[4]

○ Careful review of prescription, over-the-counter medications, and herbal therapies.

○ Thorough social history, including history of alcohol consumption, illicit drug use (e.g., intravenous and intranasal), sick contacts and exposure history, well water consumption, tattoos, piercings, recent travel, dietary history including an unusual diet (e.g., raw oyster, mushroom), sexual and menstrual history, occupational and environmental history, and transfusion history.

○ Family history of jaundice may be present in Gilbert's syndrome, Dubin-Johnson syndrome, and hereditary hemolytic syndromes. Hemochromatosis, Wilson's disease, and α_1-antitrypsin deficiency are autosomal-recessive disorders. Other hepatobiliary disorders, including primary sclerosing cholangitis, primary biliary cirrhosis, and autoimmune hepatitis, may also have a genetic component.

Physical Examination

• The physical examination should **focus on stigmata of liver disease** as well as **signs suggestive of systemic diseases** that commonly affect the liver. This includes jaundice, palmar erythema, temporal wasting, spider nevi, caput medusa, gynecomastia, ascites, hepatosplenomegaly, abdominal tenderness, and encephalopathy. Certain liver diseases can also have particular findings on physical examination such as the Kayser-Fleischer rings of Wilson's disease and xanthelasmas (fatty nodules around the eyes) in primary biliary cirrhosis.

Differential Diagnosis

• A **nonhepatic source** must be considered in any patient with abnormal liver chemistries. When a **hepatic source** is suspected, it is helpful to divide the pattern of abnormality into one of three broad categories: hepatocellular injury, cholestasis, and infiltrative processes.

• **Hepatocellular injury**

○ Hepatocellular injury typically manifests with modest to profound elevations in serum aminotransferases. AP and bilirubin may or may not be elevated, depending on the nature and severity of the injury. As a general rule, the highest elevations in transaminases are seen with ischemic and acute viral hepatitis. In ischemic hepatitis or herpes simplex hepatitis, transaminase levels >10,000 can be noted (see also Chapter 18). Toxic injury is also typically associated with marked elevations in AST and ALT. Less-marked elevations in transaminases are seen with chronic viral hepatitis and cirrhosis. The PT can be prolonged with hepatocellular injury, depending on the extent of hepatocellular necrosis and subsequent hepatic synthetic dysfunction. Albumin is normal in acute injury but can decrease in chronic disorders when synthetic function is significantly impaired. Table 9-2 lists the common causes of hepatocellular injuries. The initial evaluation should include testing for the most likely causes. Specific biochemical testing often reveals the etiology. Imaging with ultrasound or abdominal computed tomography (CT) may be useful in identifying structural causes. For patients with unexplained abnormal transaminases, liver biopsy should be considered, especially if the levels remain elevated for >6 months (Table 9-3).

- **Cholestasis**
  - Cholestatic injury typically produces moderate to profound elevations in AP, often with hyperbilirubinemia (elevations in bilirubin may be absent in certain clinical situations, such as with partial biliary obstruction). PT may be prolonged but responds to parenteral vitamin K administration. Depending on the nature of the cholestasis, serum transaminases may or may not be elevated. In early total common bile duct obstruction, AST and ALT may rise before AP. Evaluating a patient with cholestatic injury with routine liver chemistries can be particularly challenging. Once a nonhepatic source of elevated AP has been excluded, selection of other studies is directed by the degree of AP elevation. Table 9-4 lists the common causes of cholestasis. Ultrasound is the best initial study, because it allows visualization of the liver parenchyma and biliary tree (Fig. 9-1). Depending on the ultrasound findings, further evaluation may include abdominal CT, endoscopic retrograde cholangiopancreatography, or liver biopsy.
- **Infiltrative process**
  - Infiltrative liver injury is seen most commonly with granulomatous diseases, including sarcoidosis and metastatic disease to the liver. The predominant feature is an elevation in AP and, to a lesser extent, elevated bilirubin. Unlike with cholestatic liver injury, PT prolongation would not be expected in infiltrative injury because intestinal absorption of vitamin K is not affected. Table 9-5 lists the common causes of infiltrative liver disease. Imaging with either ultrasound or abdominal CT, often followed by liver biopsy, forms the basis for evaluating infiltrative processes.

Diagnostic Testing

- Diagnostic testing should be directed toward identifying the most likely causes of the abnormal liver chemistries on the basis of a detailed history and physical examination. The pattern of laboratory abnormalities (hepatocellular, cholestatic, infiltrative, or mixed) is also critical in focusing the differential diagnosis and directing the evaluation toward the most likely cause of the abnormalities.
- For chronic (6+ months) mild to moderate elevations (less than five times the upper limit of normal), evaluate for the most common causes (alcohol abuse, hepatotoxic medications and herbals, hepatitis B, hepatitis C, NASH, and hemochromatosis). See Table 9-3 and Figure 9-1 for more details.

Laboratories

- **Initial laboratory testing for chronic, mild to moderate elevations** may include hepatitis B surface antigen and antibody, hepatitis B core antibody, hepatitis C antibody, and serum iron and total iron binding capacity to screen for hemochromatosis.[5] Alcoholic hepatitis is suggested by an AST:ALT ratio of >2. NASH does not have a specific diagnostic laboratory test but is usually diagnosed on the basis of history, examination, and radiologic imaging. Unlike with alcoholic liver disease, the AST:ALT ratio in NASH is usually <1.

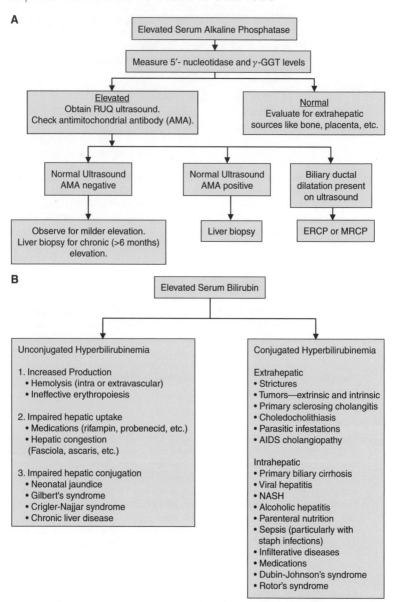

FIGURE 9-1 **A:** Algorithm for elevated serum alkaline phosphatase. **B:** Algorithm for elevated serum bilirubin. AMA, antimitochondrial antibody; ERCP, endoscopic retrograde cholangiopancreatography; γ-GGT, gamma-glutamyl transpeptidase; MRCP, magnetic resonance cholangiopancreatography; NASH, nonalcoholic steatohepatitis; RUQ, right upper quadrant.

- If initial laboratory testing is unrevealing, consider testing for less common but frequently seen disorders associated with abnormal liver chemistries. For example, nonhepatic sources of elevated aminotransferases include muscle disorders, thyroid disease, celiac disease, and adrenal insufficiency. Other less common hepatic sources of elevated liver chemistries include autoimmune hepatitis, primary biliary cirrhosis, primary sclerosing cholangitis, Wilson's disease, α_1 antitrypsin deficiency, and so forth. See Chapters 19 and 20 for more details.

Imaging
- The choice of imaging to evaluate the cause of abnormal liver chemistries depends on the most likely causes as determined by the history, physical examination, and initial laboratory investigation. It is reasonable to start with an **abdominal ultrasound** to evaluate the liver parenchyma, structural causes or mass lesions, and to visualize the biliary tree. The addition of Dopplers to the ultrasound examination can evaluate for suspected Budd-Chiari syndrome or portal hypertension. Ultrasound is noninvasive, portable, and is relatively inexpensive compared with other imaging modalities such as computed tomographic scans, magnetic resonance imaging (MRI), and so forth. Limitations of ultrasound include that it is operator-dependent and visualization can be limited by patient obesity and bowel gas. An **abdominal computed tomographic scan** also evaluates the hepatic parenchyma and biliary tree but is not operator-dependent or as limited by bowel gas or patient obesity. Use of IV contrast is needed to evaluate for malignancy. In particular, a triple-phase contrast CT to identify arterial washout is an excellent tool to evaluate for hepatocellular carcinoma. However, **MRI** is the most accurate imaging technique for identifying hepatocellular carcinoma, hemangiomas, focal nodular hyperplasia, hepatic iron overload, and focal fatty infiltration. Both CT and MRI are limited by lack of portability, increased cost, and need for contrast for the best visualization in most situations.[6]

Diagnostic Procedures
- **Liver biopsy** should be considered in patients with chronically (>6 months) elevated serum liver chemistries. The decision must be individualized to each patient's age, pattern of liver chemistry abnormalities, and associated comorbid conditions. Biopsies performed in patients with negative serologic markers are most likely to demonstrate a pattern of steatosis or steatohepatitis, occasionally associated with fibrosis.

TREATMENT

- Treatment of abnormal liver chemistries is directed toward the suspected or confirmed cause of the abnormalities. In suspected **drug-induced liver injury,** an initial first step is to discontinue nonessential medications and consider alternatives for potentially hepatotoxic medications. If **viral hepatitis** is identified, treatment decisions depend on whether the patient has acute or chronic disease and whether or not the patient has developed hepatic fibrosis or cirrhosis. Patients with suspected **nonalcoholic fatty liver disease or NASH** should have diet and exercise recommended and aim to lose 5% to 10% of their body weight over 6 to 12 months. These patients should be followed to confirm improvement in liver chemistries in response to weight loss. When

alcoholic liver disease is suspected on the basis of history, labs, and other studies, complete alcohol avoidance should be recommended and supportive services such as Alcoholics Anonymous or one-on-one counseling should be offered. In most cases of liver disease, patients should be offered immunization against viral hepatitis A and hepatitis B to protect them from future superimposed liver injury. Further details on the treatment of acute and chronic liver diseases can be found in Chapters 18 to 20.

ADDITIONAL RESOURCES

AGA technical review on the evaluation of liver chemistry tests. http://www.gastrojournal.org/article/S0016-5085(02)00241-X/fulltext

American Association for the Study of Liver Diseases (AASLD) Practice Guidelines. http://www.aasld.org/practiceguidelines/Pages/default.aspx

MELD score calculator of survival probability of a patient with end-stage liver disease. http://www.mayoclinic.org/meld/mayomodel6.html

REFERENCES

1. Green RM, Flamm S. AGA technical review on the evaluation of liver chemistry tests. *Gastroenterology.* 2002;123:1367–1384.
2. Schiff ER, Sorrell MF, Maddrey WC. *Schiff's Diseases of the Liver.* 10th ed. Philadelphia: Lippincott William & Wilkins; 2007.
3. Sharpe PC. Biochemical detection and monitoring of alcohol abuse and abstinence. *Ann Clin Biochem.* 2001;38:652–664.
4. Hay JE. Liver disease in pregnancy. *Hepatology.* 2008;47:1067–1076.
5. Pratt DS, Kaplan MM. Evaluation of abnormal liver-enzyme results in asymptomatic patients. *N Engl J Med.* 2000;342:1266–1271.
6. Goessling W, Friedman LS. Increased liver chemistry in an asymptomatic patient. *Clin Gastroenterol Hepatol.* 2005;3:852–858.

Ascites

10

Mrudula V. Kumar

GENERAL PRINCIPLES

- Ascites is the most common complication of cirrhosis of the liver.
- This is associated with a mortality rate of 15% in 1 year and 44% in 5 years.[1]
- Once ascites develops in the setting of end-stage liver disease, 1-year survival rate drops by as much as 50%.
- Development of ascites is one criterion used in determining the need for liver transplantation.

Definition

- Ascites is defined as an abnormal accumulation of serous fluid in the peritoneal cavity.

Etiology

- The **most common cause is portal hypertension due to cirrhosis of the liver.**
  - Liver disease accounts for ~80% of cases.[2]
  - Within 10 years of a diagnosis of cirrhosis, 50% of patients will develop ascites.
  - The portal pressure usually needs to exceed 12 mm Hg for ascites to develop.
- **Other hepatic causes** include chronic hepatitis, severe alcoholic hepatitis without cirrhosis, and hepatic vein obstruction (Budd-Chiari syndrome)[2] (Table 10-1).
- **Nonhepatic causes** include generalized fluid retention associated with systemic diseases (heart failure or nephrotic syndrome), peritoneal disorders (carcinomatous or infectious peritonitis), and certain systemic disorders (connective tissue disorders)[2] (Table 10-1).

Pathophysiology

- Altered hepatic architecture from advanced liver disease increases sinusoidal pressure in the fibrotic liver. This leads to increased hydrostatic pressure in the liver and splanchnic bed and accumulation of fluid in the peritoneum. Peripheral vasodilation from increased levels of arterial nitric oxide leads to renal protective mechanisms through the renin-angiotensin-aldosterone system. This results in avid renal sodium retention and contributes to fluid accumulation.[3]
- Ascites caused by right-sided heart failure is rather uncommon. When this occurs, chronic passive liver congestion leads to hepatocellular damage and fibrosis when sustained for a long time. Circulatory compromise and activation of antinatriuretic, renin-angiotensin, and sympathetic nervous systems can participate in fluid accumulation.[3]

TABLE 10-1	CAUSES OF ASCITES

High SAAG (≥1.1 g/dL)	Low SAAG (<1.1 g/dL)
Cirrhosis	Peritoneal carcinomatosis
Alcoholic hepatitis	Peritoneal tuberculosis
Congestive heart failure	Pancreatitis
Liver metastases	Nephrotic syndrome
Portal vein thrombosis	Protein-losing enteropathy
Budd-Chiari syndrome	Serositis
Veno-occlusive disease	Malignancy
Myxedema	Pelvic inflammatory disease
	Chylous ascites

SAAG, serum ascites albumin gradient.

SAAG is the simple numerical difference between serum and ascites albumin levels measured in grams per deciliter.

- Patients with nephrotic syndrome can have hypoproteinemia and anasarca, which can be associated with ascites.
- In peritoneal carcinomatosis, proteinaceous material exuded into the peritoneal cavity produces an osmotic gradient with movement of fluid from the intravascular space.
- Hepatocellular carcinoma can cause portal hypertension from replacement of normal liver parenchyma, leading to ascites.
- Cancer-induced hypercoagulable states can cause hepatic or portal venous thrombosis and subsequent ascites.
- Peritoneal infections can lead to proteinaceous exudates and subsequent movement of fluid into the peritoneal cavity.
- Pancreatic ascites can result from a pancreatic enzyme leak into the peritoneal cavity in acute severe pancreatitis. Intraperitoneal irritation and inflammation ensue, further potentiating fluid accumulation.
- Obstruction of the thoracic duct in lymphoma or after surgical trauma can lead to accumulation of chyle in the peritoneal cavity—this is termed chylous ascites.
- Serositis from connective tissue disorders can result in peritoneal inflammation and inflammatory fluid collection.

Classification

- **Ascites from portal hypertension is identified by its low albumin content.** The standard criterion used to make this determination is a measure of the difference between serum and ascites albumin concentrations (**serum ascites albumin gradient, SAAG**). The value is >1.1 g/dL in ascites from portal hypertension.
- This calculation has been shown to be 97% accurate in predicting portal hypertension.[1]
- SAAG scores of <1.1 indicate alternate etiologies for ascites, including hypoalbuminemia, chylous ascites, ovarian disease, tuberculous peritonitis, or peritoneal carcinomatosis (Table 10-1).

Associated Conditions

- Patients with ascites are at risk for spontaneous bacterial peritonitis (SBP), hepatorenal syndrome (HRS), and hepatic hydrothorax.[2]
  - ○ SBP is discussed later under Complications section.
  - ○ HRS is a clinical diagnosis based on the development of progressive renal failure in cirrhosis[4] (see Chapter 20)
    - ■ HRS can be subdivided into two categories: type I and type II.
    - ■ Type I is rapidly progressing and defined by a doubling of the initial serum creatinine or a 50% reduction of creatinine clearance in <2 weeks.
    - ■ Type II is a slower form that is a common cause of death in end-stage liver disease.
- Hepatic hydrothorax occurs in as many as 13% of patients with ascites.[5]
  - ○ It is typically right sided.
  - ○ Defects in the diaphragm permit passage of ascites from the abdominal cavity into the pleural space.

DIAGNOSIS

- The **two main purposes of sampling ascitic fluid** via diagnostic paracentesis are as follows:
  - ○ To identify the etiology of new-onset ascites
  - ○ To evaluate for SBP in patients with known ascites presenting with abdominal or nonspecific symptoms

Clinical Presentation[6]

- A thorough history and physical examination are essential for an accurate diagnosis of new-onset ascites.
- In the 20% of patients with a nonhepatic cause of ascites, the history should focus on uncovering conditions such as malignancy, heart failure, tuberculosis, or renal disease.

History

- Patients often state that they notice an increase in their abdominal girth. This may be manifested as weight gain or increase in belt size. Concurrent peripheral edema involving the feet and ankles may be seen.
- Ascites is not usually painful, but tense ascites may be uncomfortable and can cause shortness of breath.
- Because most cases of ascites are due to liver disease, patients should be asked about risk factors for liver disease (see Chapters 18 to 20).

Physical Examination

- The abdomen may be protuberant with bulging flanks. However, small ascites volumes may be difficult to identify by physical examination alone.
- Shifting dullness on percussion in two different positions (supine and left lateral) may suggest the presence of ascites.
- A fluid wave may be noted if ≥500 mL of fluid is present, though this may not be very accurate.
- Physical examination findings suggestive of chronic liver disease include jaundice, palmar erythema, spider angiomas, jugular venous distension, white nails, Dupuytren's contracture, testicular atrophy, and gynecomastia.

- A firm nodule in the region of the umbilicus (Sister Mary Joseph nodule), though not common, may indicate malignant ascites.

Diagnostic Testing

Laboratories

- **Ascitic fluid should be analyzed for the following:**
  - ○ **Albumin.** This is needed for the SAAG calculation.
  - ○ **Cell count and differential.** This helps determine whether the ascitic fluid is infected.
  - ○ **Total protein.** Protein levels of <1.0 g/dL indicate high risk for SBP. Protein levels can be high in secondarily infected ascites resulting in peritonitis.
  - ○ **Culture.** Fluid should be inoculated directly into blood culture bottles, which can increase the sensitivity of ascitic fluid **culture,** although yields are low.
  - ○ **Gram's staining** can be performed if the fluid is turbid or if there is high suspicion for infection.
  - ○ **Other optional tests** include lactate dehydrogenase (LDH), glucose, amylase, triglyceride levels, cytology, flow cytometry, mycobacterial smear, and culture. The need for these additional tests is dictated by the clinical presentation. The level of LDH is high, whereas that of glucose is low in peritonitis from secondarily infected ascites. Amylase levels are high in pancreatic ascites, and triglyceride levels can be extremely elevated in chylous ascites. Cytology is useful when peritoneal carcinomatosis is suspected. Tuberculosis or lymphoma may be associated with high lymphocyte counts and may require mycobacterial culture or flow cytometry for further confirmation.
- **An ascitic fluid neutrophil count of >250 cells/μL or total white blood cell count of >500 cells/μL indicates the presence of SBP.**
  - ○ This warrants initiation of empiric antibiotic therapy.
- The most important parameter in stratifying diagnostic workup is **the SAAG.** The SAAG, as described earlier, is the numeric difference between the serum and ascites albumin levels in grams per deciliter. A **SAAG of ≥1.1 g/dL is indicative of ascites related to portal hypertension with a specificity of 97%.**

Imaging

- **Ultrasonography** is the easiest and most sensitive technique for the detection of ascitic fluid.[6] Even small fluid collections can be accurately identified.
  - ○ Ultrasonography is also useful for localizing the most ideal site for abdominal paracentesis, especially when the ascitic volume is not large.
  - ○ Small amounts localize in the right perihepatic space, the posterior subhepatic space, and the Douglas pouch (rectouterine pouch).
- Plain abdominal films can demonstrate elevation of the diaphragm in the presence of massive ascites, but this is typically not necessary for the diagnosis of ascites.
- Ascites is demonstrated well on computed tomographic scan images, but computed tomography is not needed for diagnosis in most instances.

Diagnostic Procedures

- A **diagnostic paracentesis** should be performed in new-onset ascites or in any patient with known ascites with any abdominal or systemic symptom bringing them to medical attention, because manifestations of SBP can be subtle and nonspecific.

- Very few contraindications exist for diagnostic paracentesis. Paracentesis is a safe procedure that can be performed even in patients with coagulopathy and thrombocytopenia.[7]
- There are **no data to support administration of blood products prior to the procedure.**
- Fluid should be obtained in a sterile fashion. The **left lower quadrant is the preferred location.** A diagnostic paracentesis should be part of large-volume paracentesis performed for relief of abdominal distension.
- **Complications** are rare and are reported only in about 1% of patients, mostly consisting of abdominal wall hematomas. Hemoperitoneum is a rare complication. Introduction of secondary infection is clinically feasible, but likelihood is significantly reduced if aseptic precautions are utilized. Entry of the paracentesis needle into the bowel occurs in fewer than 1 in 1000 cases.

TREATMENT

- **Management of ascites depends on the etiology,** especially when it is caused by a process other than chronic liver disease, such as peritoneal disease (malignancy, infection, inflammation), leakage of digestive secretions (biliary or pancreatic), or lymphatic obstruction (chylous).
- If a specific etiology is identified, treatment can be directed toward the offending cause. For instance, a low-fat diet with medium-chain triglyceride supplementation can reduce the flow of chyle into the lymphatics in chylous ascites.
- Ascites is **managed in a stepwise fashion,** starting with abstinence from alcohol and dietary sodium restriction and escalating to pharmacologic therapy, large-volume paracentesis, transjugular portosystemic shunt, and liver transplantation as necessary.

Medications

- The initial pharmacologic management of ascites from portal hypertension consists of oral **furosemide** and **spironolactone.**[8]
  - The goal of diuretic therapy should be a weight loss of 1 kg/day in patients with edema and 0.5 kg/day without edema until ascites is adequately controlled.
  - Both agents are initiated simultaneously to prevent potassium derangements and to achieve desired diuresis efficiently.
  - Recommended starting doses are furosemide 40 mg/day and spironolactone 100 mg/day. The dose can be increased every 3 to 5 days to a maximum of 160 mg/day of furosemide and 400 mg/day of spironolactone.
  - Side effects may limit the ability to achieve maximum doses. Diuretics may need to be withheld in patients with renal dysfunction or hypovolemia. Patients are carefully monitored for signs of intravascular volume depletion, renal insufficiency, and decompensation of liver disease. Diuretic therapy should not be initiated when the serum creatinine level is unstable because of the risk of precipitating hepatorenal syndrome.
  - For minimal ascites, spironolactone can be used as single therapy.
  - If intolerable gynecomastia results from the use of spironolactone, amiloride or triamterine can be substituted.
- **Intravenous diuretics should be avoided in cirrhotic patients,** as these agents can precipitate renal failure. Oral furosemide has good bioavailability and should be adequate in most instances.

- Recent research has focused on the treatment of refractory ascites with **aquaretics—vasopressin V2-receptor antagonists** that promote excretion of electrolyte-free water (still awaiting approval by the FDA).[9]

Other Nonpharmacologic Therapies

- **Serial large-volume paracentesis** (removal of >5 L) is often used for ascites that is refractory to medical therapy.
  - Large-volume paracentesis is a fast, convenient, and safe technique.
  - The use of albumin remains controversial, given limited evidence in decreasing mortality and the high cost.[1] However, this option may minimize the likelihood of cardiovascular collapse and renal failure and should be considered in high-risk patients or when >5 L of fluid is expected to be removed.
  - Complications include postparacentesis hypotension, bleeding, local leakage of ascites, and infection. Perforation and death are unusual.
- **Transjugular intrahepatic portosystemic shunt (TIPS)** is currently the most effective method of managing ascites refractory to diuretics and large-volume paracentesis. TIPS consists of a conduit created between the hepatic vein and the intrahepatic portion of the portal vein, which decompresses portal pressure.[2,10]
  - TIPS is placed to reduce portal pressure in patients with complications related to portal hypertension.[11]
  - It is also used in cases of variceal bleeding, Budd-Chiari syndrome, and hepatic hydrothorax.
  - Absolute contraindications for TIPS include right-sided heart failure, polycystic liver disease, and severe hepatic failure.
  - Relative contraindications consist of active infection, severe encephalopathy poorly controlled with medical therapy, and portal vein thrombosis.
  - A study found that the VIATORR polytetrafluoroethylene-covered stent had lower rates of shunt insufficiency and hepatic encephalopathy.[12]
  - Complications include hemorrhage from capsular tears, new-onset or worsening of hepatic encephalopathy (occurs in about 25% and is directly related to shunt diameter), heart failure, and early shunt thrombosis.
  - TIPS does not alter the extrahepatic anatomy, therefore remaining an effective, nonsurgical bridge to liver transplantation.

Surgical Management

- The **peritoneovenous shunt** is an alternative for patients with medically intractable ascites.
  - This is a megalymphatic shunt that returns the ascitic fluid to the central venous system.
  - Improves short-term survival in cancer patients with refractory malignant ascites.
  - AASLD guidelines suggest considering peritoneovenous shunting for patients with refractory ascites who are not candidates for paracentesis or TIPS.[11]

Diet

- All patients should comply with a **low-sodium diet** (2000 mg/day) to ultimately avoid reaccumulation of fluid.
- Patients should be cautioned to **avoid salt supplements containing potassium chloride**, because use of these products can lead to life-threatening hyperkalemia, especially in association with aldosterone antagonists.

- Fluid restriction is used only if persistent hyponatremia is present (serum sodium <125 mmol/L).

COMPLICATIONS

- The most important complication of ascites is the development of **SBP**[2] (see Chapter 20).
  - ○ SBP is seen in ~12% of patients with ascites at the time of admission.
  - ○ Diagnosis is made with >250/mL polymorphonuclear cells in the ascites or growth of organisms in a culture of ascitic fluid.
  - ○ Second- and third-generation cephalosporins (cefotaxime 1 g IV q8h or ceftriaxone 1 g IV q24h) for 5 days have proven effective in the management of SBP.
  - ○ As for prophylaxis, there is conflicting evidence, but it is reasonable to consider daily norfloxacin administration in high-risk groups (GI bleed, ascitic fluid protein levels <1 g/dL, previous episode of SBP).
    - ■ Norfloxacin 400 mg daily or ciprofloxacin 750 mg weekly can be used for prophylaxis.
- **Hepatic hydrothorax** is an uncommon manifestation of cirrhotic patients with ascites.
  - ○ The diagnosis is established clinically by finding a serous transudate.
  - ○ Management is problematic and often does not respond to medical therapy.
  - ○ Treatment includes therapeutic thoracentesis, peritoneovenous and pleurovenous shunting, TIPS, and liver transplant.

REFERRAL

- If worsening ascites is part of progressive decompensation of chronic liver disease, a workup for assessing candidacy for liver transplantation may be warranted.

REFERENCES

1. Runyon B. AASLD practice guidelines: management of adult patients with ascites due to cirrhosis: an update. *Hepatol.* 2009;49:2087–2107.
2. Ginès P, Angeli P, Lenz K, et al. EASL clinical practice guidelines on the management of ascites, spontaneous bacterial peritonitis, and hepatorenal syndrome in cirrhosis. *J Hepatol.* 2010;53:397–417.
3. Arroyo V. Pathophysiology, diagnosis and treatment of ascites in cirrhosis. *Ann Hepatol.* 2002;1:72–79.
4. Francoz C, Glotz D, Moreau R, et al. The evaluation of renal function and disease in patients with cirrhosis. *J Hepatol.* 2010;52:605–613.
5. Kiafar C, Gilani N. Hepatic hydrothorax: current concepts of pathophysiology and treatment options. *Ann Hepatol.* 2008;7:313–320.
6. Runyon B. Approach to the patient with ascites. In: Yamada T, ed. *Textbook and Atlas of Gastroenterology* [CD-ROM]. Philadelphia, PA: Lippincott Williams & Wilkins; 1999.
7. Salerno F, Guevara M, Bernardi M, et al. Refractory ascites: pathogenesis, definition and therapy of a severe complication in patients with cirrhosis. *Liver Int.* 2010;30:937–947.
8. Ginès P, Cárdenas A. The management of ascites and hyponatremia in cirrhosis. *Semin Liver Dis.* 2008;28:43–58.
9. Okita K, Sakaida I, Okada M, et al. A multicenter, open-label, dose-ranging study to exploratively evaluate the efficacy, safety, and dose-response of tolvaptan in patients with decompensated liver cirrhosis. *J Gastroenterol.* 2010;45:979–987.

10. Narahara Y, Kanazawa H, Fukuda T, et al. Transjugular intrahepatic portosystemic shunt versus paracentesis plus albumin in patients with refractory ascites who have good hepatic and renal function: a prospective randomized trial. *J Gastroenterol.* 2011;46:78–85.
11. European Association for the Study of the Liver. EASL clinical practice guidelines on the management of ascites, spontaneous bacterial peritonitis, and hepatorenal syndrome in cirrhosis. *J Hepatol.* 2010;53(3):397–417.
12. Tripathi D, Ferguson J, Barkell H, et al. Improved clinical outcome with transjugular intrahepatic portosystemic stent-shunt utilizing polytetrafluoroethylene-covered stents. *Eur J Gastroenterol Hepatol.* 2006;18(3):225–232.

Malnutrition

11

Gowri Kularatna and Shelby A. Sullivan

GENERAL PRINCIPLES

- Assessment of nutritional status is an important aspect in the care of all patients. Nutritional status represents effectiveness of nutrient intake in maintaining body composition and meeting metabolic demands.
- The best overall approach to evaluating nutritional status involves a thorough clinical and physical examination, a nutritional history, and appropriate laboratory studies.
- To effectively manage a patient's nutritional status, familiarity with the basic principles of clinical nutrition is imperative.

Definition

A state of over- or undernutrition can be called malnutrition. For the purposes of this chapter, malnutrition will refer to the state of undernutrition, where nutrient intake is not adequate to meet the body's metabolic demands.

Epidemiology

- Undernutrition is prevalent in hospitalized patients, occurring in 20% to 70% of patients at admission or during hospital course. In the outpatient setting, unintentional weight loss is encountered in up to 13% of the elderly and 50% to 60% of nursing home residents.
- Malnutrition is frequently underdiagnosed by both practitioners and trainees. Studies have found that only 40% of malnourished patients have documentation of their nutritional status and that trainees recorded measurements of nutritional status in <33% of malnourished patients.[1]

Pathophysiology

- In terms of nutritional status, the body is made up of **lean body mass** (LBM) and **fat mass**.
  - LBM is the body's total mass minus the fat mass and includes muscle, organs, fluid, bones, and minerals.
  - Fat, in the form of adipose tissue triglyceride, is the body's major fuel reserve.
  - In times of stress, the body tries to preserve LBM; however, as fat stores run out, visceral protein mass is mobilized to meet metabolic needs, which include acting as gluconeogenic precursors and wound healing.
- Multiple changes occur in the body as a result of negative energy balance.
  - Initially, there is a decrease in resting energy expenditure (REE).
  - There is also a decrease in protein synthesis, particularly in persons with disease compared with healthy controls. This impaired protein synthesis can lead to a decrease in intestinal cell mass and, consequently, atrophy of the

mucosa. Studies have shown variable degrees of mucosal atrophy associated with malnutrition, but these changes can normalize after refeeding.

- In most cases, malnutrition is multifactorial. Nutritional disturbance in hospitalized patients typically results from reduced food intake (prescribed by physicians, critical illness, dysphagia) and increased metabolic demands (burns, inflammatory states, fluids lost through drains). Unintentional weight loss is also commonly caused by malignancy, and gastrointestinal (GI), endocrine, cardiovascular, and pulmonary disorders.

Associated Conditions

- Multiple consequences occur as the result of malnutrition in hospitalized patients.
  - Increased length of hospital stay, mortality, and susceptibility to infection; poor wound healing, increased frequency of decubitus ulcers; and impaired cardiopulmonary function.
- As little as 5% unintentional weight loss in 1 month can be clinically significant and a weight loss of ≥20% can impair most physiologic body functions.[2]

DIAGNOSIS

- Multiple tools have been developed to assist in nutritional assessment, including the Subjective Global Assessment, Mini Nutritional Assessment, Nutrition Risk Score, Nutrition Risk Index, and Geriatric Risk Index. Studies have been done to validate these tools in assessing for malnutrition, but no gold standard exists.
- The best overall approach involves a thorough nutritional history and physical examination.

Clinical Presentation

Nutritional History

Nutritional assessment includes the following[2]:

- Identification of preexisting malnutrition before acute presentations
  - The presence of mild (<5%), moderate (5% to 10%), or severe (>10%) unintentional weight loss in the last 6 months should be determined. Unintentional weight loss of >10% is associated with a poor clinical outcome.
- Relevant medical and surgical history
- Medications
- Social habits
- Focused dietary history (should assess changes in diet and, if present, the reasons for the changes)

Physical Examination

Physical examination should include an assessment of the following[2]:

- Hair, skin, eyes, mouth, dentition, and extremities
- Fluid status
- Stigmata of protein calorie malnutrition or vitamin and mineral deficiencies
  - Temporal muscle wasting, sunken supraclavicular fossae, and decreased adipose stores are easily recognized signs of malnutrition.

TABLE 11-1	BODY MASS INDEX–BASED ENERGY REQUIREMENTS FOR HOSPITALIZED PATIENTS

BMI, kg/m²	Energy Requirements, kcal/kg/day
<15	36–45
15–19	31–35
20–29	26–30
>30	15–25

BMI, body mass index.

Adapted from Klein S. A primer of nutritional support for gastroenterologists. *Gastroenterology.* 2002;122(6):1677–1687.

- Calculate body mass index (BMI) (BMI = weight in kilograms/height in meters squared) with a weight obtained in the hospital (Table 11-1).

Diagnostic Testing

Laboratory Assessment

Historically, concentrations of several plasma proteins (e.g., albumin, transferrin, prealbumin) and total lymphocyte count have been used to determine the degree of protein malnutrition and to predict clinical outcomes. However, in many cases, inflammation and injury, not malnutrition, are responsible for low levels of these markers and for the increased incidence of morbidity and mortality. As such, these parameters have poor sensitivity and specificity and will not be discussed further in this chapter.

TREATMENT

Calculating the Nutrient Requirement

- Nutritional requirements are determined by the body's energy demands or **total energy expenditure (TEE)**.
  - TEE = REE (70% TEE) + thermal effect of food (digestion, 20% TEE) + physical activity (10% TEE)
  - At times of illness or trauma, the resting energy requirement can increase by as much as 50%. Although it is often not feasible to measure energy expenditure directly in hospitalized patients, a number of predictive equations have been devised to estimate macronutrient requirements.
- The simplest approach to estimating the caloric needs of a hospitalized patient is based on BMI (Table 11-1).
  - The general rule is that caloric requirement is inversely proportional to BMI, because LBM (which includes organ mass) is the main determinant of energy expenditure. Because organs do not significantly hypertrophy with increasing adiposity, energy expenditure per kilogram body mass progressively declines with increasing adiposity but increases with lower body weights.

○ In critically ill, insulin-resistant patients, a lower energy dose should be used to avoid the deleterious effects of hyperglycemia.

○ In overweight patients, an adjusted body weight (see the following formula) should be used to avoid overfeeding.

■ Adjusted body weight = ideal body weight + 0.25 (actual body weight − ideal body weight)

○ Individual protein requirement depends on multiple factors, including the overall nutritional state, energy requirement, and nonprotein caloric intake.

■ The recommended protein intake is 0.8 g/kg/day in healthy adults.

■ Normal weight medically ill patients require 1.0 to 1.5 g/kg/day of protein; however, in patients experiencing large protein losses from burns, wounds, or fistulas, 2 to 2.5 g/kg/day of protein may be required.[2,3]

Nutritional Support

• Loss of LBM is tightly associated with mortality and therefore the goal of nutritional support is to prevent significant weight loss and preserve LBM until recovery from the underlying illness has been achieved.[2]

• Patients most likely to benefit from nutritional support are those with baseline malnutrition in whom a protracted period of starvation would otherwise occur.

• No absolute indications exist for nutritional support. A careful assessment of the patient's clinical condition and expected outcome help to determine the need for nutritional support.

• Factors that must be accounted for include amount of intake, amount of available endogenous stores (adipose tissue), lean muscle mass, and the rate of catabolism.[3]

• Individuals who are severely malnourished at the outset of an illness often require immediate nutritional support, whereas patients with adequate stores can tolerate longer periods without significant nutritional intake.

• In general, well-nourished hospitalized patients do not require nutritional support for 7 to 10 days, whereas malnourished and critically ill patients may need nutritional support initiated within 48 to 72 hours of admission.

• The decision to initiate nutritional support must be individualized and the type of support carefully chosen.[3]

Enteral Nutrition

• Enteral nutrition is infusion of a nutrient liquid formulation into the upper GI tract that can provide complete nutritional requirements.

• Preserves GI tract barrier function and should be used when possible.

• Mechanical obstruction, paralytic ileus, bowel ischemia, unstable GI bleeding, and high-output enteric fistulas are relative contraindications for enteral feedings.

• Enteral nutrition can be used with caution and careful monitoring in the setting of severe pancreatitis, and it may be associated with fewer complications than parenteral nutrition.[3,4]

Methods of Enteral Nutrition

• **For short-term support (<30 days), nasogastric or nasoenteric tubes** are preferred.

- Gastrostomy or jejunostomy tubes are indicated if the duration is expected to be >30 days.
  - Underlying condition and local expertise should dictate percutaneous, radiologic, or surgically placed gastrostomy tubes.
- Tube feeds should be started at a low dose (150 to 200 mL) every 4 to 6 hours and increased by 50 to 100 mL each feeding until the feeding goal is reached. Each feeding should be followed by a water flush. The amount of water flush depends on the patient's volume status.[2]
- With nasogastric tube feeding, a single elevated residual volume is an indication to recheck the residual volume in 1 hour. The feeding should not automatically be stopped, however.[5]
- Patients' upper body should remain upright or elevated by at least at 30 degrees during bolus tube feeds and for 2 hours after to avoid aspiration.[5]

Postpyloric or Small Bowel Feeding
- Small caliber nasojejunal feeding tubes can be placed past the ligament of Treitz for short-term postpyloric or small bowel feeding and percutaneous, surgical, or radiographic jejunostomy tubes can be placed for long term feeding.[5]
- Small bowel feeds are associated with a decreased risk of aspiration, better tolerated by patients with impaired motility, and have less pancreatic stimulation and are often used in the setting of severe acute pancreatitis.
- Small bowel feeds are given as a continuous pump-controlled infusion and typically start with 10 to 30 mL/hour and are increased in small increments (10 mL/hour every 8 to 12 hours) until the feeding goal is reached. Again, these tubes should be flushed with water every 4 hours to avoid tube occlusion.
- Bolus feeds should not be used with small bowel feeding tubes to prevent fluid shifts, abdominal distension, and diarrhea.[5]

Choosing an Enteral Formula
- Standard tube feeding formulas (Ensure, Osmolite, Isocal) are sufficient for most patients.
  - They are free of gluten and lactose and are isotonic.
  - They contain 1.0 cal/mL, and intake of 1500 to 2000 mL/day provides 100% of carbohydrates, protein, fat, vitamins, and minerals.
- Use of disease-specific and elemental formulas (monomeric and oligomeric) is controversial because these formulas are more expensive than standard formulas.[2]

Parenteral Nutrition

- Parenteral nutrition (PN) is the infusion of a nutritional liquid formulation through a central or peripheral venous catheter that can provide complete nutritional requirements.
- PN may be given if the GI tract is not accessible or functional, as occurs in patients with bowel obstruction, diffuse peritonitis, short gut syndrome, or malabsorption. In some cases, prolonged ileus or severe pancreatitis may also require PN.
- PN can be administered via a peripheral vein, but the nutrition formula cannot exceed 900 mOsm/kg (e.g., 10% dextrose, 2% amino acids, and electrolytes). This generally provides inadequate calories and therefore hyperosmolar solutions are used, which require central venous access. The optimal location of the

tip of the central venous catheter is at the junction of the superior vena cava and the right atrium.[6]

Composition and Administration of Parenteral Nutrition
- PN solution can be purchased commercially or can be made by the hospital pharmacy.
- Total number of calories and amount of protein are determined using the guidelines described in the "Calculating the Nutrient Requirement" section seen earlier.
- Lipid content of the PN ideally provides 20% to 30% of the daily calories; a 20% lipid emulsion yields 2.0 kcal/mL. The carbohydrate component is dextrose and provides the remainder of the calories; it contains 3.4 kcal/g.[2,6]
- Electrolytes, minerals, trace elements, and a multivitamin preparation are generally added to the parenteral solution. Note that *iron* is not generally part of the standard additives.
- Initiate PN at one-half to two-thirds of the total volume over the first 24 hours to avoid large fluid shifts and hyperglycemia. The volume is then advanced as tolerated. Once the volume goal has been reached, the rate of infusion can be increased and PN can be infused over 10 to 14 hours.
- Cyclic (rather than continuous) infusion of PN improves quality of life and decreases incidence of hepatobiliary complications. Shortened infusion time, however, can lead to periods of hyperglycemia.
- During initiation of nutrition support, close monitoring is indicated, with frequent measurement of vital signs, daily weights, intake and output, as well as the following:
  ○ Blood glucose checks every 6 to 8 hours.
  ○ Comprehensive metabolic panel should be checked daily until feeds are at goal and then twice weekly.
  ○ Complete blood cell count may be checked once weekly.

COMPLICATIONS

Complications of Tube Feedings

Tube feeding is a relatively safe procedure, and complications usually can be avoided or adequately managed. In addition to the complications of percutaneous tube placement (infection, bleeding, inadvertent colonic placement), patients may experience the following complications[2,5,7]:

- **Aspiration.** To limit the risk of aspiration, the head of the patient's bed should be raised ≥30 degrees during feeding and for 2 hours afterward. Intermittent or continuous feeding regimens, rather than the rapid bolus method, should be used. Gastric residuals should be checked regularly, and all patients should be observed for signs of feeding intolerance. Jejunal access is helpful either in patients with recurrent tube feeding aspiration (not oropharyngeal) or in critically ill patients at risk for impaired gastric motility.
- **Diarrhea.** To minimize the incidence of diarrhea, it is advisable to use an isosmotic, lactose-free formula and to advance tube feeds slowly. Decreasing the rate of the feeds, switching to continuous tube feeds, and adding fiber to the formula can be helpful. It is important to remember to check for antibiotic-associated diarrhea in these high-risk patients and to look for sorbitol in other

orally administered medications. If these measures fail and infectious causes have been ruled out, an antidiarrheal agent may be appropriate.

- **Hyperglycemia.** Adequate blood glucose monitoring is necessary when starting enteral nutrition. Initially, sliding scale regular insulin can be used to control blood glucose concentrations. Once the feedings have reached 1000 kcal/day, intermediate duration insulin given every 12 hours can be used in conjunction with sliding scale regular insulin for blood glucose control.
- **Small bowel necrosis.** Patients who require pressor support to maintain an adequate blood pressure are at risk for small bowel necrosis with small bowel feeds. The early signs of bowel ischemia are not specific and include bloating, loss of bowel sounds, abdominal pain, and ileus. If enteral nutrition is necessary in a patient with hypotension, he or she should be carefully monitored for any signs of early bowel ischemia.

Complications of Parenteral Nutrition
Mechanical Complications

- **Central line placement.** Complications related to **central line** placement include pneumothorax, brachial plexus injury, subclavian or carotid artery puncture, hemothorax, and chylothorax.
- **Thrombosis or pulmonary embolism.** This can occur secondary to central venous catheter use. Radiologically evident subclavian vein thrombosis occurs commonly (25% to 50%), but clinically significant manifestations (e.g., upper extremity edema, superior vena cava syndrome, or pulmonary embolus) are rare. Inline filters should be used with all PN solutions.
- **Infectious.** Complications are most commonly caused by *Staphylococcus epidermidis* or *Staphylococcus aureus.* In immunocompromised patients, gram-negative rods and *Candida* species are also a major concern.

Metabolic Complications

- **Hyperglycemia.** Blood glucose levels >200 mg/dL should be managed by minimizing the dextrose to <200 g/day as well as adding 0.1 unit of regular insulin for each gram of dextrose in PN. Blood glucose levels should be checked frequently and sliding scale insulin (SSI) used to control hyperglycemia. If blood glucose levels remain elevated despite SSI, additional insulin should be added to the PN solution, equal to 50% of the SSI from the previous 24 hours. If this fails, an intravenous (IV) insulin drip or further reduction in PN carbohydrate dose may be required.[2]
- **Hypertriglyceridemia.** Triglyceride levels >1000 mg/dL can cause or exacerbate acute pancreatitis and have been associated with thrombocytopenia. The levels should be checked at baseline and at least once during lipid emulsion infusion to ensure adequate clearance. Most practitioners reduce or eliminate lipids in the emulsion with serum triglyceride levels >400 mg/dL. Remember, the sedative propofol is administered in a 10% (1.1 kcal/mL) lipid emulsion and should be counted as part of the lipid calories.
- **Hepatobiliary.** Complications include elevated levels of serum transaminases and alkaline phosphatase. In addition, steatosis, steatohepatitis, lipidosis, cholestasis, fibrosis, and cirrhosis can occur. Although these abnormalities are usually benign and transient, more serious and progressive disease can develop in a small subset of patients, usually after 16 weeks of PN. Biliary complications

typically occur with PN administered for longer than 3 weeks and include acalculous cholecystitis, gallbladder sludge, and cholelithiasis.

- **Metabolic bone disease.** Osteomalacia or osteopenia may be seen with long-term (>3 months) total PN.

Refeeding Syndrome

Refeeding syndrome refers to the massive fluid and electrolytes shifts that can occur when a severely malnourished patient is initiated on nutritional support, leading to volume overload, cardiovascular collapse, and death.[2,8]

- **Electrolyte depletion** is the most dangerous complication of initial refeeding.
  - ○ With the administration of a carbohydrate load, serum levels of phosphorous, potassium, and magnesium rapidly fall, because of insulin-mediated transcellular shifts in the face of whole-body electrolyte depletion.
  - ○ Hypophosphatemia can lead to respiratory muscle paralysis and cardiovascular collapse.
  - ○ The rapid fall in potassium and magnesium levels can lead to cardiac dysfunction and arrhythmias.
- **Volume overload** (secondary to fluid administered with the nutritional supplement and insulin-mediated sodium retention) is the characteristic of refeeding syndrome and may progress quickly to congestive heart failure.
- **Cardiac abnormalities** include prolongation of the QT interval, which, combined with plasma electrolyte abnormalities, lead to an increased risk of ventricular arrhythmias and sudden cardiac death during the first week of refeeding.
- **Thiamine deficiency** can lead to acute beriberi, which, in turn, can lead to lactic acidosis, impaired sensory perception, edema, and heart failure.
- The best approach to refeeding syndrome is prevention by starting feeds slowly and aggressively supplementing potassium, magnesium, and phosphate in patients with normal renal function.[2,8]
  - ○ Initial feeding should start at 15 kcal/kg/day and can advance slowly as tolerated.
  - ○ Serum levels should be checked at least once a day.
  - ○ Thiamine should be supplemented at 50 to 100 mg/day for 3 days.
  - ○ To prevent fluid overload, initial fluid intake and sodium should be limited, and patient weight should be monitored daily. Weight gain in excess of 0.25 kg/day or 1.5 kg/week should be treated as volume overload; fluid intake should be reduced and diuretics used as necessary.
- Electrocardiogram should be obtained at baseline, and patients should be monitored on telemetry during early refeeding.

REFERENCES

1. Singh H, Watt K, Veitch R, et al. Malnutrition is prevalent in hospitalized medical patients: are housestaff identifying the malnourished patient? *Nutrition.* 2006;22:350–354.
2. Klein S. A primer of nutritional support for gastroenterologists. *Gastroenterology.* 2002; 122(6):1677–1687.
3. McClave SA, Martindale RG, Vanek VW, et al. Guidelines for the provision and assessment of nutrition support therapy in the adult critically ill patient: Society of Critical Care Medicine and American Society for Parenteral and Enteral Nutrition. *JPEN J Parenter Enteral Nutr.* 2009;33:277–316.

4. Gramlich L, Kichian K, Pinilla J, et al. Does enteral nutrition compared to parenteral nutrition result in better outcomes in critically ill adult patients? A systematic review of the literature. *Nutrition.* 2004;20(10):843–848.
5. Kirby DF, Delegge MH, Fleming CR. AGA technical review on tube feeding for enteral nutrition. *Gastroenterology.* 1995;108:1282–1301.
6. Koretz RL, Lipman TO, Klein S. AGA technical review on parenteral nutrition. *Gastroenterology.* 2001;121:970–1001.
7. MacFie J. Enteral versus parenteral nutrition. *Br J Surg.* 2000;87(9):1121–1122.
8. Kraft DM, Btaiche IF, Sacks GS. Review of the refeeding syndrome. *Nutr Clin Pract.* 2005;20:625–633.

Esophageal Disorders

12

Jonathan Seccombe and C. Prakash Gyawali

GASTROESOPHAGEAL REFLUX DISEASE

GENERAL PRINCIPLES

Definition

- The Montreal consensus defines gastroesophageal reflux disease (GERD) as "a condition which develops when the reflux of stomach contents causes troublesome symptoms and/or complications."
- Symptoms are "troublesome" if they are frequent and have an adverse affect on a patient's well-being.[1]

Epidemiology

- The true prevalence of GERD is difficult to ascertain because clinical diagnosis is relatively subjective, and not all patients with GERD undergo confirmatory testing.
- Various studies have estimated the prevalence of patients in the Western world with GERD to be as high as 20%, with 30% to 40% of the population reporting at least occasional symptoms consistent with GERD.[2]

Pathophysiology

- Several mechanisms underlie abnormal reflux, all of which result in the failure of the gastroesophageal junction to prevent gastric contents from entering the esophagus.
- The gastroesophageal junction is composed of the lower esophageal sphincter (LES), the crural diaphragm, and the phrenoesophageal ligament.
- Under most circumstances, GERD is related to transient, inappropriate LES relaxations. Less frequently, the gastroesophageal junction may be mechanically compromised, with decreased LES resting tone, a hiatus hernia, or both.
- Regardless of the mechanism, the acid and enzymes present in gastric contents directly injure the lining of the esophagus. Significant mucosal damage can occur when the esophagus is exposed to a pH value <4 for a prolonged period of time, because the esophageal mucosa does not have protective mechanisms against acid and pepsin as in the stomach.[3]

Risk Factors

- Alcohol intake
- Caffeine intake
- Obesity
- Smoking

- Impaired esophageal peristalsis
- Impaired salivation
- Poor gastric emptying
- Hypersecretion of gastric acid (as seen in Zollinger–Ellison syndrome)

DIAGNOSIS

Clinical Presentation

- The evaluation of GERD has three important aspects:
  - **Any "alarm symptoms" should be elicited.** These include dysphagia, weight loss, occult or overt gastrointestinal bleeding, symptoms lasting more than 5 years, symptoms unresponsive to proton pump inhibitors (PPI), and age more than 45 years.[3] Alarm symptoms indicate the need for invasive investigation, typically with upper endoscopy.
  - **The severity of GERD should be assessed.**
  - **Cardiac diseases should be excluded,** especially when chest pain is a presenting symptom.

History

- The duration, frequency, and severity of heartburn should be determined.
- Patients with GERD commonly report an "acidic" taste in the mouth and nocturnal wheezing or coughing.
- Other symptoms that may suggest GERD include hoarseness, chronic sore throat, or apnea.
- Behaviors that increase reflux should be sought, including smoking, caffeine use, large meals, and recumbency after eating.
- The presence of "alarm symptoms" should be determined.

Physical Examination

- The physical examination should include an assessment of body habitus and the evaluation of the stool for occult blood.

Diagnostic Testing

- Many clinicians advocate an **empiric trial of a PPI orally** as the initial step in suspected GERD. A symptomatic response to PPI confers a high degree of certainty of the diagnosis of GERD.
- In the presence of alarm symptoms, uncertainty of diagnosis, or inadequate response to PPI, further workup is necessary.

Laboratories

- A **complete blood count** (CBC) may reveal a microcytic anemia if bleeding occurs from esophagitis, cancer, or an erosion.

Imaging

- Barium swallow is a low-yield examination in GERD. A barium swallow is not indicated for the diagnosis of GERD. Barium studies are best used for characterization of anatomic relationships at the gastroesophageal junction prior to antireflux surgery, especially for evaluating hiatus hernias and their relationship to the gastroesophageal junction and the diaphragmatic hiatus; other uses could include better definition of tight strictures, or detection of subtle strictures where a barium pill swallow may have value.

Diagnostic Procedures

- The sensitivity of endoscopy as a diagnostic test for GERD is low, as the likelihood of finding visible esophagitis is only around 50% in treatment-naïve patients. The likelihood of esophagitis is extremely low when patients have already received PPI therapy.
- **Esophageal pH studies** involve measurement of intraluminal esophageal pH over a 24- or 48-hour period.
  - Catheter-based pH studies consist of placement of a thin catheter through the nostril with the pH recording site 5 cm above the proximal margin of the LES. Recordings last 24 hours.
  - Wireless pH studies involve attachment of a pH capsule 6 cm above the squamocolumnar junction, which corresponds to 5 cm above the LES. Recordings can last 48 hours or longer.
  - Catheter-based pH-impedance studies are now available, which can detect both acidic and nonacidic reflux events.
  - Generally, an elevated acid exposure time (pH <4 for >4–5% of the time) is considered abnormal, and suggestive of GERD.
  - Patients are asked to record their symptoms during the study. The pH recording can then be analyzed to determine whether symptoms correlate with reflux events. Simple proportions of symptoms associated with reflux events to overall symptoms reported (symptom index) can be used as a tool to record symptom reflux correlation. Statistical tests that also take the time at risk for reflux, reflux events, and reflux events without symptoms into consideration may provide more robust designation of symptom association.[4]
  - Testing is performed off PPI therapy when the diagnosis of reflux disease is in question. Adequacy of reflux control or assessment of ongoing symptoms despite adequate therapy in well diagnosed GERD patients can be best determined with a pH impedance study while on maximal PPI therapy.

TREATMENT

- The goal of treatment is to alleviate symptoms, heal esophageal damage, and prevent complications.

Medications

- **Proton pump inhibitors,** administered once daily, can heal erosive esophagitis and relieve heartburn.
  - In terms of efficacy, all PPIs are more effective than H2-blockers or motility agents in healing esophagitis.
  - The PPI can be administered twice daily with improved therapeutic benefit if once daily dosing is unsuccessful in relieving the symptoms of GERD, or if patients have severe erosive esophagitis, strictures, or ulcers.
  - Common side effects of PPI therapy include headache, diarrhea, constipation, and abdominal pain.

- **H2 receptor blockers** can be used to step down patients with minor or uncomplicated GERD, after effective symptom relief with PPI therapy. These agents are not recommended for patients with erosive esophagitis, Barrett's esophagus, strictures, or severe symptomatic GERD. If symptoms recur with the step-down approach, management will need to be stepped back up to PPI use.
  - There is no evidence that adding a nocturnal H2-blocker to twice daily PPI therapy has any lasting clinical or histopathologic benefit.[5]
- **Antacids** are the most rapidly acting agents but are not an appropriate long-term management option in patients with GERD.

Surgical Management

- Surgical management is reserved for patients with well-documented GERD who do not respond to maximal medical therapy or do not wish to remain on lifelong PPI.
- The surgical procedure most often performed is laparoscopic **Nissen fundoplication.** Partial fundoplication (Toupet, Dor) can be performed when esophageal hypomotility coexists. Roux-en-Y gastric bypass surgery is also an effective antireflux measure in obese patients.
- Surgery is as effective as properly dosed PPI with less incidence of pulmonary aspiration. However, it entails more morbidity and mortality.[6]
- Estimates suggest that 30% of patients resume PPI therapy within 5 years of undergoing antireflux surgery.[1]
- The most common complaints following surgery are an inability to belch, increase in flatulence, and increased bowel symptoms. New transit symptoms (dysphagia, regurgitation) can develop in a minority of patients; the risk seems highest when transit symptoms predate surgery.

Lifestyle/Risk Modification

- Lifestyle modification is not recommended in isolation, but rather in conjunction with pharmacologic therapy.
- Patients are encouraged to decrease consumption of alcohol, caffeine, and acidic foods that aggravate symptoms, such as onions and tomatoes.
- Patients should avoid the use of medications that lower LES tone whenever possible, such as calcium channel blockers, β-blockers, nitrates, and anticholinergic drugs.
- Other recommendations include weight loss, smoking cessation, avoidance of meals within 3 hours of bedtime, and elevation of the head end of the bed while supine.

SPECIAL CONSIDERATIONS

- The American Gastroenterological Association, in a survey of more than 1000 patients on PPI therapy for GERD, found that 38% had residual symptoms and 47% of those with residual symptoms took additional medications to control their symptoms.[5]
- **Causes of PPI failure** include
  - Incorrect medication dose timing
  - Residual pathologic acid secretion
  - Rapid PPI metabolism

  ○ Hypersecretory state
  ○ Hiatal hernia
  ○ Defective esophageal mucosal barrier
  ○ Reflux of nonacid material from the stomach or duodenum
  ○ Underlying dysmotility
  ○ Underlying eosinophilic or infectious esophagitis
- Patients who fail twice daily PPI therapy should undergo upper endoscopy; persisting symptoms on PPI constitutes an alarm symptom. Random biopsies from the proximal and distal are recommended to exclude eosinophilic esophagitis.
- If the esophagogastroduodenoscopy (EGD) is normal, pH or pH/impedance testing can define and quantitate esophageal acid exposure, and determine symptom–reflux association. Ideally, testing is performed off PPI therapy if the diagnosis of reflux disease is in question.
- If the EGD and pH/impedance testing are both normal, the patient likely does not have significant reflux disease. Alternate explanations for symptoms could include functional heartburn or chest pain.[5]

COMPLICATIONS

- Complications of long-standing or incompletely treated GERD include esophageal stricture, hemorrhage, Barrett's esophagus, and adenocarcinoma. It is important to note that these complications can occur in asymptomatic patients.
- The risk of developing esophageal adenocarcinoma in Barrett's esophagus is approximately 0.5% per year.[1] However, endoscopic monitoring of patients with chronic GERD symptoms may not necessarily reduce the risk of malignancy.[1]

ESOPHAGEAL MALIGNANCIES

GENERAL PRINCIPLES

- **Squamous cell carcinoma** and **adenocarcinoma** represent the two most common malignancies of the esophagus.
- **Barrett's esophagus** consists of replacement of normal squamous distal esophageal mucosa with intestinal type epithelium, also known as intestinal metaplasia. Dysplasia can develop within intestinal metaplasia, conferring a higher risk for adenocarcinoma compared with the general population, despite the fact that development of adenocarcinoma is relatively infrequent.

Epidemiology

- In the United States, squamous cell carcinoma is decreasing in incidence, but the risk remains elevated in African American men.[3]
- The incidence of adenocarcinoma has risen over the past 20 years.[7]
- Both diseases have a strong male predilection with a high mortality rate. Most patients have regional and distant lymph node metastases at time of diagnosis.

Pathophysiology

- **Squamous cell carcinoma**
  - This develops from carcinogenic exposure in susceptible individuals.
  - The most common locations of disease are the proximal and distal esophagus.
- **Adenocarcinoma**
  - Adenocarcinoma develops as a consequence of accumulation of genetic mutations within dysplastic intestinal metaplasia.
  - Most cases develop near the gastroesophageal junction.
- **Barrett's esophagus**
  - Defined as metaplasia of normal esophageal stratified squamous epithelium in the distal esophagus to specialized intestinal-type epithelium.
  - Barrett's esophagus occurs in approximately 10% of patients with GERD.[7]
  - Patients with Barrett's esophagus have a risk of developing esophageal adenocarcinoma that is approximately 100 times higher compared to patients without this condition.[7]

Risk Factors

- **Squamous cell carcinoma**
  - Chronic tobacco use
  - Chronic alcohol use
  - History of mediastinal or breast irradiation
  - Human papillomavirus 16 or 18 infection
  - Chronic ingestion of hot liquids
  - Achalasia
- **Adenocarcinoma**
  - Barrett's esophagus
  - GERD
  - Obesity
  - Scleroderma

DIAGNOSIS

Clinical Presentation

- A thorough history and physical should be performed.
- Patients are questioned for a history of **dysphagia** or **unintentional weight loss.**
- **Risk factors,** especially the use of tobacco or alcohol, are queried.
- The physical examination is **typically normal.** Cachexia may develop from poor nutritional intake in advanced cancer.

Diagnostic Testing

- Once malignancy is suspected, diagnostic testing must be initiated in a timely manner.

Laboratories

- Laboratory tests provide little information to aid in the diagnosis of esophageal malignancies.
- A CBC may reveal a microcytic anemia if bleeding has occurred.
- A low albumin may suggest malnutrition related to chronic dysphagia.

Imaging
- A **barium swallow** may reveal a mass in the esophageal lumen of compression from adjacent structures. However, endoscopy is generally recommended as the first diagnostic test in new onset dysphagia.
- If malignancy is diagnosed, **computed tomography (CT)** and **positron emission tomographic (PET) scanning** is often useful to evaluate for distant metastases.

Diagnostic Procedures
- **Upper endoscopy** (EGD) allows for the visualization of the esophageal lumen and biopsy of lesions suspicious for malignancy or Barrett's esophagus.
- EGD is the gold standard for diagnosis.

TREATMENT

- For both squamous cell carcinoma and adenocarcinoma of the esophagus, the standard of care with curative intent is surgery alone or in combination with radiation and chemotherapy.
- Mounting evidence suggests that adjuvant chemotherapy followed by surgery may be effective therapy.
- Severe dysphagia may be relieved with palliative beam radiation therapy or endoscopic stent placement.

MONITORING/FOLLOW-UP

- **Once** Barrett's esophagus is diagnosed, repeat endoscopic biopsies should be performed in 1 year's time. If no dysplasia is noted on histopathology at either endoscopic procedure, further surveillance can be performed in 3 years' time.
- If **low-grade dysplasia** is discovered, follow-up is recommended in 6 months. Stable low-grade dysplasia on two consecutive surveillance procedures 6 months apart can be followed up in 1- to 2-year intervals.
- If **high-grade dysplasia** is found, the patient should be referred for endoscopic ablation or esophagectomy.[7] In patients with severe surgical risks or those declining invasive therapy, surveillance can be repeated in 3-month intervals.
- A proportion of patients referred to surgery with high-grade dysplasia may have undetected adenocarcinoma.

OUTCOME/PROGNOSIS

- Five-year survival rates for both squamous cell carcinoma and adenocarcinoma of the esophagus remain poor at 10% to 15%.[3]
- However, a cure is possible with early diagnosis. This is the basis for endoscopic surveillance for high-grade dysplasia and carcinoma in situ in patients with Barrett's esophagus.

INFECTIOUS ESOPHAGITIS

GENERAL PRINCIPLES

- Infectious esophagitis is **most commonly seen in the immunosuppressed patient.**
- Fungal and viral diseases are the most common agents in this patient population.
- There are rare instances where infectious esophagitis is encountered in immunocompetent hosts.

Epidemiology

- Since the recognition of acquired immunodeficiency syndrome (AIDS) in the 1980s, the incidence of infectious esophagitis has increased, and the causal organisms have shifted over the past 20 years.
- Approximately 30% of patients with HIV infection have symptoms of infectious esophagitis during the course of their disease.[8]

Etiology

- **Fungal Esophagitis**
  - Candidiasis is the most common infectious disease of the esophagus in patients with HIV, accounting for 70% of cases.[8]
  - The most common species is *Candida albicans,* but other species of *Candida* have been implicated.
  - Other fungi, such as *Histoplasma capsulatum,* can cause esophagitis, but these infections are rare.
  - In AIDS patients that present with multiple infectious pathogens simultaneously, *Candida* is almost always one of the causal organisms.
- **Viral Esophagitis**
  - The most common viral cause of esophagitis in patients infected with HIV is cytomegalovirus (CMV). The risk of infection with CMV is low in patients with CD4 counts >100.[8]
  - Varicella zoster virus (VZV) can cause a devastating esophagitis in severely immunocompromised hosts. VZV esophagitis is rare in immunocompetent patients but can be seen in children with chicken pox or adults with herpes zoster.
  - Herpes simplex virus (HSV) is an uncommon etiology of viral esophagitis in both immunosuppressed and immunocompetent patients.
  - Other viruses, such as human papillomavirus and Epstein–Barr virus, can infect the esophagus, but are extremely rare.
- **Bacterial Esophagitis**
  - Bacterial infection of the esophagus in HIV patients is rare.
  - Causal organisms include *Mycobacterium avium* complex, *Mycobacterium tuberculosis, Nocardia, Actinomyces,* and *Lactobacillus.*
- **Idiopathic Esophagitis**
  - Idiopathic esophageal ulceration (IEU) is common in patients with a CD4 count <50.[8]
  - The etiologic agent of this disease has not been determined, although HIV itself has been implicated.

Risk Factors
- HIV or AIDS
- Ongoing treatment with chemotherapy
- Immunosuppressive therapy following organ transplantation

DIAGNOSIS

Clinical Presentation
- Clinical presentation often varies depending on the causal organism.

History
- **Candidiasis**
  - Dysphagia is the most common symptom.
  - Patients will often have thrush.
  - Odynophagia, fever, nausea, and vomiting are less common.
- **Cytomegalovirus**
  - Odynophagia and chest pain are the most common symptoms.
  - Dysphagia is uncommon.
  - Patients may also have a low-grade fever, nausea, and vomiting.
- **Herpes simplex virus**
  - Most commonly present with both dysphagia and odynophagia, as well as chest pain and fever.
- **Varicella zoster virus**
  - Presentation is similar to that of HSV.
  - The characteristic skin lesions of chickenpox in children and zoster in adults may be helpful in diagnosis.
- **Idiopathic esophageal ulceration**
  - Almost all patients with IEU present with severe odynophagia and, as a result, are malnourished and dehydrated at presentation.

Physical Examination
- The patient's vital signs may reveal fever and orthostatic hypotension from dehydration.

Diagnostic Testing

Laboratories
- An elevated **white blood cell (WBC) count** may suggest infection, although this finding is variable in patients with immunodeficiency.
- The **CD4 count** in useful in determining which causal pathogen is most likely involved in patients with AIDS (Table 12-1).

Diagnostic Procedures
- EGD is typically only recommended in Candida esophagitis if a patient fails empiric antifungal therapy or if symptoms include weight loss, dehydration, or fever.
- **EGD can distinguish between the types of esophageal infections** by gross or histologic appearance of the lesions:
  - **Candidiasis**—Multiple adherent, white or yellow, "cottage cheese" plaques are easily seen on endoscopy. Brushings or biopsies reveal yeast or budding hyphae.

TABLE 12-1	ETIOLOGY OF INFECTIOUS ESOPHAGITIS IN HIV OR AIDS
CD4 Count	Typical Organisms Involved
>200	HSV, VZV
100–200	Candida, HSV
50–100	Candida, CMV, HSV
<50	Idiopathic esophageal ulceration[10]

CMV, cytomegalovirus; HSV, herpes simplex virus; VZV, varicella zoster virus.

- CMV—Large, well-demarcated ulcers are visualized on gross examination and immunohistochemistry staining of biopsy specimens aids in the diagnosis.
- VZV—Multiple vesicles and confluent ulcers are seen on EGD. Cytology is difficult to distinguish from HSV and often requires immunohistochemistry or culture.
- HSV—Characterized by small, superficial ulcers in early disease and by diffuse esophagitis in later stages. Cytology reveals giant cells and ground-glass nuclei.
- IEU—Well-circumscribed, often large, ulcers are seen on gross examination. Biopsies are useful primarily to rule out other infectious etiologies.[9]

TREATMENT

- Treatment **focuses on eradicating the causal organism.**
- Many clinicians recommend an empiric course of fluconazole to treat *Candida* esophagitis in patients with AIDS and dysphagia, but without other symptoms.

Medications
- **Candidiasis**
  - The first-line agent is fluconazole 200 mg loading dose followed by 100 mg daily for 5 to 10 days.[9]
  - In patients with azole-resistant *Candida,* the oral dose of fluconazole may be increased, or treatment with intravenous (IV) amphotericin can be initiated.
  - Severe, refractory cases may not improve until treatment of HIV is undertaken to raise the CD4 count.
- **Cytomegalovirus**
  - First line therapy is IV ganciclovir 5 mg/kg q12h if the patient is not pancytopenic.
  - Alternate therapy consists of IV foscarnet 60 mg/kg q8h.
  - Regardless of the regimen, treatment continues until healing occurs, usually up to 1 month.
  - Approximately 30% of patients relapse.[10]

- **Herpes simplex virus**
  - ○ First-line therapy is acyclovir 5 mg/kg IV q8h for 7 to 14 days or 400 mg by mouth 5 times a day for 14 to 21 days.[9]
  - ○ Other effective agents include famciclovir, valacyclovir, and ganciclovir.
- **Varicella zoster virus**
  - ○ First line therapy is acyclovir 5 mg/kg IV q8h for 7 to 14 days.[9]
- **Idiopathic esophageal ulceration**
  - ○ The mainstay of treatment for idiopathic esophageal ulceration is corticosteroids.
  - ○ If the patient cannot tolerate PO intake, then IV formulations are used.
  - ○ Given that corticosteroids predispose patients to *Candida* infection, many clinicians prescribe fluconazole twice weekly for prophylaxis.
  - ○ Thalidomide can be used in refractory cases.

SPECIAL CONSIDERATIONS

- Many of these diseases have high recurrence rates and warrant **prophylaxis.**
  - ○ Primary prophylaxis of *Candida* is not recommended. However, secondary prophylaxis with fluconazole 100 mg weekly is recommended in patients with multiple recurrences.
  - ○ Although primary prophylaxis of CMV is recommended in patients with CD4 < 100, there is no evidence that it decreases the incidence of gastrointestinal disease.
  - ○ Primary prophylaxis for HSV is not recommended. However, secondary prophylaxis with acyclovir 600 mg daily by mouth is recommended in patients with a history of recurrent disease.[10]
  - ○ Thalidomide can be used in refractory cases.

EOSINOPHILIC ESOPHAGITIS

GENERAL PRINCIPLES

- During the last few decades, there has been a sharp increase in the number of patients with esophageal eosinophilia who were thought to have GERD but did not respond to traditional medical or surgical management.
- A unique disease termed **eosinophilic esophagitis** is identified in many of these patients.

Definition

- Although eosinophilic infiltration of the esophagus can be seen secondarily in association with other conditions such as GERD, eosinophilic esophagitis is now recognized as a primary diagnosis.
- Eosinophilic esophagitis is a clinicopathologic disease characterized by
  - ○ Symptoms of food impaction and dyphagia in adults, and feeding intolerance or GERD in children.
  - ○ More than 15 eosinophils/high power field on pathologic examination.
  - ○ Exclusion of other disorders with similar clinical or pathologic findings, especially GERD.[11]

Epidemiology

- For unclear reasons, there seems to be an increasing incidence of eosinophilic esophagitis that is not solely accounted for by increasing recognition.
- Disease occurs in all age groups but symptoms usually appear either in early childhood, adolescence, or before the fourth decade of life.[12] Males comprise 70% of cases.[13]

Pathophysiology

- The pathogenesis of eosinophilic esophagitis is unknown.
- There is some thought that the disease process originates from an immune-mediated response to a swallowed allergen.[13]
- Once eosinophils have infiltrated the esophageal mucosa, their presence appears to trigger a self-sustaining cascade of inflammatory mediators.

Risk Factors

- There seems to be an increased incidence of eosinophilic esophagitis in pediatric patients with a history of asthma, allergic rhinitis, eczema, and food or environmental allergies. This association has not been fully studied in the adult population.
- There is also a reported association of eosinophilic esophagitis in adults with eosinophilic gastroenteritis and peripheral eosinophilia.

DIAGNOSIS

Clinical Presentation

- A thorough history and physical examination should be performed.

History

- Questions regarding the risk factors listed above should be elicited.
- The most common presenting symptoms are dysphagia, heartburn, and chest pain.
- Less common presenting symptoms include a history of food impaction or symptoms consistent with esophageal dysmotility.
- Patients may have a diagnosis of GERD in the past but have failed high-dose PPI.

Physical Examination

- No physical examination findings are specific to or indicative of this diagnosis.

Diagnostic Criteria

- Generally speaking, the diagnosis is most often made on the basis of the presence of characteristic clinical features, the presence of eosinophils on biopsy, and exclusion of other possible diagnoses (e.g., GERD, parasitic and fungal infections, Crohn's disease, allergic vasculitis, and other connective tissue diseases).

Differential Diagnosis

- The differential diagnosis for esophageal eosinophilia includes:
  - GERD
  - Eosinophilic esophagitis

- ○ Eosinophilic gastroenteritis
- ○ Crohn's disease
- ○ Connective tissue disease
- ○ Hypereosinophilic syndrome
- ○ Infection
- ○ Drug hypersensitivity response[11]

Diagnostic Testing

- Typically, a thorough history and physical is not enough to make a definitive diagnosis and further evaluation is warranted.

Laboratories

- A **CBC** can be performed to evaluate for peripheral eosinophilia, although this phenomenon is more frequently seen in the pediatric population.[14]

Imaging

- A **barium swallow** may add further data regarding a patient's anatomy and assessing for dominant strictures, but is not required in the routine management of this disease.

Diagnostic Procedures

- **EGD with biopsies** along the length of the esophagus should be performed to confirm the diagnosis of eosinophilic esophagitis.
  - ○ Gross mucosal abnormalities include longitudinal furrowing, friability, edema, longitudinal shearing, whitish exudates, raised white specks, "crepe paper mucosa," narrow caliber esophagus, rings, felinization, and transient or fixed rings.[11]
  - ○ The esophageal mucosa is grossly abnormal by endoscopy in more than half of patients.
  - ○ Biopsy specimens should be obtained regardless of the gross appearance of the esophageal mucosa. In a study of 381 children with eosinophilic esophagitis, 30% had a grossly normal esophagus.[11]
  - ○ Biopsies should be obtained in the stomach and duodenum to determine whether the disease is confined to the esophagus or is a manifestation of another process, such as eosinophilic gastroenteritis or inflammatory bowel disease.
- Patients will have normal pH monitoring of the distal esophagus in contrast to GERD.
- Some physicians have suggested **allergen skin testing** in order to avoid potential precipitating foods or allergens.

TREATMENT

- Currently, there is no universally accepted treatment regimen for this disease.

Medications

- Medications are the mainstay of treatment for eosinophilic esophagitis.

First Line

- Currently, the most commonly accepted course of treatment is **topical corticosteroids.**

- One of the primary studies supporting the use of topical steroids in this manner involved the use of fluticasone.
- Patients were instructed to swallow rather than inhale the medication.
- Relief of dysphagia was seen in all study participants within the initial week of treatment.[14]

Second Line

- **Systemic corticosteroids** have been shown to have significant benefit in pediatric patients.
- However, symptoms recur quickly on cessation and, given the deleterious side effects of long-term systemic corticosteroid use, this remains a poor treatment option.
- Systemic steroids are an option when urgent symptom relief is required (severe dysphagia, dehydration, weight loss, stricture, etc.).

Third Line

- A humanized anti–IL-5 antibody, **mepolizumab,** has been studied over the past few years and preliminary results show that it is effective in improving the clinical and pathologic disease in patients with eosinophilic esophagitis.[13]
- This medication may replace those listed above if future studies demonstrate its safety and efficacy in adults and children.

Lifestyle/Risk Modification

- **Avoidance of known food and environmental allergens** may provide relief in patients with eosinophilic esophagitis.
- In one study, 26 of 35 patients showed significant improvement clinically and histologically after initiating a diet free of the 6 most common allergenic foods (dairy, eggs, wheat, soy, peanuts, fish/shellfish).[11]
- **Elemental, amino acid–based formulas** have been shown to be extremely effective in the pediatric population but usually have to be administered by gastrostomy or nasogastric tubes and are quite costly.

COMPLICATIONS

- Chronic inflammation from eosinophilic esophagitis can lead to proximal esophageal strictures as well as mucosal rings, esophageal ulceration, and esophageal polyps.
- Some patients with significant dysphagia and strictures require esophageal dilation to relieve symptoms.
- While there is a risk of perforation, this procedure is relatively safe and the dysphagia often resolves for several months.

OUTCOME/PROGNOSIS

- The prognosis of eosinophilic esophagitis is not well described although the consensus is that it does not appear to limit life expectancy.[11]
- Esophageal metaplasia or malignancy has not been reported in patients with eosinophilic esophagitis, even in adults with advanced disease.[11]

ESOPHAGEAL STRICTURES

GENERAL PRINCIPLES

- Esophageal strictures often arise as complications of other disease processes.
- Any type of chronic inflammation can lead to esophageal strictures.

Etiology

- **Peptic strictures**
  - Peptic strictures are relatively common, occurring in approximately 10% of patients with GERD.[15]
  - Stricturing occurs typically in the distal esophagus, often just proximal to the squamocolumnar junction.
- **Schatzki's rings**
  - This process often occurs in the distal esophagus, at the squamocolumnar junction. By definition, Schatzki's rings have squamous mucosa on the proximal aspect, and gastric columnar mucosa on the distal aspect.
  - Schatzki's rings can be associated with GERD, pill esophagitis, and hiatal hernias.[16]
  - Intermittent, nonprogressive solid food dysphagia can occur, sometimes termed "steakhouse syndrome."
- **Plummer–Vinson syndrome**
  - Characterized by anemia, upper esophageal webs, and dysphagia.
  - Typically seen in middle-aged women.[17]
- **Other causes** of esophageal narrowing
  - Caustic ingestion
  - After band ligation for varices
  - Esophageal infections
  - Repetitive vomiting
  - Esophageal neoplasms
  - Radiation therapy
  - Pill induced esophageal inflammation ("pill esophagitis")
  - Esophageal trauma (e.g., instrumentation, NG tube)
  - Crohn's disease

Risk Factors

- GERD
- History of esophageal infections
- Crohn's disease

DIAGNOSIS

Clinical Presentation

- A careful history is crucial in the assessment of dysphagia.
- In addition to helping rule out diseases other than stricture, the type of dysphagia and regurgitation can often localize the sire and involvement of disease.

History
- Key points of the history should include
  - Onset and duration of symptoms

○ Association of dysphagia with types of food
○ Description of regurgitated material if present
○ History of weight loss
○ History of GERD
○ Evaluation for other risk factors listed above

Physical Examination
- Physical signs of weight loss, dehydration, and malnutrition help to assess severity of disease.

Diagnostic Testing
- Management of suspected esophageal stricture involves several different diagnostic modalities.

Laboratories
- Laboratory studies are **generally not useful** in the workup of stricture.
- Anemia may support the diagnosis of esophageal inflammation, neoplasia, Plummer–Vinson syndrome.[17]
- A low albumin concentration may reflect nutritional deficiency.

Imaging
- **Barium swallow** is a useful test in the workup of suspected stricture, ring, or web, especially when the lesion is subtle and not recognized on an upper endoscopy.[15] Barium swallow is not recommended as the initial test in new onset dysphagia, as endoscopy provides both definitive diagnosis and therapy of strictures. If radiologic findings demonstrate a narrowing of the esophagus, dilation at endoscopy is warranted.

Diagnostic Procedures
- **EGD** permits the operator to directly visualize the stricture, web, or ring. Further, biopsies can be performed to further evaluate the etiology, and dilation allows therapy of the stricture.

TREATMENT

- **Peptic Stricture**
  ○ Aggressive acid control with high-dose proton pump inhibitor can cause regression of the stricture.
  ○ Dilation is often required, and is performed endoscopically.
  ○ Limited data exists on the benefit of stent placement for benign strictures and carries the risk of stent migration.[16] Currently, stent placement is not considered routine with benign strictures.
  ○ Occasionally, dysphagia is not relieved by maximal medical therapy, and surgery is required.
- **Schatzki's Ring**
  ○ Patients with mild disease should be advised to chew their food carefully.
  ○ Patients with more severe disease are at an increased risk for food bolus impaction and benefit from passage of an endoscopic dilator.
  ○ Refractory cases may require pneumatic dilation, electrocautery incision, or surgical repair.

    ○ All patients with Schatzki's rings should be evaluated for GERD and started on PPI therapy, if indicated.[16]

MONITORING/FOLLOW-UP

- Patients with Plummer–Vinson syndrome have an increased risk of developing squamous cell carcinoma of the esophagus.
- It is unclear whether they should undergo screening EGD.[17]

ESOPHAGEAL MOTILITY DISORDERS

GENERAL PRINCIPLES

- Motility disorders of the esophagus can involve both the striated and smooth muscle of the esophagus.
- These diseases can result in extreme morbidity for patients.

Definition
- Swallowing involves two types of muscular activity:
  - ○ It is initiated by neural impulses from the central nervous system, controlling voluntary, striated muscles of the oropharynx.
  - ○ It is completed by the involuntary contraction of the smooth muscle of the esophagus in a coordinated sequence.
- Dysfunction at either step can cause dysphagia.

Etiology
- **Striated muscle dysfunction** can be affected by:
  - ○ Cerebrovascular accident
  - ○ Myasthenia gravis
  - ○ Polymyositis
  - ○ Parkinson's disease
  - ○ Amyotrophic lateral sclerosis
- Causes of **smooth muscle failure** include:
  - ○ Invasive cancer
  - ○ Infectious (Chagas' disease)
  - ○ Neurologic (achalasia, diffuse esophageal spasm, nutcracker esophagus)
  - ○ Autoimmune (scleroderma)[18]

Pathophysiology
- In **striated muscle,** neuromuscular dysregulation results in the loss of a coordinated swallow and can lead to oropharyngeal dysphagia, regurgitation, and pulmonary aspiration.
- **Smooth muscle dysfunction** is caused by the loss of inhibitory neurons in the esophagus leading to disorganized peristalsis (mainly in the form of loss of sequencing of peristalsis, simultaneous waves, exaggerated wave amplitude, and prolonged wave duration) and increased LES tone with abnormal sphincter relaxation during swallows.

DIAGNOSIS

Clinical Presentation

- The most common symptoms of esophageal motor disorders are dysphagia and chest pain
- In contrast, patients with oropharyngeal dysphagia often present with drooling, regurgitation of food immediately after swallowing, and pulmonary aspiration.

History

- As with strictures, the **type, duration, and severity of dysphagia** are important to address with a good history.
- A **description of regurgitated contents** is useful in differentiating esophageal versus oropharyngeal causes.
- Patients with diffuse esophageal spasm (DES) or nutcracker esophagus often present with **intermittent chest pain** exacerbated by hot or cold items. Given that the chest pain sometimes radiates to other parts of the body, it is important to rule our myocardial ischemia in this population.
- The history should focus on **conditions that can cause motility disorders,** such as cerebrovascular accident, amyotrophic lateral sclerosis, and myasthenia gravis.
- A **history of travel** to Central and South American countries may warrant workup for Chagas' disease.

Physical Examination

- The physical examination should include a thorough **neurologic examination** as well as assessment of **nutritional status.**

Diagnostic Testing

- Barium swallow and esophageal manometry are very useful in diagnosing esophageal motility disorders. Well-defined motor disorders such as achalasia can also be identified on endoscopy.

Imaging

- **Barium Swallow:**
  - In patients with achalasia, barium swallow often reveals a characteristic "bird's beak" tapered distal esophagus with proximal dilatation. This appearance can also occur with neoplastic compression of the lower esophagus (pseudoachalasia).[18]
  - In patients with DES, barium swallow demonstrates the typical "corkscrew" or "rosary bead" appearance.[18]
  - Nutcracker esophagus often appears normal on barium swallow

Diagnostic Procedures

- **High-resolution manometry** utilizes pressure sensors along the length of the esophagus allowing for measurement of intraluminal pressure as a continuum along the length of the entire esophagus. This allows for the construction of colored topographic Clouse plots.[19] Disease-specific findings include the following:
  - In achalasia, esophageal manometry reveals a lack of primary peristalsis and increased LES tone. If patients have simultaneous and repetitive contractions, the disease is termed *vigorous achalasia*. High-resolution manometry has identified three types of achalasia, type I with low amplitude esophageal

body pressure compartmentalization, reflecting esophageal dilation; type II, with high amplitude pressure compartmentalization; and type III with spastic features in ≥20% sequences. All forms are associated with elevated LES postswallow residual pressures.

○ Manometry in DES reveals >20% simultaneous contractions involving the smooth muscle esophagus.

○ Nutcracker esophagus is defined by elevated distal esophageal peristaltic amplitude >180 mmHg.[18]

- **EGD**
  ○ In suspected cases of achalasia, EGD should always be performed to exclude mass lesions as a cause of pseudoachalasia.
  ○ EGD is typically normal in patients with DES or nutcracker esophagus.

TREATMENT

- Treatment regimens differ for each class of dysmotility.

Medications

- In achalasia, **endoscopic botulinum toxin injection** of the LES may temporize symptoms till more effective therapy is available, or can be used as sole therapy in elderly patients where more effective modalities are contraindicated because of comorbidities. Effective therapy requires repeated injection, as efficacy wanes after a median of 9 to 12 months.[18]
- Patients with DES and nutcracker esophagus can be treated with **nitrates** and **calcium channel blockers** for symptomatic relief. Spastic disorders have a perceptive component to symptomatology, presumably from coexistent visceral hypersensitivity, that may require **neuromodulator therapy** (e.g., low-dose tricyclic antidepressants, particularly for chest pain). Obstructive symptoms (dysphagia, regurgitation) may improve with botulinum toxin injection if abnormal LES relaxation can be demonstrated. **PPI therapy** can also be included in the regimen, if acid reflux is thought to contribute to symptoms.
- The medical treatment of scleroderma should involve aggressive acid control with high-dose PPI.

Other Nonpharmacologic Therapies

- **Endoscopic pneumatic dilation** of the LES to 30 to 40 mm disrupts the LES, and is effective in achalasia patients, often offering immediate relief. Esophageal perforation can occur in 2% to 5%, requiring emergent surgery in some instances.
- Endoscopic dilation is typically not useful in DES and nutcracker esophagus.

Surgical Management

- **Laparoscopic surgical myotomy** of the LES with partial fundoplication may offer definitive resolution of achalasia symptoms, with the added benefit of protection against reflux with the fundoplication.
- This procedure offers durable efficacy compared with medications and botulinum toxin injection.
- The choice between surgical myotomy and pneumatic dilation depends on institutional expertise.

MONITORING/FOLLOW-UP

- Patients with achalasia have an increased risk of squamous cell esophageal carcinoma (developing in 2% to 7%) and there is debate whether regular surveillance EGD should be performed.[20]

REFERENCES

1. Kahrilas PJ, Shaheen NJ, Vaezi MF, et al. AGA medical position statement on the management of gastroesophageal reflux disease. *Gastroenterology.* 2008;135:1383–1391.
2. Falk GW. Gastroesophageal reflux disease and Barrett's esophagus. *Endoscopy.* 2001; 33(2):109–118.
3. Goyal RK. Diseases of the esophagus. In: Fauci AS, Braunwald E, Isselbacher KJ, et al, eds. *Harrison's principles of internal medicine.* New York, NY: McGraw-Hill; 1998:1588–1596.
4. DiPalma JA. Management of severe gastroesophageal reflux disease. *J Clin Gastroenterol.* 2001;32(1):19–26.
5. Dellon ES, Shaheen NJ. Persistent reflux symptoms in the proton pump inhibitor era: the changing face of gastroesophageal reflux disease. *Gastroenterology.* 2010;139(1):7–13.
6. Lundell L, Miettinen P, Myrvold HE, et al. Continued follow-up of a randomized clinical study comparing antireflux surgery and omeprazole in gastroesophageal reflux disease. *J Am Coll Surg.* 2001;192:172–181.
7. Heath EI, Forastiere AA, Limburg PJ, et al. Adenocarcinoma of the esophagus: risk factors and prevention. *Oncology.* 2000;14(4):507–514.
8. Bonacini M, Young T, Laine L. The causes of esophageal symptoms in human immunodeficiency virus infection: a prospective study of 110 patients. *Arch Intern Med.* 1991;151: 1567–1572.
9. Bonacini M. Medical management of benign oesophageal disease in patients with human immunodeficiency virus infection. *Dig Liver Dis.* 2001;33(3):294–300.
10. Wilcox CM, Monkemuller KE. Diagnosis and management of esophageal disease in the acquired immunodeficiency syndrome. *South Med J.* 1998;91(11):1002–1007.
11. Furata GT, Liacouras CA, Collins MH, et al. Eosinophilic esophagitis in children and adults: a systematic review and consensus recommendations for diagnosis and treatment. *Gastroenterology.* 2007;133:1342–1363.
12. Noel RJ, Putnam PE, Rothenberg ME. Eosinophilic esophagitis. *N Engl J Med.* 2004; 351:940.
13. Furata GT, Straumann A. Review article: the pathogenesis and management of eosinophilic oesophagitis. *Aliment Pharmacol Ther.* 2006;24:173–182.
14. Straumann A, Simon HU. Eosinophilic esophagitis: escalating epidemiology? *J Allergy Clin Immunol.* 2005;115:418.
15. Shiflett DW, Gilliam JH, Wu WC, et al. Multiple esophageal webs. *Gastroenterology.* 1979; 77:556.
16. Spechler SJ. AGA technical review on treatment of patients with dysphagia caused by benign disorders of the distal esophagus. *Gastroenterology.* 1999;117(1):233–254.
17. Hoffman RM, Jaffee PE. Plummer-Vinson syndrome. *Arch Intern Med.* 1995;155:2008–2011.
18. Adler DG, Romero Y. Primary esophageal motility disorders. *Mayo Clin Proc.* 2001; 76(2):195–200.
19. Kahrilas PJ, Sifrim D. High-resolution manometry and impedance-pH/manometry: valuable tools in clinical and investigational esophagology. *Gastroenterology.* 2008;135:756–769.
20. Streitz JM, Ellis FH, Gibb SP, et al. Achalasia and squamous cell carcinoma of the esophagus: analysis of 241 patients. *Ann Thorac Surg.* 1995;59:1604–1609.

Gastric Disorders

13

Amit Patel and C. Prakash Gyawali

PEPTIC ULCER DISEASE

GENERAL PRINCIPLES

- Gastric disorders, especially peptic ulcer disease (PUD), are among the most common illnesses encountered by both internists and gastroenterologists.
- PUD accounts for a significant portion of health care expenditures and can lead to potentially life-threatening complications.

Definition

- PUD is characterized by the denudation of mucosa extending into the muscularis propria layer from exposure to gastric acid.
- Lesions <5 mm in diameter are called *erosions,* whereas lesions >5 mm in diameter are called *ulcers.*
- PUD most commonly occurs in the gastric antrum or duodenal bulb; duodenal ulcers are more common than gastric ulcers in Western countries.

Epidemiology

- PUD is a worldwide problem; the current global annual incidence rate of physician-diagnosed PUD is estimated to be ~0.1% to 0.2%.[1]
- Although the incidence of PUD has fallen since the 1950s with improved hygiene and socioeconomic conditions and decreased *Helicobacter pylori* infection rates, the number of hospital admissions for PUD-related complications does not appear to have decreased.[2]
- The mortality rate of PUD has remained stable over the past two decades and comes mostly from the four major complications of PUD—hemorrhage, perforation, penetration to adjacent organs, and gastric outlet obstruction.
- Duodenal ulcers are slightly more common in men than in women, but gastric ulcers occur with equal frequency in both genders.
- Duodenal ulcers present at a slightly younger age range than gastric ulcers: ages 25 to 55 years versus ages 40 to 70 years, respectively. This difference likely derives from the increased use of nonsteroidal anti-inflammatory drugs (NSAIDs), which are associated primarily with gastric ulcers, especially in the elderly population.

Etiology

- Table 13-1 lists etiologies of peptic ulcers. *H. pylori*–associated PUD and NSAID-associated PUD account for >90% of PUDs.
- In patients in whom *H. pylori,* NSAID use, Crohn's disease, and Zollinger-Ellison syndrome have been ruled out, no apparent etiology is found in as many as 50% of cases, termed idiopathic PUD.[3] Many of these could still represent partially treated *H. pylori* and NSAID etiologies that have not been

TABLE 13-1 ETIOLOGY OF PEPTIC ULCERS

Most Common

Helicobacter pylori–associated
NSAID-associated

Other

Idiopathic
Zollinger-Ellison syndrome
Gastroduodenal Crohn's disease
Viral infection
Chemotherapy
Radiation therapy
Vascular insufficiency

NSAID, nonsteroidal anti-inflammatory drug.

determined from routine clinical evaluation and investigation. Other factors include increased acid output and rapid gastric emptying, which have been associated with idiopathic PUD.

- *Helicobacter pylori*–associated PUD
  - *H. pylori* is a gram-negative bacillus that lives in the mucous layer overlying gastric epithelium, leading to inflammation. It can also be found within epithelial cells and attached to mucous cells.
  - *H. pylori* infection is associated with lower socioeconomic status and is typically acquired in childhood.[4]
  - *H. pylori* infection has been traditionally associated with up to 90% of duodenal ulcers and 70% to 90% of gastric ulcers. The incidence of *H. pylori* infection in PUD is decreasing in the United States. Recent studies have shown that 20% to 50% of ulcers in the United States are not associated with *H. pylori,* though the proportion of *H. pylori*–negative ulcers elsewhere in the world remains much lower.[3]
  - In the case of duodenal ulcers, *H. pylori* is thought to infect the non–acid-secreting gastric antrum or ectopic gastric mucosa in the duodenum, thus stimulating gastrin release and leading to increased acid production from the more proximal acid-secreting fundic mucosa (relatively spared from inflammation). This increased gastric acid secretion can result in an increased duodenal acid load and ulceration.[5]
  - Conversely, *H. pylori* infection that damages the acid-producing mucosa of the stomach can lead to hypochlorhydria or achlorhydria, and subsequent gastric ulceration.
  - Therefore, gastric ulcers are typically associated with normal or reduced levels of acid secretion, whereas duodenal ulcers are generally characterized by increased levels of acid secretion.
  - Although it does not appear to have a predominant virulence factor, the ability of *H. pylori* to induce gastritis likely stems from a combination of factors.[6]
    - The organism secretes a urease enzyme that breaks down urea in the stomach to produce ammonia, which neutralizes the acidic gastric environment and thereby protects the bacteria.

- This urease activity provides the basis for many of the laboratory tests used to evaluate for *H. pylori* infection.
- *H. pylori* infection is also thought to increase the permeability of the gastric mucous layer to pepsin and acid.
- Finally, the bacterium produces a cytotoxin (CagA) that may also contribute to its pathogenicity.
  - *H. pylori* is a risk factor for gastric adenocarcinoma (which develops in 0.1% to 3% of infected patients) and gastric mucosa–associated lymphoid tissue (MALT) lymphoma (in <0.01% of infected patients).
- **NSAID-associated PUD**
  - NSAID use has been associated with 30% to 75% of *H. pylori*–negative ulcers and 15% of *H. pylori*–positive ulcers. It is the second most common cause of PUD after *H. pylori* infection.
  - The rate of serious gastrointestinal (GI) complications in patients taking long-term NSAIDs is 7.3 per 1000 patients per year for osteoarthritis and 13 per 1000 patients per year for rheumatoid arthritis.[7]
  - NSAIDs have a direct toxic effect from acidic composition and from the ability to decrease hydrophobicity of gastric mucus, allowing epithelial injury by acid and pepsin.
  - The predominant mechanism of NSAID-associated PUD is inhibition of endogenous prostaglandin synthesis. Therefore, enteric-coated, parenteral, or rectal NSAIDs present the same risk for ulcers as their oral counterparts. Administration of NSAIDs with food does not decrease ulcer risk.
  - Suppression of prostaglandin synthesis is mediated through inhibition of the cyclooxygenase (COX)-1 enzyme, a "housekeeping" enzyme that maintains integrity of the gastric mucosa where it is constitutively expressed.
  - Inhibition of prostaglandin synthesis decreases mucous production, bicarbonate secretion, mucosal perfusion, epithelial proliferation, and mucosal resistance to injury. These changes impair the integrity of the mucosa, allowing damage by harmful factors such as NSAIDs, pepsin, bile salts, and acid.
  - COX-2–selective NSAIDs are less likely to cause GI complications because COX-2 enzyme, which mediates NSAID anti-inflammatory effects, is not expressed in gastric mucosa.[7]
  - NSAID use can cause a spectrum of lesions ranging from superficial erosions to ulcers that bleed or perforate. These affect any area of the stomach, but the gastric antrum is most frequently involved. Endoscopic evidence of mucosal damage has been found in up to two-thirds of patients who use NSAIDs and frank ulceration has been found in 10% to 25%.
  - Superficial lesions include petechiae and erosions, likely from direct toxic effects of NSAIDs and may occur within hours of NSAID administration. These are typically confined to the mucosa where they do not cause complications.
  - NSAID-associated ulcers can be complicated by hemorrhage and perforation. These complications occur with similar frequency among duodenal and gastric ulcers. Risk of hemorrhage is highest in the early treatment period in first-time users but can occur at any time during the course of treatment.
  - Platelet dysfunction may contribute to the tendency toward hemorrhage, especially with acetylsalicylic acid (ASA).

- **Zollinger-Ellison syndrome**
  - ○ Uncontrolled acid hypersecretion in the setting of gastrin-producing endocrine tumors (gastrinoma) of the pancreas or duodenum, termed Zollinger-Ellison syndrome, accounts for only 0.1% of all peptic ulcers. The syndrome includes multiple peptic ulcers, severe erosive esophagitis, and secretory diarrhea.
  - ○ The increased gastrin levels cause histamine release from enterochromaffin-like cells in the gastric mucosa. The histamine then binds to histamine receptors on parietal cells, causing hypersecretion of hydrochloric acid. Peptic ulcers develop, as the normal defense mechanisms against acid are overwhelmed by the high gastric acid output.
  - ○ Ulcers typically form in the duodenal bulb but may also be seen in the distal duodenum and jejunum, and multiple ulcers are commonly seen.
  - ○ Diarrhea may also develop because of gastric acid–mediated damage to the small bowel mucosa resulting in net intestinal secretion. The excessive volume of gastric secretion may be contributory.
  - ○ The diagnosis should be suspected in any patient with multiple ulcers in unusual locations or in patients with a family history suggestive of multiple endocrine neoplasia type I.
  - ○ An elevated gastrin level suggests the diagnosis in patients who make gastric acid. This can be assessed by aspirating a small volume of gastric secretions through a nasogastric tube or at endoscopy and testing the pH using litmus paper. A secretin stimulation test or formal fasting gastric acid output analysis help confirm the diagnosis.

Pathophysiology

- Although the pathophysiology of PUD is not entirely understood, it is believed to arise from an imbalance between gastric mucosal protective factors (provided in part by prostaglandins) and destructive influences that include *H. pylori,* pepsin, NSAIDs, bile salts, and acid.

Risk Factors

- Table 13-2 displays a list of known risk factors associated with PUD. The two major risk factors for PUD are *H. pylori* infection and NSAID use.
- Risk factors for the development of NSAID-associated PUD include concomitant corticosteroid use, anticoagulants, and older age (Table 13-3). Corticosteroids alone are not a risk factor for PUD.
- The role of *H. pylori* infection in NSAID-associated PUD remains incompletely defined. It is generally believed, however, that *H. pylori* and NSAIDs may act synergistically to induce PUD.[8]

TABLE 13-2	RISK FACTORS FOR PEPTIC ULCER DISEASE	
Infection with *Helicobacter pylori*	Having a first-degree relative with peptic ulcer disease
NSAID use	Emigration from a developing nation
Smoking	African American or Hispanic ethnicity

NSAID, nonsteroidal anti-inflammatory drug.

TABLE 13-3	RISK FACTORS FOR NSAID-ASSOCIATED PEPTIC ULCER DISEASE
Increasing NSAID dose	Prior peptic ulcer disease
Concomitant bisphosphonate use	Poor overall health
Concomitant anticoagulant use	Older age
Concomitant corticosteroid use	Female gender

NSAID, nonsteroidal anti-inflammatory drug.

DIAGNOSIS

- In patients who present with symptoms that are suggestive of PUD, the diagnostic approach should attempt both to locate the anatomic abnormality and to explore its cause (often beginning with determining whether *H. pylori* infection is present).

Clinical Presentation

History

- History alone is unreliable in diagnosing PUD. Approximately two-thirds of patients who report dyspepsia have nonulcer or functional dyspepsia, and up to 40% of patients with active PUD have no abdominal pain, or "silent ulcers".[9]
- The classic symptom complex of a patient with a **gastric ulcer** includes pain that occurs 5 to 15 minutes after oral intake and is relieved with fasting. For this reason, patients with gastric ulcers may learn to avoid food and thus lose weight.
- In contrast, patients with **duodenal ulceration** may have pain that occurs when acid is secreted in the absence of a food buffer and is temporarily relieved with eating but returns 1 to 2 hours later. However, this temporal relationship between pain and meals can be nonspecific, and the relief afforded by food can also be found in nonulcer dyspepsia.
- Because of the potential for duodenal ulcers to result in right upper quadrant pain, the presentation may mimic that of acute cholecystitis or a biliary colic.
- Perforation of a peptic ulcer may be heralded by an acute change in symptoms and sudden onset of severe diffuse abdominal pain.
- Chronic PUD can lead to scarring and gastric outlet obstruction, when nausea, vomiting, or weight loss may be prominent.
- Patients should be carefully questioned about NSAID and ASA use, including over-the-counter NSAIDS, even if patients have discontinued NSAID use.
- NSAID-associated ulcers are more likely than other forms of peptic ulcers to be painless and present initially with bleeding rather than dyspepsia.

Physical Examination

- In the absence of complicated PUD, the physical examination is not very helpful. Patients may have epigastric tenderness; however, the sensitivity (~65%) and specificity (~30%) of epigastric tenderness on palpation are very limited.[9]
- Patients with perforated peptic ulcers usually exhibit signs of peritonitis.
- Patients with bleeding ulcers may have fecal occult blood, melena, or hematemesis. If patients are hemodynamically compromised, they may be tachycardic or hypotensive.
- Bleeding may be the presenting sign in up to 15% of PUD cases.[10]

TABLE 13-4   DIFFERENTIAL DIAGNOSIS FOR UPPER ABDOMINAL PAIN

Peptic ulcer disease	Functional dyspepsia
Carbohydrate malabsorption	Granulomatous diseases
Biliary pain	Crohn's disease
Malignancy (gastric, esophageal, pancreatic)	Hepatoma
Gastroparesis	Medications
Electrolytes (hypercalcemia, hyperkalemia)	Ischemic bowel disease
Chronic abdominal wall pain	Gastroesophageal reflux disease
Parasites (giardia, strongyloides)	Systemic (diabetes mellitus, connective tissue diseases)

Differential Diagnosis

- Table 13-4 lists a differential diagnosis for upper abdominal pain.
- Of note, it is difficult to differentiate functional or nonulcer dyspepsia from PUD on the basis of clinical examination. There are no diagnostic tests for functional dyspepsia, rendering it a diagnosis of exclusion.
- Many medications can cause dyspeptic symptoms, including NSAIDs (with or without ulceration), iron, theophylline, and digitalis.
- Granulomatous diseases, including sarcoidosis, eosinophilic granuloma, and Wegener's granulomatosis, may also present, albeit rarely, with dyspeptic symptoms.

Diagnostic Testing

Laboratories

- Routine laboratory studies are usually unremarkable. **Complete blood cell count** testing may show iron-deficiency anemia from chronic fecal occult blood loss or anemia from acute blood loss.
- Patients in whom PUD is established or suspected should be tested for *H. pylori* infection, as it represents the major risk factor for PUD and can represent a contributing factor in ulcers with other causes, such as NSAID use.
  - **Serologic tests for IgG antibodies to *H. pylori***
    - Serology diagnoses *H. pylori* infection rather than the presence of PUD per se.
    - Because of high sensitivity, serologic tests are more accurate in areas with a high prevalence of *H. pylori.*
    - The most common serologic tests are laboratory-based enzyme-linked immunosorbent assay (ELISA) tests; the accuracy of ELISA testing can extend up to 95%.
    - Less commonly used serology tests are based on immunochromatography and Western blot.
    - Serologic testing is simple and inexpensive, but antibodies to *H. pylori* can remain positive for 1 to 2 years after eradication of the infection, so it is difficult to evaluate *H. pylori* infection with serology after treatment.[10]
  - **Stool antigen testing** can be more accurate than serology and can detect *H. pylori* only 1 week after discontinuation of proton pump inhibitor (PPI) therapy.

○ **Urease assays** test for the presence of the urease enzyme, which is produced in high amounts by *H. pylori*.

  ■ These tests include noninvasive urea breath testing as well as biopsy urease tests.

  ■ They can be used to diagnose active infection and to confirm eradication of infection.

  ■ False-negative results can occur in the setting of treatment with PPI, histamine 2 (H_2)-receptor blockers, antibiotics, or bismuth-containing medications. Therefore, PPI should be held for 7 to 14 days before testing.

  ■ In addition, urease breath testing to confirm eradication of *H. pylori* infection should be held until at least 4 to 6 weeks after completing treatment.

  ■ The two forms of the urea breath test are the ^{14}C-urea breath test and the ^{13}C-urea breath test.

  ■ These two breath tests use urea that has been labeled with a radioactive (^{14}C) or nonradioactive (^{13}C) isotope.

  ■ Labeled urea is given orally to the patient, and in the presence of urease, the urea is broken down into ammonia and labeled CO_2. After absorption of CO_2 into the circulation, it is expelled into the breath, and $^{13}CO_2$ can be detected by mass spectroscopy and $^{14}CO_2$ by scintillation counting.

  ■ Radioactive urea breath testing is contraindicated in pregnant women and in children.

  ■ The theoretical advantage of urea breath testing over biopsy urease tests is a decreased number of false-negative tests deriving from sampling error.

  ■ Biopsy urease tests may be obtained via endoscopy and are discussed later.

• **Culture** is not generally performed because it is expensive, time-consuming, and difficult. Culture should not be considered unless a patient does not respond to eradication treatment and there is concern about antibiotic resistance.

• **Histology** may be obtained via endoscopy and is discussed later.

• Measurement of **serum gastrin levels** and/or **secretin stimulation testing** may be performed if Zollinger-Ellison syndrome is suspected.

Imaging

• Given the advantages of endoscopy, **upper GI radiography** has a limited role in the diagnosis of PUD.

• A radiographic diagnosis of PUD requires demonstration of barium within an ulcer niche, but the sensitivity of barium radiography for detecting PUD depends on the radiologist, and radiography can miss up to half of all duodenal ulcers.[11]

Diagnostic Procedures

• **Upper endoscopy** (esophagogastroduodenoscopy, or EGD) is the most accurate diagnostic test for PUD.

• Decisions regarding EGD for patients with symptoms of PUD should be based on patient symptoms and the risk of gastric cancer. EGD should be performed in patients who have signs or symptoms worrisome for gastric cancer ("alarm symptoms"), including anorexia, dysphagia, epigastric mass, severe vomiting, weight loss, anemia, advanced age, or family history of upper GI cancer.

• Patients with significant dyspepsia, acute GI bleeding, fecal occult blood, or abdominal pain of unclear etiology should also undergo EGD.

• In patients with a high suspicion of PUD, consideration may be given to performing noninvasive testing, such as serology or urease breath testing without endoscopy, especially if the patient is young and otherwise healthy, as these noninvasive tests are more cost-effective than EGD.

- **Biopsy urease testing** is the best endoscopic method of diagnosing *H. pylori* infection.
  - Biopsy urease tests include the CLOtest, PyloriTek, and Hp-fast.
  - Most of these tests involve a pH-sensitive dye that changes color because of an increase in pH secondary to the production of ammonia from urea.
  - In addition to false-negative results in the setting of prior treatment with PPI, false-negative results can also occur if blood from recent or active bleeding is present.
  - If it is not possible to hold PPI before testing, biopsy samples should be taken from both the antrum and the fundus to increase the likelihood of a positive result.
- **Endoscopic biopsies** are indicated in gastric ulcers because of the risk of malignancy, or in cases of PUD in which urease testing might be falsely negative (i.e., in the setting of PPI use before endoscopy).
- In the case of gastric ulcers, biopsy samples should be obtained from around the ulcer crater and edges to rule out malignancy, but they should also be obtained from other areas of the stomach to test for *H. pylori* infection.
- Biopsy may be less sensitive in the setting of bleeding ulcers, so other sampling-independent testing, such as serology, should be performed.
- Patients with a gastric ulcer should undergo follow-up EGD at 8 to 12 weeks to document ulcer healing and exclude malignancy in most instances, as follow-up endoscopy improves survival.[12]
- Duodenal ulcers do not require biopsy or repeat EGD because of the extremely low risk of malignancy.

TREATMENT

Medications

- Medications used to treat PUD include antisecretory drugs and mucosal protectants such as sucralfate and prostaglandin analogues.
- Antisecretory drugs include H_2-receptor antagonists, and PPI.
  - **H_2-receptor antagonists**
    - H_2-receptor blockers inhibit acid secretion by blocking the binding of histamine to its receptor on the parietal cell. They inhibit both basal and food-induced acid secretion.
    - The H_2-receptor blockers available in the United States include cimetidine, famotidine, nizatidine, and ranitidine.
    - This class of medications is well tolerated, although doses should be adjusted in patients with renal insufficiency. They have largely been replaced by PPIs.
    - In general, when used in the treatment of PUD, H_2-receptor blockers are most effective when administered between dinner and bedtime.
  - **Proton pump inhibitors**
    - These medications are prodrugs that, when activated by acid, bind to and inhibit the parietal cell H^+/K^+ adenosine triphosphatase (ATPase).
    - Because they require acid for activation, they are most effectively taken before or with a meal and in the absence of other antisecretory drugs.
    - PPIs pose a theoretical risk of inducing enterochromaffin-like cell hyperplasia and carcinoid tumors, but these medications have been used safely

TABLE 13-5	TREATMENT REGIMENS FOR *HELICOBACTER PYLORI* ERADICATION

PPI PO BID; amoxicillin, 1000 mg PO BID; clarithromycin, 500 mg PO BID

PPI PO BID; amoxicillin, 1000 mg; metronidazole 500 mg PO BID

PPI PO BID; bismuth subsalicylate, 525 mg PO QID; metronidazole, 500 mg PO QID; tetracycline, 250 mg PO QID

PPI PO BID; metronidazole 500 mg PO TID; bismuth subsalicylate two tablets TID or QID; tetracycline 500 mg PO TID

Ranitidine bismuth citrate, 400 mg PO BID for 28 days; clarithromycin, 500 mg PO BID for 14 days

PPI, proton pump inhibitor.

With the exception of ranitidine bismuth citrate, treatment duration is 14 days.

in the United States for the past decade without a notable increase in the incidence of carcinoid tumors.

- **Misoprostol**
  - Misoprostol is a prostaglandin analogue.
  - It is approved by the US Food and Drug Administration for prophylaxis of NSAID-induced peptic ulcers.
  - Because of its mechanism of action, misoprostol can cause diarrhea or spontaneous abortion.
- **Treatment of *Helicobacter pylori*–associated PUD**
  - Treatment requires both antisecretory and antibiotic therapy, as the **eradication of *H. pylori* infection with antibiotics** significantly lowers the 12-month ulcer recurrence rate from upward of 60% in patients treated with antisecretory therapy alone to <5%.[13]
  - *H. pylori*–associated ulcers may heal spontaneously but frequently recur if the infection is not eradicated.
  - Many regimens have been developed for *H. pylori* eradication, mostly through trial and error, and accepted treatment regimens are listed in Table 13-5. Some regimens are relatively inexpensive but require dosing four times daily, which may decrease compliance.
  - Effective regimens typically involve more than one antibiotic to maximize the likelihood of eradication and prevent the spread of antimicrobial resistance; monotherapy is inadequate. Amoxicillin and clarithromycin are pH-dependent antibiotics that work more effectively in combination with antisecretory drugs. If this "triple therapy" fails, a salvage course of bismuth-containing "quadruple therapy" can eradicate *H. pylori* infection in an additional three-fourths of patients. Second-line antimicrobials, such as levofloxacin, rifabutin, and furazolidone, are often utilized next or in the case of penicillin allergies.
  - The success rates of these recommended regimens for eradicating *H. pylori* infection appear to have decreased to 70% to 85% with increasing antibiotic resistance.[14] Treatment failure may be secondary to noncompliance or antibiotic resistance, which occurs most commonly with metronidazole in the United States.
  - With regard to the course of **antisecretory medications,** duodenal ulcers should be treated for 4 weeks and gastric ulcers should be treated for 8 weeks. In

cases with ulcers >1 cm, complicated PUD, unsuccessful *H. pylori* eradication, or *H. pylori*–negative PUD, it is reasonable to treat with a longer course of antisecretory therapy. Otherwise, maintenance antisecretory therapy after treatment of *H. pylori* infection is not cost-effective and is generally unnecessary.

○ In patients with uncomplicated PUD, confirmation of eradication is not required because recurrence would most likely also be uncomplicated. However, testing for *H. pylori* eradication should be performed in patients with recurrent symptoms, complicated PUD, gastric MALT lymphoma, or early gastric cancer. Because of the high rate of bleeding recurrence in untreated *H. pylori*–positive bleeding ulcers, testing for eradication is critical.

○ Confirmation of cure can be performed by urea breath testing, but it should be done at least 4 to 6 weeks after completion of *H. pylori* therapy and 2 weeks after finishing PPI treatment to avoid false-negative results. Serology is less useful to document eradication, as the antibodies to *H. pylori* may remain positive for 1 to 2 years after successful eradication.

- **Treatment of NSAID-associated PUD**
  ○ Consideration must be given to **stopping the offending drug,** as continuation of NSAID use delays ulcer healing. However, discontinuing the NSAID is not always practical, and in these cases, GI toxicity may be reduced by decreasing the dose or switching to a less gastrotoxic medication. Concomitant corticosteroid, anticoagulant, or bisphosphonate therapy should also be discontinued if possible.
  ○ Direct treatment of NSAID-induced PUD is **acid suppression with a PPI.**
  ○ Even with continued NSAID use, acid suppression with PPI therapy results in 85% of NSAID-induced gastric ulcers and >90% of duodenal ulcers healing within 8 weeks, whereas acid suppression with conventional doses of H_2-receptor blockers heals ~70% of gastric and duodenal ulcers within 7 weeks. In this manner, PPI therapy is indicated for NSAID-associated PUD and should be continued as long as the patient is being treated with NSAID to reduce the risk of ulcer recurrence.[15]
  ○ The following patients require gastroprotection with either PPI or misoprostol during NSAID use: history of a prior ulcer, severe concomitant disease, concomitant warfarin or corticosteroid use, or elderly (>65 years).

Lifestyle/Risk Modification

- Withdrawal of potential contributing agents such as NSAIDs, cigarettes, and excess alcohol is indicated.
- Patients should be instructed to avoid foods that precipitate dyspepsia, although no particular dietary recommendations are necessary.

SPECIAL CONSIDERATIONS

- **Stress ulcers** develop in the stomach and duodenum under situations of severe physiologic stress and intensive care unit (ICU) admission, such as mechanical ventilation, coagulopathy, renal failure, head injuries, burns, and multiple trauma. Pathophysiology involves relative mucosal ischemia and poor mucosal protection from intraluminal acid when splanchnic blood supply is shunted to more important organs during physiologic stress. Erosions and ulcers are demonstrated to form frequently within the first 2 to 3 days of ICU admission, but complications (bleeding, perforation) are relatively rare in the present day, attributed to better ICU care, attention to hemodynamic stability, and stress ulcer prophylaxis. Patients at risk can be administered intravenous H2-receptor antagonists by infusion; PPIs have also been demonstrated to provide equivalent protection. Sucralfate has also been used successfully as a prophylactic agent. If bleeding ensues, management is similar to that of nonvariceal upper GI bleeding from peptic ulcers (Chapter 6).

COMPLICATIONS

- **Hemorrhage**
  - Hemorrhage can occur in ~15% of patients with peptic ulcers. See Chapter 6 for further discussion on management of GI bleeding from PUD.
  - NSAID-associated ulcers are overrepresented among hemorrhagic ulcers.
  - Hemorrhage can present as either an acute event with hemodynamic shock or as a slow intermittent blood loss with chronic anemia.
  - If necessary, endoscopic intervention can be utilized to locate the source of bleeding and achieve hemostasis with thermal or laser coagulation, injection sclerotherapy, or mechanical compression with clips.
  - The administration of intravenous PPIs in acute hemorrhage decreases rebleeding rates, the need for blood transfusions, and mortality rates.[16]
- **Perforation** should be suspected in patients with PUD who suddenly develop severe diffuse abdominal pain and other manifestations of peritoneal irritation. Plain abdominal radiography may reveal free air under the diaphragm. Emergent surgery is often indicated for perforation.
- **Obstruction** of the gastric outlet can develop from ulcers in the duodenal bulb and/or pyloric channel, and patients can present with nausea and vomiting. Management typically involves nasogastric tube placement with measurement of the gastric residual, EGD to facilitate diagnosis (with balloon dilation in patients who do not respond to medical therapy), and intravenous PPI therapy.
- **Penetration** occurs when an ulcer penetrates through the bowel wall without any free perforation or leakage of luminal contents into the peritoneal cavity. Most commonly, ulcers penetrate into the pancreas, gastrohepatic omentum, biliary tract, or liver, but only a small proportion become clinically apparent.

GASTRIC ADENOCARCINOMA

GENERAL PRINCIPLES

- In the early 1900s, gastric cancer represented the most common cancer in the United States, but since then, the incidence has decreased dramatically, possibly related to the popularization of refrigeration. Nevertheless, each year >21,000 patients in the United States have a diagnosis of gastric cancer, of whom >11,000 are expected to die.[17]
- As recently as the 1980s, gastric cancer represented the leading cause of cancer deaths worldwide. Of note, *H. pylori* infection appears to be associated with an approximately sixfold increase in the risk of gastric cancer.[18]
- Table 13-6 outlines risk factors for gastric cancer.

TABLE 13-6	RISK FACTORS FOR GASTRIC ADENOCARCINOMA
Helicobacter pylori infection	Prior gastrectomy
Chronic atrophic gastritis	Blood type A
Pernicious anemia	Family history of gastric cancer
Gastric adenoma	Low socioeconomic status

DIAGNOSIS

- Many patients with gastric cancer are asymptomatic or present with **nonspecific symptoms** that can include indigestion, epigastric discomfort, anorexia, early satiety, and weight loss. By the time symptoms have been investigated, many gastric cancers are advanced.
- The **physical examination** may reveal an epigastric mass, ascites, occult blood in stool, or lymphadenopathy.
- An enlarged left supraclavicular lymph node (Virchow's node) or periumbilical lymph node (Sister Mary Joseph's node) represents a metastatic site.
- **Laboratory evaluation** is of limited use but may demonstrate iron-deficiency anemia from chronic blood loss from the cancer.
- **Diagnosis is best made with EGD,** as it allows for direct visualization as well as tissue sampling. Most gastric cancers are exophytic or fungating masses, but some manifest as nonhealing ulcers or with perforation of the gastric wall.
- All gastric ulcers should be aggressively biopsied to exclude malignancy, and repeat EGD should be performed at 8 to 12 weeks to document healing in any patient with a gastric ulcer.
- Once the diagnosis of gastric adenocarcinoma is established, staging should be performed with endoscopic ultrasonography or abdominal computed tomographic scanning to determine whether surgical resection is an option.

TREATMENT

- **Surgical resection** offers the only chance for cure.
- However, ~60% of gastric cancers are deemed unresectable because of local or metastatic spread at the time of diagnosis.
- Depending on location, partial or total gastrectomy may be performed.
- Even with complete resection, 5-year survival rate is only ~20%.
- **Palliative chemotherapy** can be given to patients who are not surgical candidates, but the median survival is only 6 to 9 months.

GASTROINTESTINAL STROMAL TUMORS

GENERAL PRINCIPLES

- Gastrointestinal stromal tumors (GIST) represent 1% to 2% of all malignant GI tumors. Before the molecular definition of GIST in 1998, these lesions were commonly unrecognized and unreported.

- Despite the increasing recognition of GIST, its true incidence remains unknown, although it has been estimated to be ~15 cases per million persons in the United States.
- The median occurrence is in the fifth decade of life, and GIST is found more commonly in women than in men.
- In 1998, the pathophysiology of GIST was discovered to involve mutations in *KIT* signaling pathways leading to tumor proliferation. The definition of GIST has subsequently been narrowed to include a subset of tumors arising from the interstitial cells of Cajal, >90% of which exhibit KIT mutations.
- GIST can be found throughout the GI tract, although 60% to 70% arise in the stomach.

DIAGNOSIS

- Patients may complain of nonspecific symptoms, such as nausea, vomiting, or early satiety. GIST may also be discovered incidentally on endoscopy or imaging.
- Alternatively, GIST lesions may present after achieving a large size and causing mass effect or obstruction, or with acute upper GI hemorrhage.

TREATMENT

- **Surgical resection** represents the treatment of choice for localized tumors.
- However, if the tumor has metastasized, **chemotherapy** remains an option.
- GIST harbors impressive resistance to traditional cytotoxic chemotherapy agents, but the introduction of the tyrosine kinase inhibitor imatinib mesylate has increased the median survival of patients with advanced GIST from 20 to 60 months.[19]

GASTRIC LYMPHOMA

GENERAL PRINCIPLES

- The GI tract represents the predominant site of primary extranodal lymphomas.
- GI lymphomas are most commonly found in the stomach (almost three-fourths of cases) in developed countries. More than 90% of gastric lymphomas are either diffuse large B-cell type or MALT type.
- MALT lymphomas comprise 40% of gastric lymphomas and arise from the transformation of B cells in the marginal zone of the stomach in response to *H. pylori* infection.
- Although *H. pylori* infection is a risk factor, the incidence of MALT in *H. pylori*–infected individuals is between 1 in 30,000 to 1 in 80,000.

DIAGNOSIS

- The most common presenting symptoms are abdominal pain and dyspepsia; B-type symptoms are rare.
- Diagnosis is typically established via EGD with biopsies.

TREATMENT

- Up to three-fourths of patients with low-grade MALT lymphomas experience complete regression after **eradication of *H. pylori* infection.**[20]
- For patients who do not respond to *H. pylori* eradication, radiation, chemotherapy, and surgery represent effective therapeutic options.

REFERENCES

1. Sung JJ, Kuipers EJ, El-Serag HB. Systematic review: the global incidence and prevalence of peptic ulcer disease. *Aliment Pharmacol Ther.* 2009;29:938–946.
2. Post PN, Kuipers EJ, Meijer GA. Declining incidence of peptic ulcer but not of its complications: a nation-wide study in The Netherlands. *Aliment Pharmacol Ther.* 2006;23:1587–1593.
3. McColl KE. *Helicobacter pylori*-negative non-steroidal anti-inflammatory drug-negative ulcer. *Gastroenterol Clin North Am.* 2009;38:353–361.
4. Woodward M, Morrison C, McColl K. An investigation into factors associated with *Helicobacter pylori* infection. *J Clin Epidemiol.* 2000;53:175–181.
5. El-Omar EM, Penman ID, Ardill JES, et al. *Helicobacter pylori* infection and abnormalities of acid secretion in patients with duodenal ulcer disease. *Gastroenterology.* 1995;109:681–691.
6. McColl KE. *Helicobacter pylori* infection. *N Engl J Med.* 2010;362:1597–1604.
7. Wolfe MM, Lichtenstein DR, Singh G. Gastrointestinal toxicity of nonsteroid anti-inflammatory drugs. *N Engl J Med.* 1999;340:1888–1899.
8. Huang JQ, Sridhar S, Hunt RH. Role of *Helicobacter pylori* infection and non-steroidal anti-inflammatory drugs in peptic-ulcer disease: a meta-analysis. *Lancet.* 2002;359:14–22.
9. Moayyedi P, Talley NJ, Fennerty MB, et al. Can the clinical history distinguish between organic and functional dyspepsia? *JAMA.* 2006;295:1566–1576.
10. Malagelada JR, Kuipers EJ, Blaser MJ. Acid peptic disease: clinical manifestations, diagnosis, treatment, and prognosis. In: Goldman L, Ausiello DA, eds. *Cecil Textbook of Medicine.* 23rd ed. Philadelphia, PA: WB Saunders; 2008:1013–1018.
11. Glick SN. Duodenal ulcer. *Radiol Clin North Am.* 1994;32:1259–1274.
12. Hopper AN, Stephens MR, Lewis WG, et al. Relative value of repeat gastric ulcer surveillance gastroscopy in diagnosing gastric cancer. *Gastric Cancer.* 2006;9:217–222.
13. Leodolter A, Kulig M, Brasch H, et al. A meta-analysis comparing eradication, healing and relapse rates in patients with *Helicobacter pylori*-associated gastric or duodenal ulcer. *Aliment Pharmacol Ther.* 2001;15:1949–1958.
14. Chey WD, Wong BC; Practice Parameters Committee of the American College of Gastroenterology. American College of Gastroenterology guideline on the management of *Helicobacter pylori* infection. *Am J Gastroenterol.* 2007;102:1808–1825.
15. Yeomans ND, Tulassay Z, Juhasz L, et al. A comparison of omeprazole with ranitidine for ulcers associated with non-steroidal anti-inflammatory drugs: acid suppression trial, ranitidine versus omeprazole for NSAID-associated ulcer treatment (ASTRONAUT) study group. *N Engl J Med.* 1998;338:719–726.
16. Leontiadis GI, Sharma VK, Howden CW. Systematic review and meta-analysis: proton-pump inhibitor treatment for ulcer bleeding reduces transfusion requirements and hospital stay—results from the Cochrane Collaboration. *Aliment Pharmacol Ther.* 2005;22:169–174.
17. Jemal A, Siegel R, Ward E, et al. Cancer statistics, 2006. *CA Cancer J Clin.* 2006;56:106–130.
18. EUROGAST Study Group. An international association between *Helicobacter pylori* infection and gastric cancer. *Lancet.* 1993;341:1359–1362.
19. Blanke CD, Demetri GD, von Mehren M, et al. Long-term results from a randomized phase II trial of standard- versus higher-dose imatinib mesylate for patients with unresectable or metastatic gastrointestinal stromal tumors expressing KIT. *J Clin Oncol.* 2008;26:620–625.
20. Bayerdorffer E, Neubauer A, Rudolph B, et al. Regression of primary gastric lymphoma of mucosa-associated lymphoid tissue type after cure of *Helicobacter pylori* infection, MALT lymphoma study group. *Lancet.* 1995;345:1591–1594.

Small Bowel Disorders

14

A. Samad Soudagar and Anisa Shaker

INTRODUCTION

- The small bowel is approximately 600 cm in length, with a functional surface area >600 times that of a hollow tube.
- The following three features unique to the gut enhance the surface area of the small intestine:
  - The plicae circulares, or circular folds, are visible mucosal and submucosal invaginations located predominantly in the duodenum and jejunum.
  - Villi are fingerlike projections, consisting of a layer of epithelial cells overlying the lamina propria, approximately 0.5 to 1.5 mm long, which protrude into the intestinal lumen and cover the mucosal surface.
  - Microvilli, tubular projections visualized by electron microscopy, are extensions of the apical cell membrane and compose the brush border.
- These unique mucosal features create an enormous area for digestion, absorption, and secretion.

MALABSORPTION

GENERAL PRINCIPLES

- Small bowel disorders, pancreatic exocrine insufficiency, and cholestatic liver disease account for most causes of malabsorption.
- Table 14-1 lists the most common causes of malabsorption. Cholestatic liver diseases are discussed in Chapter 19. Pancreatic disorders are discussed in Chapter 21.

Definition

- Malabsorption is usually considered an interruption of normal digestion, absorption, and transport of a number of nutrients and minerals.
  - Malnutrition, diarrhea, steatorrhea, electrolyte abnormalities, and weight loss are frequent consequences.
  - Clinical manifestations of small bowel disorders often reflect deficiencies of various macro- and micronutrients.

Pathophysiology

- Various disease processes (including celiac disease, Whipple's disease, tropical sprue, small bowel bacterial overgrowth, radiation or chemotherapy–induced injury, see subsequent sections) interfere with mucosal luminal digestion, absorption, and nutrient transport.
- The small bowel is primarily responsible for absorbing much of the daily dietary carbohydrates, proteins, electrolytes, and essential nutrients.

TABLE 14-1   CAUSES OF MALABSORPTION

Small Intestine Disorders	Pancreatic Exocrine Insufficiency
Celiac sprue	Chronic pancreatitis
Ileal resection	Cystic fibrosis
Short bowel syndrome	Pancreatic cancer
Radiation enteritis	Cholestatic liver disease
Small bowel lymphoma	Extrahepatic biliary obstruction
Bacterial overgrowth	Intrahepatic biliary obstruction
Crohn's disease	Cirrhosis
Tropical sprue	
Whipple disease	
Acquired immunodeficiency syndrome	
Abetalipoproteinemia	
Diabetes mellitus	
Amyloidosis	

- ○ 80% of injested protein is absorbed in the jejunum and 10% in the ileum. Diffuse loss of normal jejunal mucosal function (celiac sprue, extensive surgical resection of the small bowel) can result in protein malabsorption.
- ○ Small bowel disorders can also result in malabsorption of selective nutrients. Iron, folate, calcium (duodenum), B_{12}, bile salt (ileum), and fat-soluble vitamins A, D, E, and K (proximal intestine) deficiencies can occur.

DIAGNOSIS

- Clinical features and presentation of intestinal malabsorption form the cornerstone of diagnosis and result in effects on numerous organ systems including the gastrointestinal (GI) tract and the hematopoietic, musculoskeletal, endocrine, epidermal, and nervous systems.

Clinical Presentation

- Abdominal pain, cramping, excessive flatus, diarrhea (postprandial or unremitting without prandial exacerbation).
- Weight loss despite appropriate appetite and adequate oral intake.
- Foul smelling stool with oily character with classic presentation of "floating on top of the toilet bowl."
- Specific fat-soluble vitamins malabsorption leads to various clinical findings including night blindness (vitamin A), osteopenia (vitamin D), bleeding diathesis (vitamin K), or neurologic symptoms (vitamin E).
- In addition, amenorrhea, infertility, and impotence may manifest as part of patient history.
- Physical examination findings include glossitis, stomatitis (iron, riboflavin, niacin), tetany (calcium, magnesium, vitamin D), dermatitis (vitamin A, zinc), peripheral neuropathy (B_{12} deficiency), and edema (protein-losing enteropathy).

Differential Diagnosis

- Infectious, secretory, and inflammatory causes of diarrhea must be excluded.
- Pancreatic exocrine insufficiency and hepatobiliary disease resulting in intraluminal bile salt deficiency (biliary strictures, cholestatic liver diseases) can result in intraluminal maldigestion and malabsorption.
- Associated malabsorption symptoms must be evaluated on their own accord.
  ○ For example, alternative causes of weight loss including malignancy, hormonal disorders, and inflammatory/autoimmune disorders should be evaluated.
  ○ Postprandial abdominal cramping should be evaluated for etiologies such as peptic ulcer disease, cholelithiasis, pancreatitis, and so forth.

Diagnostic Testing

Laboratories

- Laboratory test abnormalities include macrocytic (folate, Vitamin B_{12} deficiency) and microcytic (iron deficiency) anemia, elevated INR/prolonged prothrombin time (vitamin K deficiency), and decreased serum calcium (calcium malabsorption or vitamin D deficiency).
- Low serum magnesium and zinc levels, decreased serum albumin, and low cholesterol may also be found.
- **Fecal fat analysis** provides a simple, rapid, inexpensive screening test for malabsorption.[1]
  ○ Measurement includes fecal fat quantification for 48 to 72 hours while patient is on a defined intake of fat, typically 100 g/day.
  ○ Normally, >95% of dietary fat is absorbed; consequently >5 g/day of fecal fat is diagnostic of steatorrhea.
  ○ Fecal fat analysis does not distinguish among intestinal, hepatobiliary, and pancreatic causes of malabsorption, although the level of steatorrhea associated with pancreatic insufficiency (~50 g) tends to be higher than the level for intestinal disease (~20 g).[2]
- **Xylose absorption test**
  ○ This test assesses the absorptive capacity of the small intestine and determines whether a small bowel disorder is present.[1,3]
  ○ This test is usually performed for further diagnostic purposes once malabsorption is determined.
  ○ d-Xylose is a 5-carbon sugar primarily absorbed passively in the small intestine. Intraluminal digestion is not required and urinary excretion reflects the mucosa's ability to absorb it.
  ○ This test is performed by administration of 25 g of xylose orally, followed by measurement of urinary excretion, hydrogen breath testing (discussed below), or serum concentration of xylose. A 5-hour urine collection contains at least 5 g of d-xylose.
  ○ This test can therefore differentiate between pancreatic disorders (d-xylose concentration within normal limits) and true mucosal malabsorptive processes (d-xylose concentration decreased postadministration).[3,4]
- It is important to note that certain bacterial species may metabolize d-xylose causing concurrent bacterial overgrowth–mediated decreased d-xylose levels.
- Low urinary excretion will also occur when delayed gastric emptying, impaired renal function, or ascites is present.

- **Hydrogen breath tests**
  - Hydrogen breath tests are based on the principle that hydrogen is produced by bacterial fermentation of carbohydrates that have escaped absorption in the small intestine. A portion of this hydrogen diffuses into the blood stream and is subsequently exhaled by the lungs and analyzed in breath. Commonly used carbohydrates include lactose, fructose, glucose, and nonabsorbable compounds such as lactulose.[5]
  - Hydrogen breath tests can be used to diagnose disaccharidase (lactase) deficiency and lactose intolerance in association with symptoms of abdominal pain, gas, and diarrhea with lactose intake. It is also used for the evaluation of small intestinal bacterial overgrowth (SIBO) (see later).[6,7]
  - Under typical circumstances, only bacterial carbohydrate metabolism is responsible for exhaled hydrogen.
  - In disaccharidase deficiency, carbohydrates are not metabolized in the proximal small bowel lumen and travel to the distal small bowel/colon where they are metabolized by colonized bacteria releasing hydrogen.
- Exhaled hydrogen is measured after the patient is given 25 to 50 g of oral lactose dissolved in water.
- Hydrogen (H_2) levels in end-expiratory breath samples are measured every 15 minutes for up to 3 hours.
- An increase of >20 ppm over basal values for two time points indicates lactose malabsorption. A positive test usually peaks at 2 to 4 hours.
  - False negative results can occur in setting of colonic flora that do not produce hydrogen, delayed gastric emptying, or prolonged orocecal transit time. False-positive results can occur from oral flora substrate fermentation and hydrogen production. Antibiotic use and fiber intake can also alter the results.
  - An early hydrogen peak within 1 hour of ingestion of lactulose may indicate SIBO.
- The lactulose hydrogen breath test suffers from similar false positive and false negative results as disaccharidase deficiency work up.
  - It is usually performed with an oral load of 10 g lactulose or glucose in a dose of 50 to 75 g dissolved in water with subsequent hydrogen breath level measurement as above.
- Interpretation of these tests is not uniform; reported sensitivity and specificity of the lactulose hydrogen breath test in detecting SIBO is 68% and 44%, respectively, and for the glucose breath test 62% and 83%, respectively.[5]
- The gold standard remains aspiration of the small bowel contents and subsequent culture. This is not used clinically for diagnosing SIBO.

Imaging
- Traditional imaging for small bowel pathologic processes can be performed with **barium small-bowel follow-through** examinations, **single- or double-contrast intubated enteroclysis**, and **computed tomography** (CT) cross-sectional imaging.
- **Capsule endoscopy, push endoscopy,** and **double-balloon endoscopy** are newer techniques that have been developed to examine the small bowel in its entirety.
- Cross-sectional imaging techniques provide good visualization of both superimposed bowel loops and extraluminal findings and complications.
- The emergence of **CT** and **magnetic resonance (MR) enterography** has led to further improvements in the noninvasive evaluation of the small bowel.

- ○ **MR enterography** advantages include the lack of ionizing radiation, improved soft tissue contrast, and the ability to provide real-time and functional evaluation.[8]
- ○ Such imaging will likely prove more useful in patients requiring routine surveillance screening, for instance, those with familial adenomatous polyposis or Peutz-Jeghers syndrome.
- ○ Cross-sectional imaging advances have been made with the development of **CT enterography.**[9]
- ○ Advantages of this technique include superior temporal and spatial resolution compared with MR, more widespread access, and less cost.
- Indications for cross-sectional imaging of the small bowel continue to evolve but include evaluation of obscure GI bleeding, the presence and activity of Crohn's disease, and suspected neoplasia.

Diagnostic Procedures

- **Endoscopic biopsy**
  - ○ Biopsy of the small intestine is extremely useful in patients with suspected malabsorption.
- Specific histologic findings allow diagnosis of the more common causes of malabsorption, such as celiac sprue, as well as more infrequent causes, such as lymphoma and amyloidosis.

CELIAC SPRUE

GENERAL PRINCIPLES

- Celiac sprue is the most frequently evaluated etiology among the malabsorptive small bowel disorders.
- Increasingly sensitive and specific serologies and tissue diagnosis are usually confirmatory.
- Symptomatic resolution is achieved with avoidance of food products containing gluten.

Definition

- Permanent intolerance to the storage proteins or *gluten* found in wheat, rye, and barley result in symptoms of malabsorption including weight loss, abdominal cramping, diarrhea, and excessive flatus.[10]

Epidemiology

- The prevalence of celiac disease in the United States is approximately 1%, with a range of 0.71% to 1.25%.
- HLA antigen class II DQ molecules DQ2 and DQ8 are necessary but not sufficient for phenotypic expression of the disease.

Pathophysiology

- A consequence of complex adaptive and innate immune responses to dietary gluten, it is characterized by chronic inflammation of the proximal intestinal mucosa mediated primarily by T-cell immunologic processes.[10]
  - ○ The adaptive immune response is mediated by gluten-reactive CD4[+] T cells, which are presented as gluten-derived peptides by HLA antigen class II molecules.

- ○ Deamidation of these peptides by tissue transglutaminase allows higher affinity binding to the binding groove of DQ2 or DQ8 when presenting specific gluten antigens to T cells.
- ○ Subsequently, T cells release helper T-cell cytokines that precipitate mucosal damage.
- ○ Additional innate immune responses are mediated and activated by intraepithelial lymphocytes and act in concert via interleukin-15 produced by enterocytes.

Risk Factors/Associated Conditions

- **High-risk populations** include the following[10]:
  - ○ First-degree relatives of patients with celiac disease (prevalence 10%).
  - ○ Patients with dermatitis herpetiformis (prevalence >90%).
  - ○ Patients with unexplained iron-deficiency anemia (prevalence 2–5%).
  - ○ Osteoporosis and bone demineralization (prevalence 1.5–3%).
  - ○ Type 1 diabetes mellitus (prevalence 2–5% in adults and 3–8% in children).
  - ○ Patients with liver disease:
  - ○ Elevated transaminase levels of unknown cause (prevalence 1.5–9.0%).
  - ○ Autoimmune hepatitis (prevalence 2.9–6.4%).
  - ○ Primary biliary cirrhosis (prevalence 0–6.0%).
  - ○ Genetic disorders (prevalence in patients with Down syndrome ranges from 3–12%).
  - ○ Autoimmune thyroid disease (prevalence 1.5–6.7%).
  - ○ Reproductive disorders (prevalence in Turner's syndrome can range from 2.1–4.1%).
- **Small intestinal lymphoma** is also noted to have increasing prevalence with celiac disease.
- Five-year abstinence from gluten normalizes risk of lymphoma.

DIAGNOSIS

Clinical Presentation

- Intestinal symptoms predominate and include characteristic malabsorption symptoms: weight loss, steatorrhea, fatigue, and abdominal cramps.
- Fatigue can also manifest secondary to iron deficiency anemia.
- Infertility, short stature, osteoporosis, and additional manifestations of malabsorption can also be present.
- **Dermatitis herpetiformis**, a pruritic blistering rash on the extensor surfaces, may be seen. Histopathology from the skin lesions, when diagnostic, provides confirmation of celiac sprue.

Diagnostic Criteria

- Current American Gastroenterology Association recommendations suggest positive serologic tests coupled with mucosal biopsy suggestive of celiac disease, supported by a positive symptomatic response to a gluten-free diet to clinch the diagnosis.[10,11]

Differential Diagnosis

- In the absence of symptomatic relief with treatment/lifestyle modifications, additional etiologies of malabsorption must be considered:
  - ○ Pancreatic exocrine insufficiency

- ○ Hepatobiliary diseases
- ○ Disaccharidase deficiency
- ○ Intestinal lymphoma
- ○ Refractory sprue
  - ■ Characterized by severe villus atrophy associated with severe malabsorption that either does not or no longer responds to a gluten-free diet.[12]
  - ■ Possibility remains that some cases of refractory sprue are not associated with gluten sensitivity.
  - ■ Refractory sprue occurs most often in older patients and may be associated with carriage of a double DQ2 allele.
  - ■ Refractory sprue may be responsive to immunosuppression or corticosteroids.
- ○ Alternative etiologies to consider include causes of enteropathy (autoimmune enteropathy, common variable immunodeficiency syndrome, tropical sprue, and eosinophilic gastroenteritis) resulting in hypoalbuminemia and massive malnutrition.

Diagnostic Testing

Laboratories

- Initially, it is important to evaluate for deficiencies in certain proximal small intestinal nutrients consistent with malabsorption (decreased fat-soluble vitamins, iron, B_{12}, folate, etc).
- **Serologic testing** with either **endomysial antibody (EMA IgA)** or **tissue transglutaminase (tTG IgA)** is appropriate as an initial screening test in suspected cases of celiac disease.[10,11]
  - ○ The reported sensitivity and specificity of EMA are close to 90% and 99%, respectively.
  - ○ The reported sensitivity and specificity for tTG IGA are 90% and >95%, respectively.
  - ○ A correlation has been shown between the sensitivities of these serologic tests and degree of histologic activity.
  - ○ **Antigliadin antibody testing** is now rarely performed, but a newer serologic test targeting antibodies against **deamidated gliadin peptide (DGP)** provides much better diagnostic accuracy.
  - ○ Sensitivity and specificity for DGP are 94% and 99%, respectively.[13]
  - ○ DGP and tTG IGA in combination improve therapeutic gain of serologic testing in celiac disease.
- If initial serologic studies are negative, other causes of malabsorption have been excluded, and suspicion for celiac disease remains, then measurement of **serum IgA levels** is appropriate.
- Prevalence of selective IgA deficiency in the celiac disease population is 1.7% to 3.0%, 10 to 15 times higher than in the general population.
- In addition, if small bowel biopsy (see later) and serologic testing remain nondiagnostic, analysis of the **HLA-DQ2/DQ8 alleles** may be helpful.
  - ○ Either or both of these alleles are uniformly seen in almost all patients with celiac disease; absence of these markers has a negative predictive value close to 100%.

Diagnostic Procedures

- As noted above, the gold standard for diagnosis, in addition to serologic tests and dietary modification, consists of a **proximal small bowel biopsy** confirming the diagnosis.
  - ○ Histologic findings on biopsy include

- atrophy/blunting of the small intestinal villi;
- hyperplasia, deepening of crypts; and
- infiltration of lamina propria and intraepithelial compartments with chronic inflammatory cells, typically lymphoplasmacytic infiltrate.

TREATMENT

Lifestyle/Risk Modifications

- Gold standard of treatment involves **lifelong adherence to a gluten-free diet.**
  - This often proves difficult, as gluten is found in several types of food.
  - Typically, wheat, rye, and barley should be removed from the diet.
  - Knowledge about dietary compliance is crucial for avoiding inadvertent ingestion of gluten and exacerbation of celiac symptoms.
  - Consultation with a dietitian is important and membership in a local celiac society is often helpful.
- Routine evaluations by physicians and dieticians are appropriate; however, no specific serologic screening testing (i.e., tTG/EMA/DGP) or time line for follow-up has been established.
- Routine serologic testing is sensitive for major but not minor dietary indiscretions and negative serologic test results do not necessarily mean improvement beyond severe or total villous atrophy.[11]
- In addition, it is important to ensure **nutrient deficiency supplementation** (e.g., iron, folate).
- **Screening for concurrent osteoporosis** with bone mineral density scans should also be performed with prolonged disease course.

SMALL INTESTINAL BACTERIAL OVERGROWTH (SIBO)

GENERAL PRINCIPLES

- Bacteria within the small bowel lumen generally consist of organisms produced by oropharyngeal flora. Several disorders can lead to profound bacterial overgrowth, causing a wide variety of malnutrition symptoms and clinical abnormalities.

Definition

- Usually defined as $>10^5$ colony-forming units/mL in the proximal small bowel.
- Abnormal, excessive proliferation of bacterial growth within the small bowel intestinal lumen can lead to impaired nutrient digestion and subsequent damage to the bowel mucosa, further hindering appropriate digestion and absorption.

Epidemiology

- SIBO is common in older adults and is often an underrecognized etiology of malabsorption.
  - In one series of adults older than 65 years who suffered from malabsorption, SIBO was the most common cause (70.8%).[14]
  - Prevalence in the asymptomatic elderly population is high (14.5% to 38%), although the significance of this in the absence of symptoms is unclear.

Etiology

- SIBO can be caused by the following:
  - **Intestinal stasis** caused by
    - intestinal motility disorders such as diabetic gastroparesis, hypothyroidism, postsurgical ileus, medication-induced (i.e., opiates), and rheumatologic/infiltrative conditions (i.e., scleroderma, amyloidosis);
    - structural lesions in the setting of inflammatory disease (i.e., Crohn's) mediated bowel strictures, radiation enteritis, postsurgical adhesions, and malignancy;
  - **fistulous, abnormal connections between small and large intestines,** often seen postsurgically in bypass patients yielding postsurgical blind bowel loops;
  - **reduced gastric acid secretion** and consequent decreased acid barrier to ingested bacteria. This can sometimes be seen in setting of excessive acid suppression, postvagotomy, impaired gastric acid secretion postgastrectomy, or in setting of pernicious anemia;
  - **immunodeficiency syndromes.**

Pathophysiology

- Direct bacterial overgrowth-mediated toxin production can damage bowel lumen epithelium, impairing digestion and absorption.
- Bacteria are also known to deconjugate bile salts, leading to earlier reabsorption and impairment of fat-soluble nutrient absorption.
- Bacteria are known to coat the bowel wall, bind certain nutrients intended for absorption (i.e., vitamin B_{12}), and reduce availability.

DIAGNOSIS

Clinical Presentation

- Presentation can be similar to other malabsorptive states, with findings of abdominal distention, cramping, excessive flatus, significant vitamin and carbohydrate malnutrition, and weight loss.
- Patients often have medical histories predisposing them to states of impaired intestinal motility, immunodeficiency, or reduced gastric acid secretion.

Differential Diagnosis

- Includes alternative etiologies of malabsorption including hepatobiliary diseases, autoimmune-mediated processes, such as celiac disease, refractory sprue, intestinal lymphoma, and infectious causes such as tropical sprue or Whipple's disease.

Diagnostic Testing

Laboratories

- Typical malabsorptive vitamin (vitamins A,D, E, K, and B_{12} and folate) and electrolyte (iron and calcium) deficiencies are noted.
- Additional findings include macrocytic or microcytic anemia, elevated prothrombin time and INR leading to bleeding diathesis.

Diagnostic Procedures

- Gold standard for diagnosis remains microbiological culture of small bowel aspirate.
  - Typical small bowel intraluminal bacteria concentrations are $<10^4$ colony-forming units per milliliter (CFU/mL), most of which are gram-positive aerobes, derived from oropharyngeal flora.
  - Thus, findings of colonic-type bacterial count $>10^5$ are typically diagnostic of SIBO.

- Because of the time-consuming, expensive, and invasive nature of small bowel aspirate culture, hydrogen breath tests using glucose or lactulose have become the method of choice.

TREATMENT

- Focus is twofold:
  - ○ Eradication of the abnormal proliferating intraluminal bacteria.
  - ○ Reversal of predisposing risk factors that precipitate SIBO.

Medications

- **Antibiotics** are typically used to treat enteric gut flora.
  - ○ **Quinolones or amoxicillin in combination with clavulanic acid or metronidazole** is routinely used.
  - ○ **Rifaximin** is increasingly used in the treatment of SIBO. This agent also has value in the management of hepatic encephalopathy.
  - ○ Repeat courses of antibiotics are often required, with probiotic use possibly allowing maintenance of bacterial growth after initial antibiotic therapy, although remission is not induced with probiotics alone.
- **Agents to augment altered intestinal motility** (e.g., metoclopramide, erythromycin) can be considered, but these agents are not uniformly beneficial, and long-term use can be associated with significant adverse effects.
- In the setting of systemic disorders associated with altered intestinal motility, attention should be focused on **treating the underlying disease etiology** (i.e., diabetic control, thyroid supplementation in setting of hypothyroidism, immunosuppressive agents in scleroderma, etc).

Surgical Management

- Reversal of structural abnormalities that can predispose intestinal stasis should be pursued.
  - ○ Elimination of postsurgical or inflammatory disease-mediated adhesions or strictures either endoscopically or surgically.
  - ○ Correction of postsurgical blind loops may prevent recurrence of bacterial overgrowth in those bowel segments.

SHORT BOWEL SYNDROME (SBS)

GENERAL PRINCIPLES

- The small bowel has significant capability to tolerate resection of large segments and yet retain adequate absorptive capabilities (up to 25% to 30% can be resected).

Definition

- Resection of large segments of small bowel (usually resulting in <200 cm of small intestine) can culminate in symptoms and presentation ranging from mild nutritional deficiencies to debilitating diarrhea and malnutrition.

Etiology

- In infants, congenital SBS can occur as a consequence of intestinal atresia and other congenital intestinal anomalies.[15,16]

- More often, SBS is an acquired condition resulting from multiple resections for refractory complications from Crohn's disease, catastrophic vascular events, trauma, intestinal adhesions, and extensive aganglionosis.

Pathophysiology

- Resection of small intestine can reduce the surface area for nutrient absorption.
  - If the resected segment length is not significant, patients remain asymptomatic and do not suffer from consequences of SBS.
  - Postsurgically, the length of remaining small bowel and continuity with the colon determines disease severity.
- Nutritional risk remains greatest for those with[15]
  - duodenostomy or jejunoileal anastomosis, with resulting <35 cm of residual small bowel;
  - jejunocolic or ileocolic anastomosis, with <60 cm of residual small bowel;
  - end jejunostomy, with <115 cm of residual small bowel; and
  - resection of the ileocolic valve.
- Intestinal adaptive response to resection involves an increase in absorptive surface area that results from crypt cell hyperplasia and increase in villus height.[15]
  - Commonly, the ileum may account for the adaptive processes lost from jejunal resection and assume, to some extent, the role of absorbing folate, iron, and calcium.
  - Ileal resection, however, cannot be compensated by jejunal hypertrophy and a resultant loss in vitamin B_{12}, bile salts, and fat-soluble vitamin resorption occurs.
  - Consequently, nutrient malabsorption depends on location and extent of small bowel resection.
- Altered intestinal motility often develops postsurgically (e.g., ileocecal valve resection) predisposing to bacterial colonization and resulting in SIBO.
- Postresection, there are alterations in the release of distal ileum and colonic hormones (glucagon-like peptide-1, neurotensin) stimulated by fat or bile salts.
  - Rapid gastric emptying may be precipitated from this process causing significant volume losses.
- In the setting of ileal compromise, further diarrhea can be precipitated by bile acid–mediated irritation of the bowel lumen.

DIAGNOSIS

Clinical Presentation

- Symptoms in patients having had recent surgical resection vary from malabsorption, weight loss, and increased frequency of bowel movements, especially postprandially, to significant malnutrition, profuse diarrhea, and dehydration.

Diagnostic Testing

- Diagnosis in these patients is relatively simple and often requires a history of prior surgical intervention, routinely for the above etiologies.

Laboratories

- Malabsorption (carbohydrate, vitamin, nutrient deficiencies) can be significant in these patients.
- In addition, significant electrolyte abnormalities, renal insufficiency, and varying degrees of acid/base disturbances result from the profound diarrhea and dehydration that occur in SBS.

TREATMENT

- Treatment is primarily supportive.[15] Principles of management include the following:
  - Appropriate hydration and volume resuscitation.
  - Adequate nutrition and supplementation with mineral and vitamins.
  - Often, supplemental enteral feeding (via nasogastric/orogastric tubes) is required on a short-term basis before possible transition to total parenteral nutrition.
- To ensure adequate time for absorption, agents such as **diphenoxylate–atropine** or **loperamide** can be used to slow intestinal motility.
- If the suspicion of concurrent SIBO is high, **antibiotics** such as quinolones, metronidazole, or rifaximin can be used.
- For possible bile acid–mediated diarrhea, **bile acid–binding agents** such as cholestyramine may provide additional relief.
- **Growth factor administration** is sometimes recommended in patients with refractory SBS who receive minimal symptom control with conservative, supportive management.
  - Growth factors, including somatotropin, glutamine, and glucagon-like peptide 2 (GLP-2), are theorized to increase mucosal adaptation and consequent dietary absorption in post–bowel resection states.
  - Studies detailing use of these agents in various combinations have had conflicting results; consequently, no consensus exists regarding their use, which remains a controversial treatment modality.[17]

SMALL BOWEL NEOPLASMS

GENERAL PRINCIPLES

- The small bowel comprises 75% of the length of the entire GI tract and 90% of the mucosal surface. However, <2% of GI malignancies originate in the small bowel.
- Age-adjusted incidence of small bowel malignancies is 1 per 100,000 and the prevalence is 0.6%.

Classification
- Benign tumors consist of the following:
  - Leiomyomas, which are the most frequent symptomatic benign tumors of the small bowel. These occur most commonly in the sixth or seventh decade of life.
  - Other benign tumors include adenomas, lipomas, and hamartomas.
- Several malignant tumors can occur in the small bowel.
  - Adenocarcinomas account for 30% to 50% of malignant tumors.[18]
  - Annual incidence is 3.9 cases per million, with a slight male predominance, most commonly presenting in the sixth or seventh decade.
  - Carcinoids account for 25% to 30% of malignant tumors.
  - Lymphomas account for 15% to 20% of malignant tumors.
  - Depending on the series, non–Hodgkins lymphoma accounts for 18% to 24%.

Risk Factors
- Certain hereditary conditions predispose individuals to small intestinal tumors.
  - **Peutz-Jeghers syndrome** is known to cause hamartomatous polyps primarily in the jejunum and ileum.

○ **Familial adenomatous polyposis** (FAP) can be associated with small bowel adenomas, often progressing to adenocarcinoma.

○ Malignant conversion of proximal gut polyposis after prophylactic colectomy has increased in FAP patients over their lifetime, varying from 4% to 10%.[19] This may reflect an increase in survival of FAP patients.

○ **Inflammatory conditions** such as **Crohn's disease** and **celiac sprue** may also predispose patients to adenocarcinoma and lymphoma of the small bowel. There is a 20- to 40-fold increase in risk of small bowel adenocarcinoma with Crohn's disease compared with the general population.[20]

DIAGNOSIS

Clinical Presentation

• Small bowel tumors can cause intermittent abdominal pain, anemia, bleeding (either overt or occult, manifesting in the setting of chronic anemia), or structural abnormalities resulting in obstruction. Presentation can be insidious and nonspecific. In one large series, mean time to diagnosis was 7 months.

• **Symptomatic presentation is more likely to be seen with malignant tumors,** whereas benign tumors are often discovered incidentally, often at surgery for small bowel obstruction.

○ **Leiomyomas** are highly vascular tumors that can present with bleeding (65%), often from the duodenum, or with obstruction or intussusception (25%).

○ **Adenomas and adenocarcinomas,** specifically those located in the duodenum with periampullary involvement, can present with signs of obstructive jaundice when the distal common bile duct is involved. Typically, manifestations are nonspecific and occur late in the disease course.

○ **Lymphoma** often presents with abdominal pain, weight loss, abdominal mass, perforation, or obstruction.

Differential Diagnosis

• Small bowel tumors are often appreciated incidentally in the setting of unremitting abdominal pain, unexplained anemia, lower GI bleeding, and small bowel obstruction.

• Alternative etiologies for all these presenting symptoms must be considered prior to endoscopic or invasive diagnostic testing. This can include inflammatory strictures, adhesions as a cause for small bowel obstruction, and other common causes for GI bleeding (see Chapters 6 and 7).

Diagnostic Testing

Laboratories

• Patients can present with laboratory abnormalities consistent with malabsorption (see earlier) from luminal obstruction and consequent impaired nutrient absorption.

• Unexplained anemia can be seen if occult bleeding is a chronic manifestation.

• **Genetic testing** may be performed in the setting of inherited cancer syndromes. For instance, mutations of the APC gene suggest FAP and SMAD4 mutations suggest juvenile polyposis syndrome.

Imaging

• Luminal irregularities consistent with intestinal tumors can be seen in barium contrast studies, specifically with small bowel follow-through series, contrast enteroclysis, or CT/MR enterography.

Diagnostic Procedures

- **Endoscopic diagnosis with histopathologic confirmation** remains the ideal confirmatory test prior to surgical resection, when possible.
  - ○ **Leiomyomas** are most frequently found in the jejunum, followed by the ileum and the duodenum.
  - ○ Endoscopically, they appear as single, firm, grayish-white, well-defined masses with central umbilication and ulceration, often covered with normal epithelium.
  - ○ **Adenomas** can be diffusely found through the small bowel, primarily in the duodenum.
  - ○ Large size or findings of prominent villus component or atypia increase the risk for malignancy.
  - ○ **Adenocarcinomas** are most routinely found in the proximal small bowel, with the duodenum, and more specifically, the periampullary region being the most common location.
  - ○ **Lymphomas** can be diagnosed with endoscopic visualization and biopsy, but often exploratory laparotomy is required for diagnosis.

TREATMENT

- Endoscopic or surgical excision is indicated whenever possible for all tumors, particularly benign and localized small bowel tumors.
- Radiation or chemotherapy may be necessary in malignant tumors with more widespread extraluminal involvement.

Surgical/Endoscopic Management

- Adenomas should be removed or ablated as first-line treatment endoscopically if possible.
  - ○ Tumor locations dictate the method of resection. For example, duodenal polyps may be amenable to endoscopic resection, whereas periampullary tumors may require a combination of endoscopic and surgical management due to an increased risk of malignant transformation.
- Adenocarcinomas require surgery as it provides the only potential for cure.
  - ○ Specifically, pancreaticoduodenectomy (Whipple procedure) is often required for tumors of the first or second part of the duodenum.

Other Therapies

- In the setting of inadequate surgical resection or increased small bowel adenocarcinoma disease burden, **chemotherapy and radiation therapy** may be indicated. However, these modalities have not been shown to improve survival in advanced disease.
- Lymphomas often require an aggressive combination of surgical management, chemotherapy, or radiation therapy since they frequently present with advanced disease.

MONITORING/FOLLOW-UP

- When incidental adenomas are found on endoscopy, routine endoscopic surveillance is recommended to ensure complete ablation and to monitor for recurrence. Surveillance intervals vary and can range from 1 to 3 years.
- More aggressive surveillance is indicated in the setting of adenocarcinoma or lymphoma after curative management.

- Genetically predisposed individuals such as those with FAP should receive routine screening for polyposis and malignant transformation. No clear recommendations exist, but yearly endoscopy may be indicated.

OUTCOME/PROGNOSIS

- Small bowel adenocarcinoma prognosis remains dismal despite aggressive management, with an overall 5-year survival rate as low as 30%.
- Prognosis for adenomas, however, is excellent for those who lack malignant change or in which malignancy is confined to superficial layers on biopsy.

REFERENCES

1. Thomas PD, Forbes A, Green J, et al. Guidelines for the investigation of chronic diarrhea, 2nd edition. *Gut.* 2003;52(suppl 5):1–15.
2. Bai JC, Andrush A, Matelo G, et al. Fecal fat concentration in the differential diagnosis of steatorrhea. *Am J Gastroenterol.* 1989;84(1):27–30.
3. Craig RM, Atkinson AJ Jr. D-xylose testing: a review. *Gastroenterology.* 1989;97(1):246–247.
4. Craig RM, Ehrenpreis ED. D-xylose testing. *J Clin Gastroenterol.* 1999;29:143–150.
5. Braden B. Methods and functions: breath tests. *Best Pract Res Clin Gastroenterol.* 2009; 23:337–352.
6. Simrén M, Stotzer PO. Use and abuse of hydrogen breath tests. *Gut.* 2006;55:297–303.
7. Bures J, Cyrany J, Kohoutova D, et al. Small intestinal bacterial overgrowth syndrome. *World J Gastroenterol.* 2010;16(24):2978–2990.
8. Fidler J. MR imaging of the small bowel. *Radiol Clin N Am.* 2007;45:317.
9. Macari M, Megibow A, Balthazar E. A pattern approach to the abnormal small bowel: observations at MDCT and CT enterography. *AJR.* 2007;188:1344.
10. Rostom A, Murray JA, Kagnoff MF. AGA institute technical review on diagnosis and management of celiac disease. *Gastroenterology.* 2006;131:1981.
11. AGA Institute Medical Position Statement on the Diagnosis and Management of Celiac Disease. *Gastroenterology.* 2006;131:1977–1980.
12. Abdallah H, Leffler D, Dennis M, et al. Refractory celiac disease. *Curr Gastroenterol Rep.* 2007;9(5):401–405.
13. Sugai E, Vasquez H, Nachman F, et al. Accuracy of antibodies to synthetic gliadin-related peptides in celiac disease. *Clin Gastroenterol Hepatol.* 2006;4:1112–1117.
14. Elpick HL, Elpick DA, Sanders DS. Small bowel bacterial overgrowth: an under-recognized cause of malnutrition in older adults. *Geriatrics.* 2006;61:21–26.
15. Buchman AL, Scolapio J, Fryer J. AGA technical review on short bowel syndrome and intestinal transplantation. *Gastroenterology.* 2003;124:1111–1134.
16. Rubin DC. Small intestine: anatomy and structural anomalies. In: Yamada Y, Alpers DH, Kaplowitz N, et al., eds. *Textbook of Gastroenterology.* Philadelphia: Lippincott Williams & Wilkins; 2003:1561–1583.
17. Scolapio JS. Short bowel syndrome: recent clinical outcomes with growth hormone. *Gastroenterology.* 2006;130(2 suppl 1):S122–S126.
18. Delaunoit T, Neczyporenko F, Limburg P, et al. Pathogenesis and risk factors of small bowel adenocarcinoma: a colorectal cancer sibling? *Am J Gastroenterol.* 2005;100:703–710.
19. Brosens LA, Keller JJ, Offerhaus GJ, et al. Prevention and management of duodenal polyps in familial adenomatous polyposis. *Gut.* 2005;45:1034–1043.
20. Beaugerie L, Sokol H, Seksik P. Noncolorectal malignancies in inflammatory bowel disease: more than meets the eye. *Dig Dis.* 2009;27(3):375–381.

Colon Neoplasms

Nishant J. Patel and Dayna S. Early

GENERAL PRINCIPLES

Background

- More than 142,000 new cases and 51,000 deaths are attributed to colorectal cancer (CRC) in the United States each year.[1] CRC is the second leading cause of cancer death. However, mortality is progressively declining since 1990 at a rate of 3% per year.
- Prognosis is closely linked to stage at diagnosis. The 5-year survival rate for localized cancers is >90%, whereas the 5-year survival rate for those with invasive cancer is <10%.
- Nearly all CRC develops from colorectal adenomas, with a progression that occurs over 5 to 15 years.
- Screening colonoscopy and polypectomy have been shown to reduce mortality from CRC.[2] The high survival rate of patients with localized CRC and the ability to detect and resect precursor polyps make screening a vital tool in the treatment and prevention of CRC.

Epidemiology

- The prevalence of adenomatous polyps in asymptomatic patients varies from 23% to 41%.
- The lifetime incidence of CRC is roughly 5% for average risk individuals, with 90% of cases occurring after age 50 years.
- Different ethnic populations carry varying risks for developing colorectal adenomas and cancer. For example, Hawaiian-Japanese have a prevalence of adenoma as high as 50% to 60%; in contrast, Japanese living in Japan have prevalence rates of <12%. This disparity suggests that lifestyle and environmental influences are additional risk factors in the development of CRC.
- Developing countries have lower rates of CRC than North America, Australia, and Europe. This may be due to diets high in red meat and fat and low in fruits, vegetables, and fiber in developed countries.
- Distribution of polyps is fairly uniform throughout the colon. In patients older than 60 years and in women, adenomas tend to be more common in the proximal colon. In recent years, a gradual shift has occurred to greater incidence of proximal (ascending colon and cecal) CRC.

Etiology

- Adenomatous polyps are believed to develop in a stepwise fashion as a result of a series of genetic mutations. These arise in colonic crypts wherein the proliferative component of the crypt, usually confined to the base, extends through the entire crypt.[3]

- Histologically, the tubular adenoma is the most common subgroup, representing 80% to 86% of all adenomatous polyps. These lesions tend to be small and exhibit only mild dysplasia, seen microscopically as a complex network of branching adenomatous glands.
- Villous adenomas tend to have a higher degree of dysplasia, with adenomatous glands extending through to the center of the polyps, thereby appearing grossly as fingerlike projections.
- Villous (papillary) and tubulovillous adenomas are three times more likely to become malignant than tubular adenomas.
- Traditional serrated adenomas and sessile serrated adenomas share some histologic features with hyperplastic polyps. These lesions, however, are associated with CRC risk similar to classic adenomas. Sessile serrated adenomas are more common in the proximal colon, and traditional serrated adenomas are more common in the rectosigmoid colon.
- Overall, only a small percentage of colon polyps develop into carcinomas.

Pathophysiology

- CRC develops from colorectal adenomas in nearly all instances, the exception being CRC that develops in patients with idiopathic inflammatory bowel disease manifesting as colitis.
- Several studies including the National Polyp Study found that removal of adenomas resulted in a significantly lower incidence of CRC. In confirmed colon cancers, residual adenomatous tissue can be found within cancerous tissue. Additionally, surgically resected CRC may contain adjacent adenomatous polyps in one-third of cases.
- The progression from adenoma to carcinoma occurs as a result of a series of DNA mutations. However, the exact sequence of mutations necessary for malignant progression is unclear.
  - ○ Among the earliest mutations is inactivation of the adenomatous polyposis coli (APC) gene.[4]
  - ○ Other later changes include mutations of the K-ras proto-oncogene, DNA hypomethylation, 18q inactivation, and p53 (tumor suppressor gene) inactivation.[4]
  - ○ The accumulation of abnormalities results in a stepwise progression over ~10 years from normal mucosa to adenoma to carcinoma.
  - ○ Detection of these mutations from sloughed cells in stool samples as a useful screening test for early CRC detection is currently under investigation.

Risk Factors

- Several factors predict the risk of developing colorectal adenomas and cancer.
- **Older age** is the most important risk factor and is associated not only with a higher prevalence of polyps but also with multiple polyps, severe dysplasia, and larger adenoma size.
- **African Americans** have an increased risk of developing colon cancer than other races.[5]
- **Personal history of CRC or adenomatous polyps** confers additional risk.
- Inflammatory intestinal diseases, such as ulcerative colitis and Crohn's disease, can increase the risk of developing colon cancer.
- Several **genetic syndromes,** most notably familial adenomatous polyposis and hereditary nonpolyposis CRC (Lynch syndrome), substantially increase the risk of developing colon cancer (see Table 15-1).

TABLE 15-1   GENETIC SYNDROMES ASSOCIATED WITH COLORECTAL CANCER

	Genetic Mutation	Phenotype	Risk for CRC	Age to Begin Screening	Type of Screening	Other Cancers
Hereditary nonpolyposis colorectal cancer	Autosomal dominant, DNA mismatch repair genes	CRC without polyposis	75%	25 or 10 yr younger than earliest case	Colonoscopy every 1–2 yr (most CRC are right-sided)	GYN, GU, UGI tract
FAP	Germline mutation of APC gene	Hundreds to thousands of adenomatous polyps	100%	10–12, perform colectomy when polyps found	Flexible sigmoidoscopy	Duodenal (especially ampullary) and gastric
• Gardner's syndrome	Same as FAP	Same as FAP	Same as FAP	Same as FAP	Same as FAP	Desmoid tumors, osteomas, CHRPE, thyroid, adrenal, hepatobiliary tumors
• Attenuated FAP	Same as FAP	Much fewer number of adenomas	Same as FAP, slightly older	Same as FAP	Same as FAP	Same as FAP
Peutz-Jeghers syndrome	Autosomal dominant, STK11 mutation	Mucocutaneous pigmentation Hamartomatous polyps, small bowel and CRC	Up to 66%	Age 8 yr for UGI and CRC, Age 25 yr for pancreatic cancer	EGD, colonoscopy, and video capsule endoscopy every 3 yr if polyps found Endoscopic ultrasonography every 1–2 yr	Genital, breast
Familial juvenile polyposis	Autosomal dominant, SMAD4 mutation	≥10 hamartomatous/"juvenile" polyps	Up to 20%	Mid-teens	FOBT every 1–2 yr or colonoscopy every 3–5 yr Small bowel examination every 1–2 yr	Possible association with hereditary hemorrhagic telangiectasia

CHRPE, congenital hypertrophy of the retinal pigment epithelium; EGD, esophagogastroduodenoscopy; FAP, familial adenomatous polyposis; GU, genitourinary; GYN, gynecologic; UGI, upper gastrointestinal.

- **Family history** of colon cancer
  - ○ The overall colon cancer risk in those with multiple first-degree relatives or a single first-degree relative with a diagnosis before age 45 years is three to four times that of the general population.
  - ○ In patients with a single first-degree relative with CRC or adenoma diagnosed before age 60 years, risk of developing CRC increases two times that of the general population.
  - ○ Tobacco and alcohol use may increase the risk of developing colon cancer.
  - ○ Other medical conditions, including diabetes mellitus, obesity, acromegaly, ureterocolic anastomoses, and pelvic radiation, have also been associated with an increased risk of developing CRC.

Prevention

- For screening purposes, individuals are stratified into average or high risk.[6]
  - ○ Average risk individuals are those with no family or personal history of CRC or adenoma and no history of ulcerative colitis.
  - ○ High-risk populations include those with prior CRC or adenoma, family history of CRC, family history of adenoma before age 60, and ulcerative colitis.[7]
  - ○ Current recommendations do not take into account race, gender, dietary, or environmental risks modifiers.
- Screening for CRC should begin at age 50 years for average risk individuals.
- Individuals deemed to be at high risk should be screened starting at age 40, or 10 years earlier than the age of the youngest CRC diagnosis in the family, whichever is earlier.
- CRC screening is unique in that national organizations provide a "menu" of screening options from which to choose, and they generally do not endorse one screening test over another.
  - ○ Options for screening include fecal immunochemical testing (FIT), fecal occult blood testing (FOBT), flexible sigmoidoscopy (FS), double contrast barium enema (DCBE), and colonoscopy.
  - ○ These tests used alone and in combination reduce CRC incidence and mortality.
- Multiple studies have shown extremely low population screening rates, generally <50%. Extensive public education of the community has modestly increased screening rates over the past few years.

Fecal Occult Blood Testing and Fecal Immunochemical Testing

- FIT and FOBT are relatively sensitive, but nonspecific, and are associated with minimal initial cost.[8]
- As a screening test, FOBT or FIT should be performed yearly.
  - ○ Two samples from each of three consecutive stool samples should be evaluated during FOBT.
  - ○ A restricted diet and avoidance of red meat for 3 days before testing are recommended.
  - ○ Two samples from two consecutive stools should be used for FIT.
  - ○ There is no need to rehydrate the slide because this increases the false-positive rate.
  - ○ Abnormal FIT and FOBT should be further evaluated with a colonoscopy.
  - ○ A study in the United States showed that only 30% of individuals with a positive test underwent follow-up colonoscopy.

Flexible Sigmoidoscopy

- FS is very low risk and of moderate cost, but it only examines approximately one-fourth of the colon.

- Sigmoidoscopy should be offered every 5 years when used as a screening test.
- Case-controlled studies have shown a reduced mortality rate for CRC in individuals who undergo FS; however, there is no reduction in CRC risk in the uninspected proximal colon.
- Patients having FS should have a diagnostic colonoscopy if an adenoma is identified because distal adenomas (within reach of FS) are associated with high rates of more proximal adenomas.
- Up to one-half of individuals with a proximal adenoma have no distal adenoma, raising concern about the use of FS as a screening modality.

Colonoscopy

- Colonoscopy is the most sensitive and specific test, but it involves the greatest cost and carries a small risk of complications.[9]
- Colonoscopy as a screening method should be offered every 10 years.
- It is the "preferred" screening test according to the American College of Gastroenterology.
- Studies evaluating the use of screening colonoscopy in average risk individuals are lacking. By extrapolating from the FS studies, however, it is safe to say that colonoscopy is at least as good as FS at reducing the incidence or mortality from CRC.[10]
- Colonoscopy allows examination of the entire colon, despite higher risks and cost.[10]
- Detection rates of adenomas appear to be directly related to longer times for scope withdrawal.[11]

Double Contrast Barium Enema

- DCBE can be offered every 5 years.
- No randomized trials have shown a reduction in CRC mortality with DCBE screening.
- DCBE has a lower sensitivity than colonoscopy; it must be combined with FS to offer complete colonoscopic evaluation and is generally not utilized as a CRC screening tool.
- A positive result requires follow-up with colonoscopy.

Computed Tomography Colonography

- Computed tomography colonography (CTC) is still under investigation as a screening tool.[12]
- It is anticipated that screening will be recommended every 5 years.
- CTC requires oral contrast as well as colonic catharsis. A small-caliber, flexible rectal catheter is used for colonic distension, generally with CO_2.
- The colonic preparation does allow for same-day colonoscopy if colon polyps are found.
  - Patients with large polyps (>10 mm) or multiple moderate size polyps (>6 mm) are referred for colonoscopy.
  - Colonoscopy is recommended for patients with one to two polyps between 6 and 9 mm, although some advocate enrolling those patients in a CTC surveillance program every 1 to 2 years.
  - Polyps <5 mm are not reported.
- Many factors limit CTC use for screening at this time, including lower sensitivity of detecting small polyps, cost-effectiveness, bowel preparation, risks of cumulative radiation exposure, and questions regarding management of the small polyps seen on CTC.

- Intense debate rages about the wisdom of CTC surveillance for polyps 6 to 9 mm, because polyps of this size carry a small but real risk of advanced neoplasia.
- Additionally, the issue of extracolonic findings on CTC adds to the complexity and cost of the procedure.

Fecal DNA Testing

- Recent tests have been able to detect DNA shed in the stool by CRC. Since all genetic abnormalities associated with CRC are not included in the stool DNA test, false-negative results occur.
- Studies have shown fecal DNA testing to be more sensitive than guaiac tests for cancer and advanced neoplasms.[13]
- To perform the test, a full bowel movement sample must be collected from the patients and shipped with an ice pack.
- Currently, screening with fecal DNA testing is performed every 5 years, but no standardized interval has been established.
- Hypermethylation of genes associated with CRC has led to investigation of new assays, which would detect aberrant methylation in stool as a marker for cancer.[14]

DIAGNOSIS

Clinical Presentation

History

- Most patients with colonic polyps are asymptomatic but may occasionally present with occult or overt bleeding from the gastrointestinal tract.
  - Villous adenomas >3 cm can cause a secretory diarrhea, which can lead to volume depletion and electrolyte abnormalities.
- Many adenocarcinomas are asymptomatic but may occasionally present with multiple symptoms, including abdominal pain (44%), change in bowel habit (43%), hematochezia or melena (40%), weakness (20%), anemia without other gastrointestinal symptoms (11%), or weight loss (6%).[15,16]
- Symptoms can be helpful in determining the location and extent of disease.
  - Right-sided cancers may grow and become large before producing symptoms because of the larger luminal caliber of the cecum and ascending colon. Iron-deficiency anemia is often the only manifestation of right-sided cancer.
  - Tumors in the left side of the colon may present with symptoms of partial or complete obstruction, including abdominal distention, bloating, and constipation.
  - Rectal or sigmoid cancers often cause hematochezia, constipation, or thinning of the stools. Tenesmus, melena, or weight loss may also be symptoms.
- An infection with *Streptococcus bovis* or *Clostridium septicum* also warrants evaluation of the colon because 10% to 25% of these individuals have CRC.[17]
- Consequently, new onset of hematochezia, anemia, or change in bowel habits, especially in older patients, mandates colonoscopic evaluation.

Physical Examination

- Examination of the patients should focus on confirming information obtained in the history.
  - An abdomen examination should be performed to evaluate for abdominal pain, distension, mass, and bowel sounds.

○ Signs of iron-deficiency anemia would present typically as pale conjunctiva, skin, or nail beds.
- Roughly 20% of patients have distant metastatic disease at presentation, with the most common sites being regional lymph nodes, liver, lungs, and peritoneum.[18]
  ○ Thus, right abdominal pain, abdominal distension, supraclavicular adenopathy, or periumbilical nodules would signify advance disease.

Differential Diagnosis

- Not all colorectal polyps have malignant potential, but visual inspection cannot predict polyp histology; accordingly, all visualized polyps should be removed and evaluated by surgical pathology.
- Hyperplastic polyps consist of hyperplastic mucosal proliferation and are considered to have no malignant potential.
  ○ Approximately one-third of colon polyps are hyperplastic.
  ○ A subset of large hyperplastic polyps may be premalignant and are felt to progress to carcinoma through the pathway of serrated adenomas.
- Juvenile polyps (also known as hamartomas) are tumors of the mucosa; in contrast, hyperplastic and adenomatous polyps result from epithelial proliferation.
- Other polypoid lesions in the colon can include lymphoma, carcinoid, Kaposi's sarcoma, or metastatic disease.
- Symptoms of CRC are nonspecific and other colonic diseases, including diverticulosis and inflammatory bowel disease, can present with similar symptoms of abdominal pain, hematochezia, and change in bowel habits.

Diagnostic Testing

- **Diagnostic colonoscopy** is the test of choice for identifying CRC and adenomas.
- Barium enema and CTC can suggest CRC or adenoma, but only colonoscopy allows for tissue sampling of tumors and removal of adenomatous polyps.

TREATMENT

- Most polyps found with flexible sigmoidoscopy or colonoscopy can be resected completely, using electrocautery techniques.
- Current guidelines for treatment of adenomatous polyps include complete resection by colonoscopy or surgery, when necessary.[2]

Staging

- Once CRC is diagnosed, further workup, including a chest radiograph, CT of the abdomen and pelvis, complete blood cell count, chemistry panel, and carcinoembryonic antigen level, is required to determine the extent of local and distant extent of the disease.
  ○ Magnetic resonance imaging of the liver can also be used to identify hepatic metastatic lesions.
  ○ Endoscopic ultrasound is also an available technique to evaluate the invasion and nodal status in rectal cancer.
- Previously, CRC was staged with the Dukes system (modified Astler Coller). Now, staging of cancers is done using the TNM (tumor, node, metastasis) universal system (Table 15-2), which was recently updated.

TABLE 15-2	TUMOR, NODE, METASTASIS (TNM) STAGING SYSTEM FOR COLORECTAL CANCER	
Stage	**Criteria**	**Estimated 5-yr Survival (%)**
0	Tis, N0, M0	N/A
I	T1–2, N0, M0	93
IIA	T3, N0, M0	85
IIB	T4a, N0, M0	72
IIC	T4b, N0, M0	
IIIA	T1–2, N1/N1c, M0	83
	T1, N2a, M0	
IIIB	T3–4a, N1/N1c, M0	64
	T2–3, N2a, M0	
	T1–2, N2b, M0	
IIIC	T4a, N2a, M0	44
	T3–4a, N2b, M0	
	T4b, N1–2, M0	
IVA	T(any), N(any), M1a	5–7
IVB	T(any), N(any), M1b	

TX, primary tumor cannot be assessed; T0, no evidence of primary tumor; Tis, carcinoma in situ; T1, tumor invades submucosa; T2, tumor invades muscularis propria; T3, tumor invades through the muscularis propria into pericolorectal tissues; T4a, tumor penetrates to the surface of the visceral peritoneum; T4b, tumor directly invades or is adherent to other organs or structures.

NX, regional lymph nodes cannot be assessed; N0, no metastasis in regional lymph nodes; N1, metastases in one to three regional lymph nodes (N1a, metastasis in one regional lymph node; N1b, metastasis in two to three regional lymph nodes; N1c, tumor deposit(s) in the subserosa, mesentery, or nonperitonealized pericolic or perirectal tissues without regional nodal metastasis); N2, metastases in four or more regional lymph nodes (N2a, metastasis in four to six regional lymph nodes; N2b, metastasis in seven or more regional lymph nodes).

MX, presence or absence of distant metastases cannot be determined; M0, no distant metastases detected; M1, distant metastases detected (M1a, metastasis confined to one organ or site (e.g., liver, lung, ovary, nonregional node); M1b, metastases in more than one organ per site or the peritoneum).

Surgical Management

- For patients diagnosed with CRC, the treatment of choice is surgical resection.
  - The goal of surgery is removal of the affected segment of bowel as well as surrounding lymph nodes, with the extent of resection determined by the distribution of blood vessels and lymphatic drainage.
  - For patients with rectal cancers, surgical treatment depends on the location, size, and extent of involvement.
  - Therapies include low anterior resection for upper rectal cancers. Low-lying and locally advanced rectal cancers are treated with neoadjuvant chemoradiotherapy, followed by low anterior resection.
  - Abdominoperineal resection is rarely performed in the current era.

- In patients with CRC, synchronous polyps can occur in 20% to 40% of cases and synchronous cancers in 3% to 5%; thus, preoperative colonoscopy is recommended in patients before undergoing resection.
  - If the tumor is obstructing and cannot be traversed by the colonoscope, barium enema may be performed to evaluate the proximal colon.
- Patients with obstructing metastatic cancers can have palliative resection or endoscopic stenting to prevent complete obstruction.

Chemotherapy

- Prospective studies show prolonged survival and enhanced quality of life for patients with metastatic disease who receive chemotherapy.
- Adjuvant chemotherapy usually uses 5-fluorouracil and leucovorin or capecitabine (Xeloda), which is an oral fluoropyrimidine.[19]
  - Adjuvant chemotherapy has been shown to have a survival benefit and increases the probability of remaining tumor free in patients with stage III disease.
  - Adjuvant therapy in patients with stage II disease is controversial because 5-year survival rate is 80% with or without treatment.
  - It is thought that a subgroup of these patients with high-risk prognostic factors (adherence of tumor to an adjacent organ or bowel perforation) may benefit from chemotherapy.
- Irinotecan and oxaliplatin are used in combination with fluoropyrimidines for the treatment of metastatic disease.[19]
- Targeted therapies are being developed and applied for CRC, which include cetuximab (Erbitux) and bevacizumab (Avastin).

Lifestyle/Risk Modifications

- Intense interest surrounds the issue of prevention and risk reduction with lifestyle modification and supplementation.
- Currently, calcium and aspirin have been demonstrated to reduce colorectal neoplasia risk in randomized controlled trials.[20]
- Hormone replacement therapy and estrogen, statins, nonsteroidal anti-inflammatory drugs, magnesium, vitamin B_6, folic acid, and physical activity have all been thought to be protective against CRC, but data are inconclusive.[20]
- Folic acid was evaluated in a randomized, double-blind, placebo-controlled trial for secondary prevention of adenoma with negative results. The timing of folate administration appears to be important, because folate may act as a preventive agent if given before preneoplastic lesions arise, but it may increase tumor development if given after a preneoplastic lesion exists.[21]

FOLLOW-UP

- The recommended interval for repeat surveillance colonoscopy depends on the findings on the initial examination.
- Table 15-3 lists the surveillance recommendations for patients with colorectal adenomas.[22]
- Surveillance intervals after polypectomy should be based on the number, size, and histology of polyps.
- Screening intervals for individuals at high risk because of family history is generally every 5 years, unless an inherited syndrome is suspected or confirmed.

TABLE 15-3	COLONOSCOPIC SURVEILLANCE FOR COLORECTAL POLYPS	
	Risk	Repeat Colonoscopy
One or two adenomas, <1 cm, low-grade dysplasia	Low	5–10 yr
Three or more adenomas, or any adenoma ≥1 cm, or any adenoma with villous architecture, high-grade dysplasia, or both	Moderate	3 yr
Malignant polyps, large sessile adenomas, multiple adenoma	High	Complete removal is mandatory and then revert to 3-yr surveillance Consider genetic counseling when hereditary syndrome suspected
Hyperplastic polyps (unless hyperplastic polyposis syndrome and then treated as moderate risk)	None	10 yr

- Individuals with hyperplastic polyps are not at increased risk for development of CRC, and colonoscopy every 10 years is sufficient. The exceptions are individuals felt to have hyperplastic polyposis syndrome, wherein many or large hyperplastic polyps are present. These individuals should be screened similarly to individuals with adenomas.
- Surveillance after resection of CRC is generally at 1 year, followed by 3 years, and then every 5 years if no subsequent adenomas or tumors are found.
  ○ Surveillance intervals should be modified if subsequent adenomas or cancers are found, if a family history of CRC is present, or if a hereditary cancer syndrome is suspected.
- Genetic counseling is recommended for any individual in whom a hereditary cancer syndrome is suspected. Features of hereditary cancer syndromes are outlined in the Special Considerations section.

PROGNOSIS

- At diagnosis, symptomatic patients have a worse prognosis than asymptomatic patients, with a 5-year survival rate of 49% versus 71%, respectively.[23]
- CRC survival is excellent for those with limited stage disease at the time of diagnosis (Table 15-2).[24]
- The development in the past decade of new chemotherapeutic agents has led to a significant increase in treatment options for CRC and improved survival.
- Survival of patients with advanced CRC has increased from a median survival of 10 to 12 months with fluoropyrimidines only to >20 months with combination therapy (fluropyrimidine, irinotecan, and oxaliplatin or cytotoxic chemotherapy with targeted therapy).

SPECIAL CONSIDERATIONS

Hereditary Syndromes with CRC Risk

- A number of hereditary syndromes are associated with increased CRC risk and are summarized in Table 15-1. These syndromes are addressed in more detail in Chapter 24. Management of patients with these syndromes should be multidisciplinary, including genetic counselors, gastroenterologists, and colorectal surgeons.[25]

Inflammatory Bowel Disease

- Surveillance colonoscopy is effective in reducing the mortality from CRC for patients with Crohn's colitis or ulcerative colitis.
- Risk of dysplasia is associated with duration, extent, and activity of disease; current recommendations are to perform surveillance colonoscopy every 1 to 3 years on patients with pancolitis for >8 years or left-sided colitis for >15 years.
  - Patients should have random biopsies taken every 10 cm throughout the entire colon.
- Patients with ulcerative colitis may have inflammatory polyps as well as adenomas.
  - Sporadic adenomas that are not associated with active inflammation can be managed similarly to polyps in patients without ulcerative colitis.
  - Adenomas or flat lesions with dysplasia found in the setting of active inflammation should be managed by proctocolectomy.
  - The finding of high-grade dysplasia mandates colectomy, whereas low-grade dysplasia is more controversial, with many experts also recommending colectomy.

REFERENCES

1. Jemal A, Siegel R, Xu J, et al. Cancer statistics, 2010. *CA Cancer J Clin.* 2010;60:277–300.
2. Winawer SJ, Zauber AG, Ho MN, et al. Prevention of colorectal cancer by colonoscopic polypectomy. *N Engl J Med.* 1993;329:1977–1981.
3. Correa P. Epidemiology of polyps and cancer. In: Morson B, ed. *The Pathogenesis of Colorectal Cancer.* Philadelphia, PA: WB Saunders; 1978:126–152.
4. Vogelstein B, Fearon ER, Hamilton S, et al. Genetic alterations during colorectal-tumor development. *N Engl J Med.* 1988;319:525–532.
5. Back PB, Pham HH, Schrag D, et al. Primary care physicians who treat blacks and whites. *N Engl J Med.* 2004;351:575–584.
6. Winawer SJ, Fletcher RH, Miller RH, et al. Colorectal cancer screening: clinical guidelines and rationale. *Gastroenterology.* 1997;112:594–642.
7. Burt RW. Impact on family history on screening surveillance. *Gastrointest Endosc.* 1999;49:S41–S44.
8. Lieberman, D. Colorectal cancer screening in primary care. *Gastroenterology.* 2007; 132:2591–2594.
9. Lieberman DA, Weiss DG, Bond JH, et al. Use of colonoscopy to screen asymptomatic adults for colorectal cancer. *N Engl J Med.* 2000;343:162–168.
10. Rex, DK. Colonoscopy: the dominant and preferred colorectal cancer screening strategy in the United States. *Mayo Clin Proc.* 2007;82:662–664.
11. Barclay R, Vicari JJ, Doughty AS, et al. Colonoscopic withdrawal times and adenoma detection during screening colonoscopy. *N Engl J Med.* 2006;355:2533–2541.
12. Kim DH, Pickhardt PJ, Hoff G, et al. Computed tomographic colonography for colorectal screening. *Endoscopy.* 2007;39:545–549.

13. Imperiale TF, Ransohoff DF, Itzkowitz SH, et al. Fecal DNA versus fecal occult blood for colorectal-cancer screening in an average-risk population. *N Engl J Med.* 2004;351:2704–2714.

14. Nagasaka T, Tanaka N, Cullings HM, et al. Analysis of fecal DNA methylation to detect gastrointestinal neoplasia. *J Natl Cancer Inst.* 2009;101:1244–1258.

15. Speights VO, Johnson MW, Stoltenberg PH, et al. Colorectal cancer: current trends in initial clinical manifestations. *South Med J.* 1991;84:575–578

16. Steinberg SM, Barkin JS, Kaplan RS, et al. Prognostic indicators of colon tumors. The Gastrointestinal Tumor Study Group experience. *Cancer.* 1986;57:1866–1870.

17. Panwalker AP. Unusual infections associated with colorectal cancer. *Rev Infect Dis.* 1988;10:347–364.

18. Jemal A, Siegel R, Ward E, et al. Cancer statistics, 2009. *CA Cancer J Clin.* 2009;59:225–249.

19. Meyerhardt J, Mayer R. Systemic therapy for colorectal cancer. *N Engl J Med.* 2005;352:476–487.

20. Burt RW, Winawer SJ, Bond JH, et al. *Preventing Colorectal Cancer: A Clinician's Guide.* Bethesda, MD: AGA Press; 2004.

21. Cole BF, Baron JA, Sandler RS, et al. Folic acid for the prevention of colorectal adenomas. *JAMA.* 2007;297:2351–2359.

22. Winawer SJ, Fletcher RH, Rex D, et al. Colorectal cancer screening and surveillance: clinical guidelines and rationale. *Gastroenterology.* 2003;124:544–560.

23. Beahrs OH, Sanfelippo PM. Factors in prognosis of colon and rectal cancer. *Cancer.* 1971;28:213–218.

24. O'Connell JB, Maggard MA, Ko CY. Colon cancer survival rates with the new American Joint Committee on Cancer sixth edition staging. *J Natl Cancer Inst.* 2004;96:1420–1425.

25. Rhodes M, Bradbum DM. Overview of screening and management of familial adenomatous polyposis. *Gut.* 1992;33:125–131.

Inflammatory Bowel Disease

16

Heba Iskandar and Matthew A. Ciorba

GENERAL PRINCIPLES

- In 1932, Burrill Crohn, Leon Ginzburg, and Gordon Oppenheimer first described inflammatory bowel disease (IBD) as an idiopathic disorder, which they designated *terminal ileitis*. Later descriptions included *regional enteritis* and granulomatous colitis before the eventual eponym of *Crohn's disease* was adopted.
- Understanding of IBD genetics and molecular pathophysiology continues to evolve and will likely be translated into targeted and patient-centered clinical management strategies.

Definition

- IBD is a spectrum of chronic intestinal inflammation of uncertain etiology.
- **Crohn's disease** (CD) and **ulcerative colitis** (UC) comprise the two main clinical entities and are often discussed together for ease of comparison and contrast. It is possible that CD and UC constitute a continuum of disease and manifest as varying clinical phenotypes. Microscopic colitis is also included under the umbrella of IBD.

Epidemiology

- IBD is more common in well-developed areas and is particularly prevalent in Caucasian Northern Europeans and North Americans. In North America, the prevalence of IBD is 26 to 199/100,000 for CD and 27 to 246/100,000 for UC. It is rare in Asia and South America, but observed prevalence appears to be on the rise.
- In the United States, prevalence is highest in the Jewish population, particularly in Ashkenazi Jews, followed by non-Jewish Caucasians, African Americans, Hispanics, and Asians. Prevalence is higher in urban areas and higher socioeconomic classes.
- Peak incidence occurs between ages 15 and 30 years, with a second minor peak between ages of 50 and 80 years. There is no gender specificity.

Etiology

- The precise etiology of IBD has not yet been defined. Genetic, autoimmune, and environmental factors are implicated in disease development and progression.
- A leading hypothesis suggests that IBD is the result of an overly aggressive immune response to a subset of commensal enteric bacteria in a genetically susceptible host in the presence of environmental triggers.

Pathophysiology

- Although most affected patients have no family history of IBD, first-degree relatives are five times more likely to develop the disease. Twin studies show higher concordance rates of IBD, greater in CD than in UC. Both UC and CD can occur in the same family, an observation now supported by the identification of susceptibility genes associated with both conditions.

- **Molecular characteristics of IBD.**[1,2]
  - ○ Multicenter and multinational genome wide association studies (GWAS) have identified >100 genes associated with IBD. Despite low relative risk for polymorphisms in most of these genes, important pathways in disease development are linked to these polymorphisms, including **autophagy** and **defects in handling of host–microbe interactions** by the innate and adaptive immunoregulation.
  - ○ The initial events in IBD development are linked to **aberrancies of innate immunity,** whereas the chronic state has an **overactive adaptive immune response** to commensal luminal microbiota.
  - ○ CD is associated with elevated levels of tumor necrosis factor (TNF) α, interferon γ, IL-1β, and the cytokines of the IL23-TH17 pathway. Elevated levels of TNF-α, IL-17, and cytokines of the Th-2 cells are found in UC. Several of these cytokines and pathways are targets for new or investigational therapeutics.
  - ○ The gene encoding NOD2 (an intracellular sensor of bacterial peptidoglycan important in innate immunity) is associated with CD. NOD2 polymorphisms are more common in Europeans than in African Americans or Asians. NOD2 polymorphism carrier status is linked to ileal and fibrostenosing disease phenotype. In heterozygous individuals, the risk of CD is increased up to fourfold, whereas individuals with two allelic variants have an 11- to 27-fold increase of relative risk.
  - ○ Autophagy is a process by which cells degrade and control or clear intracellular pathogens and organelles. Genes directly (ATG16L1 and IRGM) or indirectly (NOD2) involved in autophagy are associated with CD.
- Colitis is a nonspecific manifestation that can result from alterations in many genes involved in the mucosal barrier epithelium or mucosal immune system, backing up the polygenic hypothesis.
- Several lines of evidence support the importance of **gene–environment interactions** in disease development and activity. Bacteria and now viruses have been implicated as important luminal factors. Genetically susceptible mice raised in sterile conditions do not develop IBD. Antibiotics have therapeutic efficacy in some forms of IBD. In CD, surgical diversion attenuates inflammation in the gastrointestinal (GI) tract distal to the ostomy.
- So far, it is estimated that only 20% of genetic variability associated with IBD susceptibility has been identified. Multiple genes have been associated with both CD and UC, supporting the overlap between them. This novel information can lead to new directly targeted therapies for IBD.

Pathologic Features
- **Crohn's disease**
  - ○ CD can affect any portion of the luminal GI tract, from mouth to anus.
  - ○ CD is characterized by chronic, progressive, potentially **transmural inflammation** with mucosal damage and fissuring that can lead to fibrosis, strictures, fistulae, and obstruction. Early disease is characterized by inflammatory activity, whereas fibrosis and structuring are more common with long-standing disease.
  - ○ There is a sharp demarcation, both macro- and microscopically, between diseased and adjacent unaffected bowel with asymmetric and discontinuous inflammatory changes.

TABLE 16-1	MONTREAL CLASSIFICATION OF INFLAMMATORY BOWEL DISEASE			
	Crohn's Disease			**Ulcerative Colitis**
Age at Diagnosis	Location	Behavior		Extent of Disease
A1: <16 yr	L1: ileal	B1: nonstricturing, nonpenetrating		E1: ulcerative proctitis, distal to rectosigmoid junction
A2: 16–40 yr	L2: colonic	B2: structuring (fibrostenotic)		E2: left sided: distal to splenic flexure
A3: >40 yr	L3: ileocolonic	B3: penetrating (fistulizing)		E3: extensive: extending proximal to splenic flexure
	L4: upper GI disease	p: perianal disease		

L4 can be added to L1, 2, or 3 as needed.

p (perianal disease) can be added to any behavior.

- Noncaseating granulomas can be seen on histopathology.
- Roughly 80% of patients have small bowel involvement, a third with exclusively ileitis (usually with terminal ileum involvement), and one-half with ileocolitis. Approximately 20% of patients have disease limited to the colon, and about one-half of these patients have rectal sparing.
- About 7% of patients have predominant oral or gastroduodenal involvement, and even fewer patients (5%) have esophageal or proximal small bowel involvement. This can be concurrent with the ileocolonic involvement. These patients are typically younger at disease onset. About a third of patients have perianal disease, including fistula and fissures.
- Extraintestinal manifestations are common, often related to inflammatory disease activity, and are more frequent with colonic involvement.
- The Montreal classification of CD uses age at diagnosis, location, and behavior to characterize the disease. This is particularly useful for CD due to its variable phenotypes. See Table 16-1.[3]
- **Ulcerative colitis**
  - UC is a chronic, relapsing, ulceroinflammatory disease limited to the colon extending proximally from the rectum.
  - UC is a systemic disorder with frequent extraintestinal manifestations, including hepatic involvement as primary sclerosing cholangitis.
  - Lesions affect predominantly the mucosa and submucosa in a circumferential and uninterrupted distribution.
  - Well-formed granulomas and fistulae are absent in UC. Islands of regenerating mucosa protrude into the lumen to create pseudopolyps.
  - The extent of disease is the basis for the most recent Montreal classification of UC. See Table 16-1.[3]

Risk Factors

- Patients who have **first-degree relatives with IBD** have an increased risk of having IBD themselves (see *Pathophysiology*).
- **Smoking**
  - Current smokers' risk of developing UC is lower, about 40% that of non-smokers. Former smokers, however, have a 1.7 times increased risk for UC over lifetime nonsmokers.
  - Smoking is associated with a twofold increased risk of CD and increases rates of disease flares. Current smoking is associated with resistance to medical therapy.
- **Concomitant infections** (intestinal and extraintestinal) can exacerbate IBD.
- **Nonsteroidal anti-inflammatory drugs** (NSAIDs) are often cited as worsening IBD, but the data are conflicting. Short courses of cyclooxygenase 2 inhibitors (e.g., celecoxib) may be safer than nonselective NSAID in patients with UC in remission.
- Appendectomy before age 20 for appendicitis or lymphadenitis may protect against developing UC but not CD.
- Stress and psychopathology do not increase the onset of IBD, but stress may increase exacerbations of IBD possibly via activation of the enteric nervous system and elaboration of proinflammatory cytokines.
- Controversy remains as to whether oral contraceptive or isotretinoin (Accutane) use puts individuals at increased risk of IBD.

DIAGNOSIS

Clinical Presentation

- **Crohn's disease**
  - Clinical manifestations of CD are more variable than those of UC because of the transmural nature and the variability of disease locations. CD may present with GI symptoms, extraintestinal symptoms, or both.
  - Ileal and colonic CD can present with chronic diarrhea, abdominal pain, weight loss, fatigue, and fever, with or without rectal bleeding (bleeding is less common than in UC). CD patients do not uniformly have diarrhea (Table 16-2).
  - Coexistent irritable bowel syndrome can contribute to symptoms of pain and diarrhea highlighting the importance of using objective measures when determining disease activity.
  - Signs can include cachexia, abdominal tenderness or mass (most commonly in the right lower quadrant), perianal fissures, fistulas, or abscess.
  - Gastric and duodenal CD may present with nausea and vomiting, epigastric pain, or gastric outlet obstruction.
  - Oral and esophageal CD can present as oral ulcers, gum pain, dysphagia, and odynophagia.
  - A proposed **severity classification** is as follows[4]:
    - **Mild-moderate disease:** Patients are able to tolerate oral intake without signs of systemic toxicity.
    - **Moderate-severe disease:** Patients have failed therapy for mild-moderate disease, or have abdominal pain, nausea, vomiting, fevers, dehydration, anemia, or weight loss of >10%.

- **Severe-fulminant disease:** Persistent symptoms after corticosteroid therapy, or the presence of high fevers, obstruction, cachexia, surgical abdomen, or abscess formation.
- **Remission:** Asymptomatic patients who have no evidence of disease after medical or surgical intervention.

- Ulcerative colitis
  - Patients with UC can have varying symptoms and signs dictated by anatomic extent and disease severity (Table 16-2).
  - **Rectal bleeding** is much more common in UC than in CD. UC can involve mucous passage, urgency, diarrhea, or fever.
  - **Tenesmus** (the constant feeling of the need to empty the bowel with false alarms), **pain, and cramping** are common.
  - The Montreal classification of symptoms severity is helpful for determining UC management[3]:
    - **Clinical remission:** asymptomatic
    - **Mild disease:** fewer than four stools a day (may be bloody) and no signs of systemic toxicity, normal erythrocyte sedimentation rate (ESR).
    - **Moderate UC:** four to six stools per day and minimal signs of systemic toxicity
    - **Severe UC:** more than six loose stools per day, pulse rate of 90 beats per minute, higher temperatures of ≥37.5°F, hemoglobin <10.5, erythrocyte sedimentation rate ≥30
  - **Fulminant colitis** was previously used to describe >10 stools a day, continuous bleeding, and tenderness or distension and dilation on imaging but is along the continuum with severe colitis.
  - **Toxic megacolon** can develop with severe systemic manifestations in addition to fulminant colitis. Potential precipitants include opiates, electrolyte abnormalities, antimotility agents, and intercurrent infectious colitis. The colon can be dilated up to 5 to 6 cm with a precipitous decrease in bowel movement frequency; rarely, the colon may not be dilated. Complications include sepsis, hemorrhage, and perforation.

- **Extraintestinal manifestations**
  - Extraintestinal complications are frequent in both CD and UC.[5] These involve almost any organ system and contribute considerably to patient morbidity (Table 16-3).
  - Extraintestinal manifestations may parallel or be independent of intestinal disease activity. These are typically associated with UC or colonic CD.
  - The presence of one manifestation increases the likelihood of having others. Extraintestinal manifestations represent autoimmune-related processes, with antibodies against antigens shared among the colon and four common locations (skin, joints, eyes, and liver).
  - **Ankylosing spondylitis and sacroiliitis** are more common in CD than in UC. Other joint manifestations include pauciarticular, asymmetric, peripheral arthritis of the larger joints and a polyarticular, symmetric arthritis of the small joints.
  - **Osteoporosis** is common and is multifactorial in origin. Steroid use, malabsorption, low intake or absorption of dietary calcium and vitamin D, low body weight, and relative hypogonadism have all been implicated.
  - **Primary sclerosing cholangitis** (PSC) is seen in about 5% of patients with UC, more commonly than in CD. Conversely, most patients with PSC have colitis.

TABLE 16-2	COMPARISON BETWEEN CROHN'S DISEASE AND ULCERATIVE COLITIS	
	Crohn's Disease	Ulcerative Colitis
Disease location	Anywhere in GI tract; terminal ileum most common	Colon only; begins in rectum
Clinical presentation	Abdominal pain or mass (right lower quadrant), diarrhea, weight loss, vomiting, perianal disease	Rectal bleeding, diarrhea, passage of mucus, crampy pain, increased bowel movement frequency/ urgency
Endoscopy	Rectal sparing, skip lesions, aphthous ulcers, cobblestoning, linear ulceration	Rectal involvement, continuous, friability, loss of vascularity
Radiology	Small bowel and terminal ileal disease, segmental, strictures, fistulae	Colon disease, loss of haustra, continuous ulceration, no fistulae
Histology	Transmural disease, aphthous ulcers, noncaseating granulomas	Abnormal crypt architecture, superficial inflammation
HLA antigen association	HLA-A2, HLA-DR1, HLA-DQw5	HLA-DR2
IBD genes	IBD-1: NOD-2/CARD-15; IL23R	IL23R
Cigarette smoking	Increases risk development, recurrence rates and complicates treatment	Current smoking decreases risk
Appendectomy	No effect	Decreases risk (if prior to onset)
Antibiotics	Some response in colonic disease	No response
p-ANCA/ASCA	ASCA associated	p-ANCA associated
PSC	Not associated	5% develop PSC

ASCA, anti-*Saccharomyces cerevisiae* antibodies; HLA, human leukocyte antigen; IBD, inflammatory bowel disease; p-ANCA, perinuclear antineutrophil cytoplasmic antibodies; PSC, primary sclerosing cholangitis.

TABLE 16-3	EXTRAINTESTINAL MANIFESTATIONS OF INFLAMMATORY BOWEL DISEASE
Manifestation	Parallels Intestinal Disease Activity
Erythema nodosum	Yes
Pyoderma gangrenosum	Yes
Peripheral arthropathy	Yes
Episcleritis or scleritis	Yes
Anterior uveitis	No
Spondyloarthropathy (ankylosing spondylitis, sacroiliitis)	No
Osteoporosis (often steroid-induced)	No
Primary sclerosing cholangitis (usually ulcerative colitis)	No
Nephrolithiasis (usually Crohn's disease)	No
Cholelithiasis (after ileal resection)	No

- ○ Rates of both **venous and arterial thromboembolism** are increased in IBD. IBD-associated hypercoagulable state can occur both dependent and independent of disease activity.
- ○ **Nephrolithiasis** can be related to ileal CD because of the formation of oxalate stones. Fat malabsorption in CD leads to increased absorption of free dietary oxalate, which then binds to available calcium ions to form kidney stones.
- ○ Generally, manifestations that parallel disease activity are managed by intensification of intestinal IBD therapy, whereas the other conditions are treated symptomatically.

History

A careful history should be obtained to include the following:

- Epidemiology and risk factors such as smoking and family history
- Disease onset and duration and severity of current symptoms
- Presence or absence of constitutional symptoms
- Extraintestinal manifestations
- Symptoms of infections, risk factors for superimposed infections
- Quality of life, impairment of daily activities
- Prior clinical course including medication and surgical history

Physical Examination

A full physical examination should be performed.

- Vital signs should be reviewed along with weight trends.
- A careful abdominal examination is essential. The abdomen should be auscultated for high-pitched or absent bowel sounds. The abdomen may be tender in both CD and UC. Right lower quadrant tenderness and fullness is classic in CD involving the terminal ileum. A palpable mass is also more common in CD than in UC. Peritoneal signs are concerning for an intestinal perforation.

- A rectal and perianal examination should be performed for evaluating skin tags, anal fissures, and fistulae or abscesses that would suggest CD rather than UC. Gross or occult blood on the examining finger may indicate active disease.
- Skin, joint, and eye examinations should also be performed to evaluate for the presence of extraintestinal manifestations (Table 16-3).

Differential Diagnosis

- The differential diagnosis of IBD is extensive (Table 16-4) and includes infectious as well as noninfectious causes. Chronic symptoms of 3 months or longer are suggestive of IBD.

TABLE 16-4	DIFFERENTIAL DIAGNOSIS OF INFLAMMATORY BOWEL DISEASE

Infectious Etiologies

Bacterial	Mycobacterial	Viral
Salmonella	Tuberculosis	Cytomegalovirus
Shigella	Mycobacterium avium	Herpes simplex
Toxigenic Escherichia coli	**Parasitic**	HIV
Campylobacter	Amebiasis	**Fungal**
Yersinia	Isospora	Histoplasmosis
Clostridium difficile	Trichuris trichura	Candida
Gonorrhea	Hookworm	Aspergillus
Chlamydia trachomatis	Strongyloides	

Noninfectious Etiologies

Inflammatory	Neoplastic	Drugs and Chemicals
Appendicitis	Lymphoma	NSAID
Diverticulitis	Metastatic carcinoma	Phosphosoda
Diversion colitis	Carcinoma of the ileum	Cathartic colon
Collagenous/Lymphocytic colitis	Carcinoid	Gold
	Familial polyposis	Oral contraceptives
Ischemic colitis		Cocaine
Radiation colitis/enteritis		Chemotherapy
Eosinophilic gastroenteritis		
Neutropenic colitis		
Behçet's syndrome		
Graft-versus-host disease		

HIV, human immunodeficiency virus; NSAID, nonsteroidal anti-inflammatory drug.

- At initial presentation and during exacerbations, it is important to rule out infectious disease. *Salmonella, Shigella, Campylobacter, Aeromonas, Escherichia coli* 0157:H7, *Clostridium difficile,* and sexually transmitted diseases can all cause bloody diarrhea.
- Findings suggestive of CD include rectal sparing; small bowel involvement; absence of gross bleeding; presence of perianal disease; and the presence of skip lesions, granulomas, or fistula (Table 16-3).
- In about 10% to 15% of patients with colonic IBD, the distinction between CD and UC cannot be made, and these are termed **inflammatory bowel disease, type unclassified (IBDU). Indeterminate colitis** is reserved for whom pathologic diagnosis cannot be made even after colectomy and full examination of the colon. In the future, combined genetic and serologic markers may assist in distinguishing CD and UC.[4]

Diagnostic Testing

- The diagnosis of IBD is made with a combination of clinical, laboratory, radiographic, endoscopic, and pathologic findings.

Laboratory Tests

- Laboratory tests can help support, but not confirm, the diagnosis in clinical presentations consistent with IBD.
- Evaluation should include a **complete blood cell** count to assess for anemia and leukocytosis. A **complete metabolic panel** evaluates for electrolyte and metabolic abnormalities related to IBD.
- Elevated levels of **C-reactive protein** are nonspecific but are observed in active IBD. This is generally higher in CD than in UC.
- **Stool studies** (*C. difficile,* culture, ova, and parasites) should be sent to evaluate for superimposed infections that may mimic IBD. Some clinicians use fecal calprotectin or lactoferrin to distinguish inflammatory from noninflammatory diarrhea.
- **Autoantibodies** have been detected in IBD patients. The two most commonly used antibody tests are **antineutrophil cytoplasmic antibodies (p-ANCA),** which is more common in UC, and **anti-*Saccharomyces cerevisiae* antibodies (ASCA),** which along with **anti-Omp C antibody and antibody against CBir1 flagellin,** are more common in CD. Combination serologic testing is available commercially and is used by some physicians to distinguish between CD and UC.

Imaging

- A **plain abdominal radiograph** is helpful in the acute setting to evaluate for toxic megacolon or bowel obstruction.
- **Small bowel follow-through** x-ray series can provide evaluation of the small bowel in CD. Typical features are luminal narrowing with "string" sign, nodularity and ulceration, a "cobblestone" appearance, and fistulae or abscess formation.
- **Air contrast barium enema** may be used to confirm the anatomic pattern and extent of disease in UC and Crohn's colitis. Barium studies may be normal despite endoscopically evident mild disease. Barium enema must be avoided in severely ill patients because of the risk of precipitating ileus with toxic megacolon.
- **Computed tomography** and **magnetic resonance enterography** are useful in evaluating specific complications (e.g., abscesses, strictures, and fistulas). Magnetic resonance enterography has the advantage of avoiding radiation

exposure and has become an imaging modality of choice at many institutions for nonemergent evaluations.

Diagnostic Procedures

- **Colonoscopy with ileoscopy and biopsy** can usually differentiate CD, UC, and disorders that mimic IBD. Colonoscopy assesses disease location, extent, and severity to confirm IBD diagnosis, obtains tissue for histologic evaluation, and assesses response to therapy.
  - Endoscopic features common to both CD and UC include pseudopolyps, loss of haustral folds, fibrotic strictures, and linear superficial scars.
  - In CD, specific endoscopic features include discrete aphthous ulcers, "cobblestoning" (formed by deep linear ulcers), discontinuous "skip" lesions, rectal sparing, and involvement of the terminal ileum.
  - In UC, endoscopy shows contiguous and circumferential involvement, beginning at the anal verge and extending proximally to a transition to normal mucosa. Erythema, loss of the fine vascular pattern, mucosal granularity, friability, and edema are seen.
  - On histopathology, aphthoid ulcers, focal crypt abscesses, and chronic transmural inflammatory infiltrates can be seen only in CD. **Noncaseating granulomas** are pathognomonic for CD but are seen in only <50% of biopsies.
  - Continuous, diffuse inflammatory infiltrate confined to the mucosa and submucosa, cryptitis, and crypt abscesses are common in UC.
- Complete colonoscopy is typically not performed in patients with severe colitis or toxic megacolon because of the increased risk of perforation. Flexible sigmoidoscopy is often performed in these circumstances to rule out a complicating superinfection with *C. difficile* or cytomegalovirus.
- **Capsule endoscopy** can be useful in diagnosing CD of the small bowel when diseased areas cannot be reached by endoscopy, but risk of intestinal obstruction exists if the capsule lodges in a tight stricture. The use of a **"patency capsule"** prior to the capsule endoscopy may help avert this complication; many centers obtain a barium small bowel follow-through series prior to a capsule study.

TREATMENT

Medications

- Medical therapy for both CD and UC includes induction and maintenance phases of therapy.[6,7]
- Choice of treatment modality takes disease location or extent, severity, complications, and extraintestinal manifestations into consideration.
- Initiation of immunosuppressant or immunomodulator therapy requires ruling out any superimposed infections.
- *5-Aminosalicylic acid compounds*
  - 5-Aminosalicylic acid (5-ASA) drugs are used for induction and maintenance of remission in mild to moderate IBD. In CD, they may have modest efficacy in delaying postoperative recurrence or treating colonic disease.
  - Available formulations in the United States are **mesalamine** (Pentasa, Asacol, Asacol HD, Apriso, Lialda), **sulfasalazine**, and **balsalazide** (Colazal), as well as **rectal mesalamine** (Canasa, Rowasa). These formulations differ in the mechanism of release of 5-ASA (Table 16-5).

TABLE 16-5 5-AMINOSALYCYLIC ACID THERAPIES

5-ASA Compound	Indication	Dosage
Diffusion dependent[a]		
Mesalamine controlled release (Pentasa)	Proximal disease Severe diarrhea (release not affected by rapid transit) Strictures Pouchitis Postoperative anastomosis	Pentasa = 2.4–4.8 g
pH dependent[b]		
Mesalamine delayed-release (Asacol) MMX (multimatrix) mesalamine (Lialda) Mesalamine delayed and extended release (Apriso)	Ileocolonic disease	Asacol = 2.4–4.8 g daily in divided doses. Asacol as 400 mg tablets; Asacol HD as 800 mg tablets Lialda = 1.2 g tablet (once-daily dosing as 2–4 tablets for a 2.4–4.8 g daily dose) Apriso = 1.5 g (0.375 g capsules, 4 capsules once daily)
Colonic bacteria dependent		
Sulfasalazine (Azulfidine)	Colonic disease (bacteria required to cleave azo-bond)	Sulfasalazine = 2–6 g daily in divided doses, usually TID
Balsalazide (Colazal) Diazo compound with 5-ASA bonded to the sulfonamide sulfapyridine (sulfasalazine) or inert carrier (balsalazide)	Universal and distal UC Colonic CD Arthropathy	Balsalazide = 6.75–13.5 g
Directly acting (topical)		
Mesalamine suppositories (Canasa) Mesalamine enema (Rowasa)	Left-sided colitis and proctitis	Canasa = 500 mg Rowasa = 4 g

CD, Crohn's disease; UC, ulcerative colitis.

[a]Timed release begins in the upper small intestine, continues through the colon.

[b]Released at pH 6–7 in terminal ileum/colon. Of note 2.4 g mesalamine = 6 g sulfasalazine = 6.75 g balsalazide.

○ Therapeutic effects of sulfasalazine are derived primarily from the 5-ASA moiety, whereas side effects are mostly caused by its sulfa moiety. Nausea, vomiting, malaise, anorexia, and headache are dose related, whereas hypersensitivity reactions (rash, fever, hemolytic anemia, agranulocytosis, hepatitis, pancreatitis, and worsening of colitis) are idiosyncratic. Nonsulfa 5-ASA derivatives are better tolerated than sulfasalazine and can be escalated to higher doses of 5-ASA.

○ In patients with colonic disease and associated peripheral arthropathy, sulfasalazine has benefit as a disease-modifying antirheumatic drug.

○ Other potential side effects of all 5-ASA drugs are diarrhea and abdominal pain. These drugs are safe in pregnancy. 5-ASA drugs should be used with caution in patients with salicylate or sulfa allergy.

○ There are reports of nephrotoxicity from interstitial nephritis with 5-ASA compounds. This is more frequent in the first year of therapy but can occur at any time. Serum creatinine level is usually measured before and monitored during treatment.

○ Topical rectal therapies are useful in induction and maintenance for ulcerative proctitis. These agents provide added benefit to orally administered 5-ASA preparations in the treatment of more extensive colitis.

○ Once remission is achieved, lower doses of sulfasalazine (2 g daily) or mesalamine (2.4 g daily) may maintain remission in UC or potentially reduce postoperative relapse rates in CD.

○ Maintenance 5-ASA treatment has been shown to reduce risk of developing colorectal cancer.

• *Antibiotics*
  ▪ Although a specific causative microorganism has not been identified in IBD, antibiotics have a role in disease therapy.
  ○ **Antibiotic use in Crohn's disease:**
  ▪ **Metronidazole** (10 or 20 mg/kg/day) **with or without ciprofloxacin** (500 mg PO BID) may be useful in the treatment of mildly active luminal CD.
  ▪ Metronidazole, ciprofloxacin, tetracycline, or combinations thereof are often used for extended periods in CD patients who have fistulas, abscesses, or perianal disease.
  ▪ Antibiotics are indicated for bacterial overgrowth, seen with small bowel strictures or after ileocolic resection.
  ▪ **Patients taking long-term metronidazole need to be monitored closely for peripheral neuropathy,** which can be irreversible. Ciprofloxacin use has been associated with tendon inflammation and/or rupture, especially in patients using concurrent steroids, age >60 years, or organ transplant recipients.
  ○ **Antibiotic use in ulcerative colitis:**
  ▪ In fulminant colitis, antibiotics reduce the risk of bacterial translocation. Otherwise, antibiotics do not have a role in the management of UC.

• *Corticosteroids*
  ○ **In UC and CD:**
  ▪ Corticosteroids have long been **used to induce remission** in moderate to severe IBD, and to treat patients who have active disease despite other simpler therapies (e.g., 5-ASA).
  ▪ Steroids are **ineffective in *maintaining* remission or *preventing* relapse,** and their use should be limited, given their numerous side effects.
  ▪ Superimposed infections, such as cytomegalovirus or *C. difficile,* and complications, including toxic megacolon or perforation, must be considered before starting steroids.

- Both **oral prednisone** (40 to 60 mg daily) and **intravenous methylprednisolone** (40 to 60 mg daily) induce remission in patients with active disease compared with placebo. Doses are typically tapered (about 5 mg/week) when a clinical response has been achieved. Tapers should be slow (over 2 to 3 months), as rapid tapers lead to return of symptoms.
- As >50% of patients treated acutely with steroids become steroid dependent or refractory, a maintenance strategy (such as an immunomodulator or a biologic agent) needs to be considered when initiating steroids.

○ In Crohn's disease:
- **Budesonide** (up to 9 mg daily) is a controlled-release corticosteroid with high local potency and lower systemic activity due to high first-pass hepatic metabolism. It is an alternative to prednisone in patients with distal small bowel disease and may reduce systemic side effects.

○ In ulcerative colitis:
- **Steroid enemas** (e.g., Cortenema) **or foams** (e.g., Cortifoam or Proctofoam) can be used to treat rectal disease.
- If tapering leads to a return of symptoms despite 5-ASA treatment, an immunomodulator or biologic should be considered.

- *Immunomodulator therapy*
  ○ Oral **azathioprine** (AZA, 2.5 to 3 mg/kg/day) and its metabolite **6-mercaptopurine** (6-MP; 1.5 mg/kg/day) are used to achieve maintenance of steroid-free remission in CD and UC, especially with recurrent disease flares as steroid-sparing agents.
  ○ In CD, these agents have a role in fistulous CD and perianal disease and in preventing postoperative relapses.
  ○ Onset of action is generally delayed for as long as 8 to 12 weeks, and full therapeutic effect can take 3 to 6 months of continued use. Time to efficacy can be shortened by starting at full-weight–based dose rather than using a titration approach.
  ○ Side effects of thiopurines:
    - Bone marrow suppression (including granulocytosis), pancreatitis, allergic reactions, hepatitis, and life-threatening infections have been reported but are usually reversible on discontinuation of therapy. Allergic symptoms, such as joint aches, fevers, nausea, and malaise, typically occur within the first 1 to 2 weeks of use; pancreatitis occurs around week 3 and leukopenia by week 4.
    - Susceptibility to early, severe leukopenia can be predicted before initiation by measuring **thiopurine *S*-methyltransferase** (**TPMT**) enzyme activity. TPMT is responsible for drug metabolism. However, TPMT testing does not substitute for monitoring blood counts. 6-MP and AZA should be avoided in patients with very low TPMT activity, and the starting dose should be lowered with intermediate activity. See Chapter 24 for further discussion.
    - **Blood counts should be followed every 7 to 10 days the first 4 weeks and after dose increases.** Once the goal dose has been reached, a complete blood cell count should be checked every 3 months. If the leukocyte count falls below 3000 cells/μL, the dose should be lowered or held.
    - An increased risk of lymphoma is reported with azathioprine or 6-MP, but the overall absolute risk still remains quite low. The risk of hepatosplenic T-cell lymphoma in young men is modestly elevated when used concurrently with anti-TNF agents.
    - Although controversial, experts feel the risk of harm to a developing fetus is low. Since active disease is associated with poor fetal outcomes,

the risks and benefits of discontinuing therapy during pregnancy should be carefully considered.

○ **Monitoring response to therapy.**

■ 6-Thioguanine nucleotide (6-TGN), the active metabolite of 6-MP, can be checked to assess for adequate therapeutic levels of the medications. Low 6-TGN levels can indicate underdosing, high metabolism, or nonadherence. Adequate levels of 6-TGN without a clinical response may indicate the need to change to other therapies.[8]

■ The second metabolite that is measured is 6-MMP, which is inactive. Patients who preferentially produce large amounts of 6-MMP can be given allopurinol to shift the metabolism toward increased production of 6-TGN. The addition of allopurinol is accompanied by a decrease in the dose of the immunomodulator to 25% of the original dose due to drug–drug interactions. If this technique is used, close monitoring of blood counts is obligatory.

○ **CD-specific immunomodulators.**

■ Subcutaneous or intramuscular **methotrexate** (25 mg weekly) is more effective than placebo in inducing remission in patients with severe CD, with trials showing an effective dose for maintenance of remission at 15 mg weekly. Current evidence is insufficient to support the use of methotrexate for UC.

○ **UC-specific immunomodulators:**

■ **Intravenous cyclosporine** (2 to 4 mg/kg/day) has been shown effective in fulminant UC, but side effects include grand mal seizures, opportunistic infection, and bowel perforation. Cyclosporine probably has little role in most cases of CD.

○ The roles of **tacrolimus and mycophenolate mofetil** in IBD therapy require further study.

• *Biologic (antibody-based) therapy*

○ TNF-α is an important cytokine in the pathogenesis of both CD and UC. Three **monoclonal antibodies against TNF** are used in CD therapy: infliximab, adalimumab, and certolizumab. Only infliximab is currently approved for therapy of UC, though trials with adalimumab met clinical endpoints, and FDA approval is anticipated for use in UC (Table 16-6).[9–15]

○ **Considerations with biologic therapy:**

■ A recent randomized trial study of biologic and immunomodulator-naive patients with CD suggests a benefit to combination therapy with infliximab and AZA for maintenance, when evaluated at 26 and 50 weeks, as compared with infliximab or AZA alone (SONIC trial).[16] Whether this concept extends to other biologics is not yet known.

■ Clinical experience with infliximab and adalimumab demonstrates that increases in dosing or dose frequency are sometimes required to maintain therapeutic effect.

○ **Important side effects:**

■ Acute infusion reactions and delayed-type hypersensitivity reactions are more common with repeat infusions of infliximab, especially after a prolonged interval since the previous infusion (over 12 weeks). Development of human antichimeric antibodies, often referred to as antibodies to infliximab, occur in 10% to 15% of cases and are associated with decreased efficacy.

■ Reactivation of latent tuberculosis can occur; therefore, a purified protein-derivative skin test must be placed and confirmed negative before therapy. Congestive heart failure has also been reported. Because of reports of

TABLE 16-6 BIOLOGIC THERAPY IN INFLAMMATORY BOWEL DISEASE

Name (Trade Name)	Target	Route	Dosing	Indications	Representative Trials
Infliximab (Remicade)	TNF (chimeric monoclonal Ab)	IV infusion	5–10 mg/kg body weight over 2 hr at weeks 0, 2, and 6 and then every 8 wk for maintenance	CD (luminal and fistulizing), UC	CD: ACCENT 1[9] UC: ACT 1 and ACT 2[10]
Adalimumab (Humira)	TNF (human Ab)	Subcutaneous	160 mg → 80 mg → 40 mg (weeks 0, 2 and then every week)	CD (luminal), likely UC in the future	Induction: CLASSIC I[11] Maintenance: CHARM[12]
Certolizumab (Cimzia)	TNF (PEGylated Fab' fragment of humanized Ab)	Subcutaneous	400 mg at weeks 0, 2, and 4 and then every 4 wk	CD (luminal)	Induction: PRECISE 1[13] Maintenance: PRECISE 2[14]
Natalizumab (Tysabri)	α₄-Integrin (selective adhesion molecule humanized IgG4 monoclonal Ab)	IV infusion	300 mg every 4 wk	CD (luminal)	ENCORE[15]

Ab, antibody; CD, Crohn's disease; IV, intravenous; UC, ulcerative colitis.

disseminated histoplasmosis, a chest radiograph can be considered in endemic areas to assess for granulomatous disease. Other mild and self-limited side effects include headache, upper respiratory infection, and nausea.

- Side effects of subcutaneously administered biologic agents include injection site reactions or pain. Other side effects, including risk for infections and lymphoma, are similar in all biologic categories.
- Natalizumab has been associated with progressive multifocal leukoencephalopathy in clinical trials. Its use is reserved for patients who have failed all other CD therapies.

○ There are multiple novel biologics currently being developed for CD. These new therapies utilize unique targets based on modern understanding of CD genetics and pathogenesis.

- *Antidiarrheal agents*
  ○ Antidiarrheal agents, such as **loperamide** (Imodium), **codeine**, or **tincture of opium** may decrease the frequency and volume of diarrhea.
  ○ These agents should be withheld if intestinal infection or severely active disease is suspected because of the risk of toxic megacolon.

Surgical Management

- **Crohn's disease**
  ○ Surgical management is often necessary for certain complications, including intractable hemorrhage, perforation, persistent obstruction from stricturing disease, abscess, or disease activity intractable to medical therapy. Abscesses often require drainage under radiographic guidance or with surgery.
  ○ Surgical resection is **not curative** in CD, with clinical recurrence rates of 10% to 15% annually. Postoperative management with immunomodulators, metronidazole, or mesalamine may lower recurrence rates. Recent studies suggest that anti-TNF therapy may also be very effective.[17]
  ○ Smoking increases recurrence rates.
  ○ **Suppurative perianal disease** is often treated surgically with the placement of **a noncutting seton** (silastic band).
  ○ **Therapeutic options for strictures** include strictureplasty, endoscopic balloon dilation, and local injection of steroids or biologic glues. All strictures should be biopsied to exclude malignancy.

- **Ulcerative colitis**
  ○ Medically refractory disease activity is the most common reason for surgery in UC. Less commonly, total colectomy is required for acutely ill patients with megacolon or systemic toxicity not responding to medical therapy within 48 hours.
  ○ **Proctocolectomy or colectomy with rectal preservation is curative** in UC. The mortality of colectomy is low even in severe cases. Advances in surgical technique allow for the creation of an ileal pouch–anal anastomosis, and a permanent ileostomy is typically not required.[18]
  ○ **Pouchitis,** or inflammation of the surgically created ileal reservoir, is the most common complication of this surgery and occurs at least in a mild form in ~50% of the population. Symptoms include increased stool frequency, urgency, hematochezia, abdominal pain, and fever, but the diagnosis is made endoscopically and histologically. First-line therapy is typically with **antibiotics** (metronidazole or ciprofloxacin); **probiotics** (such as VSL#3) may be useful for prevention. Recurrent or refractory pouchitis may represent misdiagnosed CD,

which is typically confirmed when significant inflammation is identified prox-imal to the pouch. Pouch excision is required in 5% of patients.

○ **Cuffitis** is an inflammation due to a short section of retained rectal mucosa and is treated with topical steroids or 5-ASA suppositories.

Lifestyle/Risk Modification

Diet, Nutrition, and Complementary Therapies

• No dietary factors have been shown to either cause or cure IBD. On an indi-vidual basis, certain foods may trigger symptomatic exacerbations and may need avoidance.

• In stricturing disease, a **low-residue diet** (avoidance of pulps, peels, and whole leaf vegetables) is recommended to avoid obstruction.

• Maintenance of adequate nutrition is essential in the care of CD patients. Approximately, 75% of CD patients admitted to the hospital are malnourished.

• **Nutritional deficiencies** are typically related to decreased oral intake, malab-sorption, and blood loss. Vitamin and nutrient supplementation may be needed after small bowel resection or in the setting of extensive bowel involvement. For example, patients with ileitis may need vitamin B_{12} supplementation.

○ Common deficiencies in CD include vitamins B_{12}, A, and D, calcium, potas-sium, iron, and zinc. In UC, common deficiencies are folate, vitamin D, and iron, and less commonly vitamin B_{12}. Levels should be measured. Repletion and prophylactic supplementation may be beneficial.

• To meet nutritional needs, **enteral feeding** is generally preferable to parenteral [total parenteral nutrition (TPN)]. In certain refractory situations, TPN is effi-cacious in refractory CD when used in conjunction with bowel rest and medi-cal therapy. In these instances, discontinuation of TPN may be associated with high relapse rates.

• Some **probiotics** have shown efficacy in maintenance of remission in UC (VSL#3, *E. coli* Nissle). They also have a role in the treatment of pouchitis (VSL#3). The evidence for the effective use of probiotics in CD is poor.

SPECIAL CONSIDERATIONS

• **Pregnancy in IBD**
  ○ Pregnancy has been associated with both improvement and worsening of dis-ease activity.[19]
  ○ High disease activity is associated with poor fetal outcomes, mainly preterm delivery. Thus, achieving remission prior to conception is optimal.
  ○ Medical therapy of IBD in pregnancy should be addressed by a gastroenter-ologists and obstetricians experienced with such care. The risk to benefit ratio for biologic or immunomodulator therapy should be considered.
  ○ Systemic steroids should be avoided in the first trimester but may be the therapy of choice in the third trimester. Methotrexate is a known teratogen.

• **Microscopic colitis**
  ○ Microscopic colitis (MC) consists of a group of diseases characterized by chronic, watery, nonbloody diarrhea, with largely normal endoscopic find-ings. MC is less common than CD and UC.
  ○ The two main types of MC are **collagenous colitis** and **lymphocytic colitis**, although mixed forms and variants have also been described. On histology, a

thickened subepithelial collagenous band is seen with collagenous colitis. Lymphocytic colitis is marked by a subepithelial lymphocytic infiltrate.

○ Etiology is unknown, and it is doubtful that a single pathogenetic mechanism exists.

○ Collagenous colitis has a female-to-male predominance of 9 to 15:1, whereas lymphocytic colitis has equal incidence in both genders. Onset typically occurs after age 50.

○ Collagenous colitis may be caused by abnormal collagen metabolism, particularly reduced matrix degradation rather than enhanced synthesis. Vascular endothelial growth factor may play a role in this collagen balance. Celiac disease, bacterial toxins, NSAIDs, selective serotonin reuptake inhibitors, and other drugs have been linked to the development of MC.

○ The **clinical presentation** of collagenous and lymphocytic colitis consists of progressively increasing watery diarrhea that is often refractory to over-the-counter antidiarrheal medications. Associated symptoms can include nausea, abdominal pain, and fecal urgency. Many patients have a diagnosis of a diarrhea predominant irritable bowel syndrome until colonic pathology is examined, stressing the importance of colonoscopy and random biopsies of normal appearing mucosa.

○ Although the disease course is generally benign, relapsing and remitting symptoms can be debilitating. Patients should be reassured that MC is not associated with increased mortality or an increased risk of developing colorectal cancer. NSAIDs or other drugs associated with MC should be discontinued if possible. Patients should be tested for celiac disease.

○ **Antidiarrheal agents,** such as loperamide and lomotil, can be first tried. Most cases referred to a gastroenterologist lead to a trial of **budesonide** (9 mg daily for a month, followed by a taper over next 2 months). Bismuth subsalicylate, cholestyramine, and mesalamine products are effective in some patients. In refractory cases, immunomodulators, systemic corticosteroids, and even biologic-based therapy have been tried.

REFERRAL

With advances in newer biologic therapies as well as improved understanding of existing medications, treatment of moderate or severe IBD is best orchestrated by physicians with significant experience in IBD management or in specialized centers focusing on IBD.

MONITORING/FOLLOW-UP

• **Response to therapy.**
  ○ In addition to symptomatic improvement, mucosal healing is an important endpoint, as it can indicate better long-term outcomes, including decreased rates of hospitalization and surgical resections. Routine endoscopy with biopsies is recommended.
• **Osteoporosis**
  ○ Osteoporosis is a source of significant morbidity, impaired quality of life, and costs in IBD.

- IBD itself only modestly lowers bone mineral density but increases the risk of fractures by 40% over the general population.
- Bone densitometry (DEXA) scan to read (DEXA scan) is indicated in all postmenopausal women and those with exposure to corticosteroids.
- Other useful tests include an alkaline phosphatase, calcium level (corrected for serum albumin), creatinine, testosterone level (males), and 25-OH-vitamin D level.
- All patients should be educated about the importance of regular weight-bearing exercise and avoiding smoking and excessive alcohol intake.
- Adequate intake of vitamin D (800 IU daily) and calcium (1000 to 1500 mg daily) is recommended.
- Bisphosphonates are used in patients at highest risk for fractures.

- **Malignancy**
  - Patients with UC and colonic CD are at increased risk for **colorectal cancer (CRC)** compared with the general population (see also Chapter 15). The level of risk is related to the duration, severity, and colonic extent of inflammation. Risks are higher with a family history of CRC. Because CRC is generally preceded by dysplasia, surveillance is recommended to detect and intervene when dysplasia is found.[20]
  - In patients with UC and pancolitis, CRC risk seems to increase after 8 to 10 years of symptoms. The cumulative incidence of CRC in UC is 5% to 10% after 20 years and 12% to 20% after 30 years of disease, although recent studies report lower incidences.
  - For left-sided colitis, CRC risk may increase after 15 to 20 years. Distal colitis and proctosigmoiditis probably do not increase the risk of CRC. Patients with UC with PSC have an even higher increased risk for developing CRC.
  - Surveillance colonoscopy with random biopsies is recommended beginning after 8 years of pancolitis and after 15 years of left-sided colitis and then repeated every 1 to 2 years thereafter. No screening is recommended for ulcerative proctitis.
  - Patients with an ileal pouch should undergo flexible sigmoidoscopy with biopsies every other year.
  - Colectomy is generally recommended for carcinoma, high-grade dysplasia, and multifocal low-grade dysplasia.
  - In CD, patients with long-standing colitis or age >30 years at diagnosis are at greatest risk. Recommended surveillance strategies are similar to those for UC.

- **Other health-maintenance issues.**[21]
  - IBD patients on immunomodulators and biologic therapy should be up to date in **vaccinations against preventable illnesses.** Considerations include hepatitis A/B, yearly *influenza, pneumococcus, meningococcus,* tetanus. After immunosuppressive therapy has begun, live-attenuated vaccines should be avoided.
  - Pap smears should also be performed regularly, as there is an increased risk of abnormal pap smears with thiopurine therapy. Vaccination against malignancy-associated human papillomavirus (Gardasil) should be offered.

OUTCOME/PROGNOSIS

- Both CD and UC are chronic diseases with intermittent exacerbations of mild to severe symptoms alternating with periods of varying levels of remission.
- About 10% to 20% of patients with CD will experience a very prolonged remission after initial presentation. Conversely, predictors of a severe course

include age <40 years, presence of perianal disease, initial requirement of corticosteroids, and perforating disease. CD can be associated with a modest decrease in overall life expectancy.

- The course of UC depends on extent of disease. Proctitis and distal colitis usually have a more benign course, resolving spontaneously in about 20% of cases.
- In UC, increased relapse rates are seen in younger patients (ages 20–30 years), older patients (>70 years), women, those with more than five prior relapses, and those with basal plasmacytosis on rectal biopsy. Approximately 30% undergo colectomy after 15 to 25 years of disease. Overall mortality is only slightly increased compared with the general population.

REFERENCES

1. Abraham C, Cho JH. Inflammatory bowel disease. *N Engl J Med.* 2009;361:2066–2078.
2. Xavier RJ, Podolsky DK. Unravelling the pathogenesis of inflammatory bowel disease. *Nature.* 2007;448:427–434.
3. Sastagni J, Silverberg MS, Vermeire S, et al. The Montreal classification of inflammatory bowel disease: controversies, consensus, and implications. *Gut.* 2006;55:749–753.
4. Talley NJ, Abreu MT, Achkar JP, et al. An evidence-based systematic review on medical therapies for inflammatory bowel disease. *Am J Gastroenterol.* 2011;106(suppl 1):S2–25
5. Rothfuss KS, Stange EF, Herrlinger KR. Extraintestinal manifestations and complications in inflammatory bowel diseases *World J Gastroenterol.* 2006;12:4819–4831.
6. Lichtenstein GR, Abreu MT, Cohen R, et al. American Gastroenterological Association Institute medical position statement on corticosteroids, immunomodulators, and infliximab in inflammatory bowel disease. *Gastroenterology.* 2006;130:935–939.
7. Kornbluth A, Sachar DB. Ulcerative colitis practice guidelines in adults: American College of Gastroenterology, Practice Parameters Committee. *Am J Gastroenterol.* 2010; 105:501–523.
8. Ha C, Dassopoulos T. Thiopurine therapy in inflammatory bowel disease. *Expert Rev Gastroenterol Hepatol.* 2010;4:575–588.
9. Hanauer SB, Feagan BG, Lichtenstein GR, et al. Maintenance infliximab for Crohn's disease: the ACCENT I randomised trial. *Lancet.* 2002;359:1541–1549.
10. Rutgeerts P, Sandborn WJ, Feagan BG, et al. Infliximab for induction and maintenance therapy for ulcerative colitis. *N Engl J Med.* 2005;353:2462–2476.
11. Hanauer SB, Sandborn WJ, Rutgeerts P, et al. Human anti-tumor necrosis factor monoclonal antibody (adalimumab) in Crohn's disease: the CLASSIC-I trial. *Gastroenterology.* 2006;130:323–333.
12. Colombel JF, Sandborn WJ, Rutgeerts P, et al. Adalimumab for maintenance of clinical response and remission in patients with Crohn's disease: the CHARM trial. *Gastroenterology.* 2007;132:52–65.
13. Sandborn WJ, Feagan BG, Stoinov S, et al. Certolizumab pegol for the treatment of Crohn's disease. *N Engl J Med.* 2007;357:228–238.
14. Schreiber S, Khaliq-Kareemi M, Lawrance IC, et al. Maintenance therapy with certolizumab pegol for Crohn's disease. *N Engl J Med.* 2007;357:239–250.
15. Targan SR, Feagan BG, Fedorak RN, et al. Natalizumab for the treatment of active Crohn's disease: results of the ENCORE Trial. *Gastroenterology.* 2007;132:1672–1683.
16. Colombel JF, Sandborn WJ, Reinisch W, et al. Infliximab, azathioprine, or combination therapy for Crohn's disease. *N Engl J Med.* 2010;362:1383–1395.
17. Fichera A, Michelassi F. Surgical treatment of Crohn's disease. *J Gastrointest Surg.* 2007;11: 791–803.
18. McLaughlin SD, Clark SK, Tekkis PP, et al. Review article: restorative proctocolectomy, indications, management of complications and follow-up—a guide for gastroenterologists. *Aliment Pharmacol Ther.* 2008;27:895–909.

19. Dubinsky M, Abraham B, Mahadevan U. Management of the pregnant IBD patient. *Inflamm Bowel Dis.* 2008;14:1736–1750.
20. McCabe RP, Dassopoulos T, Lewis J, et al. AGA medical position statement on the diagnosis and management of colorectal neoplasia in inflammatory bowel disease. *Gastroenterology.* 2010;138:738–745.
21. Moscandrew M, Manadevan U, Kane S. General health maintenance in IBD. *Inflamm Bowel Dis.* 2009;15:1399–1409.

Irritable Bowel Syndrome

17

Benjamin E. Cassell and Gregory S. Sayuk

GENERAL PRINCIPLES

Background and Definition

- The functional gastrointestinal disorders (FGIDs) are a group of chronic or recurrent conditions wherein alterations in bowel sensitivity, motility, or both are predominant manifestations.
- These commonly encountered conditions impose substantial burdens on patient well-being and, in turn, account for large portion of visits to both primary care physicians and gastroenterologists.
- FGIDs represent a complex interface between abnormal GI motility, visceral hypersensitivity, altered central nervous system (CNS) processing of peripheral stimuli, as well as psychosocial factors.
- Importantly, by definition, FGIDs lack identifiable structural abnormalities on diagnostic evaluations.
- FGID symptoms can arise from any portion of the GI tract (esophagus to anus), and frequently multiple FGIDs may be identified in the same individual.
- These functional syndromes, as defined by the Rome criteria,[1] are listed in Table 17-1.
  - The prototypical and most common functional GI disorder is irritable bowel syndrome (IBS), which is characterized by abdominal pain or discomfort associated with defecation or a change in bowel habit and features of disordered defecation (constipation and/or diarrhea).

Classification

- Several historical diagnostic criteria for IBS exist, with the Rome III criteria (Table 17-2) representing the most recent and encompassing criteria. It should be asserted that these criteria were devised primarily as a tool for devising clinical studies in the area.
- When applied to clinical practice, these criteria have a high positive predictive value (>95%).
- Although they are not necessary for IBS diagnosis, several supporting symptoms (Table 17-3) help to solidify the diagnosis and further characterize the disorder into IBS with constipation (IBS-C), IBS with diarrhea (IBS-D), mixed IBS (IBS-M), or unsubtyped IBS.

Epidemiology

- IBS is frequently seen in both primary care and specialty care settings and is one of the most common diagnoses seen by gastroenterologists.[2]
  - Estimates place the prevalence of IBS anywhere from 1% to 20% worldwide.
  - Systematic reviews from suggest 5% to 10% of individuals in North America are affected with IBS.[3]

TABLE 17-1	ROME III DESIGNATIONS OF FUNCTIONAL GASTROINTESTINAL DISORDERS

Functional esophageal disorders

Heartburn
Chest pain of presumed esophageal origin
Dysphagia
Globus

Functional gastroduodenal disorders

Functional dyspepsia
Belching disorders
Nausea and vomiting disorders
Rumination syndrome

Functional bowel disorders

Irritable bowel syndrome
Functional bloating
Functional constipation
Functional diarrhea
Unspecified functional bowel disorder

Functional abdominal pain syndrome

Functional gallbladder and SO disorders

Functional gallbladder disorder
Functional biliary SO disorder
Functional pancreatic SO disorder

Functional anorectal disorders

Functional fecal incontinence
Functional anorectal pain
Functional defecation disorders

SO, sphincter of Oddi.

- ○ Population surveys of adults have shown IBS to be more prevalent in women than in men, with a ratio of 3 to 4:1.
- ○ Symptom onset tends to occur before 50 years of age, but it can occur at anytime.
  - When considering a new diagnosis of IBS in older individuals, exclusion of other mimicking conditions (celiac disease, inflammatory bowel disease, small intestinal bacterial overgrowth) is essential.

TABLE 17-2	THE ROME III IRRITABLE BOWEL SYNDROME CRITERIA

Recurrent abdominal pain or discomfort at least 3 days per month in the last 3 mo associated with two or more of the following:

1. Improvement with defecation
2. Onset associated with a change in frequency of stools
3. Onset associated with a change in form (appearance) of stool

TABLE 17-3   SUPPORTIVE SYMPTOMS OF IRRITABLE BOWEL SYNDROME

Abnormal stool frequency (*abnormal* defined as more than three bowel movements per day or fewer than three bowel movements per week)

Abnormal stool form (lumpy/hard or loose/watery stool)

Abnormal stool passage (straining, urgency, or feeling of incomplete evacuation)

Passage of mucus

Bloating or feeling of abdominal distention

- As few as one in three individuals affected with IBS in the United States actually seek medical attention.
  - Still, the cost to society is considerable, accounting for ~3.6 million physician visits and $1.6 billion in direct medical costs each year.
  - Indirect costs in the form of work absenteeism may reach as high as $19 billion per annum.
- The burden on the patient is also considerable with health-related quality-of-life scores similar to patients with diabetes and worse than patients with chronic kidney disease and gastroesophageal reflux disease.[4]

Pathophysiology

- No single pathophysiologic abnormality has been found that adequately explains the manifestations of IBS.
- Given the symptomatic basis on which the diagnosis is made, it is conceivable that more than one pathophysiologic mechanism may be operative.
  - Multiple factors, including abnormalities of intestinal motility, visceral hypersensitivity, GI tract inflammatory processes, disturbances along the brain–gut axis, and psychological factors, have been examined as potentially causative in IBS.
- A portion of patients with IBS will exhibit exaggerated motility, and sensory responses to stressors, meals, and balloon inflation in the GI tract can be identified.
  - These motility responses, however, are neither uniformly identifiable in patients with IBS nor consistently detectable in the same individual.
  - Nonetheless, accelerated transit times may be seen in diarrhea-predominant IBS and slowed transit times in constipation-predominant IBS.
- IBS may result from sensitization of afferent neural pathways from the gut in such a fashion that normal intestinal stimuli induce pain.
  - IBS patients have a lower pain threshold to balloon distention of the colon than healthy volunteers, while retaining normal sensitivity to somatic stimuli.
- Intestinal inflammation has also been hypothesized as playing a role in the development of IBS, particularly as it relates to persistent neuroimmune interactions following infectious gastroenteritis ("postinfectious IBS").
  - Approximately one-third of patients with IBS report symptom onset after an episode of acute gastroenteritis.
  - Seven percent to 30% of patients presenting with an acute enteric infection go on to develop IBS-like symptoms.

○ Psychological distress (particularly somatization) seems to be an important cofactor in determining who develops persistent functional symptoms following an enteric infection.

- The role of small intestinal bacterial overgrowth (SIBO) in the development of IBS has been a focus of recent investigations.[5]
  ○ The evidence for the role of SIBO in IBS remains incompletely understood and likely is relevant to only a subset of IBS patients.[6]
- The CNS (and its interpretation of peripheral enteric nerve signals) is receiving increasing attention in investigational settings because of the potential mechanistic significance in IBS.
  ○ Differential responses of brain activation to both noxious rectal stimulation and anticipated rectal discomfort can be appreciated in patients with IBS.
  ○ These connections are both the focus of intense research and the potential target for novel therapies.
  ○ Psychological factors (anxiety, depression, somatization) are important in their potential to further modulate this afferent pain network but, by themselves, are not sufficient explanations of IBS pathogenesis.[7]
  ○ In addition to amplifying both visceral and somatic pain experiences, the patient's psychological framework may also influence illness behaviors, such as seeking health care.

DIAGNOSIS

Clinical Presentation

History and Physical Examination

- IBS is a symptom-based diagnosis founded on a reporting of abdominal discomfort and a temporal association with alterations in stool pattern, improvement with bowel movement, or both.
- IBS diagnosis requires an element of chronicity (per Rome criteria, ≥3 days per month over the preceding 3 months).
- The diagnosis of IBS should be made after organic causes have been considered, so a careful search for alarm symptoms should be conducted.
  ○ Important alarm symptoms include weight loss of ≥10 lb (≥4.53 kg), recurrent fever, persistent diarrhea, hematochezia, age >50 years, and family history of GI malignancy, inflammatory bowel disease, or celiac sprue.
  ○ A brief history of rapidly progressive symptoms suggests organic disease. The presence of any such "red flag" features warrants a more entailed investigation before establishing a diagnosis of IBS.
- Likewise, the physical examination should be focused to exclude organic disease.
  ○ Diffuse abdominal tenderness is commonly present because of the heightened visceral sensitivity noted in this population.
  ○ Physical examination alarm signs include the presence of ascites, jaundice, organomegaly, abdominal mass, adenopathy, or heme-positive stool.

Diagnostic Testing

- **Laboratory and invasive testing should be kept to a minimum,** because extensive or repetitive investigations may be costly and serve only to reinforce illness behavior.

- Initial laboratory testing should include a complete blood cell count, erythrocyte sedimentation rate, and fecal occult blood test when appropriate.
- These tests, along with a complete metabolic profile, stool culture, and *Clostridium difficile* toxin assay can be ordered if the pretest probability is high enough but likely are low yield for the majority of IBS patients.
- **Testing for celiac sprue should be considered in all IBS patients** (particularly in IBS-D and IBS-M).
- Sensitivity and specificity of glucose and lactose breath tests are inadequate to evaluate for SIBO, and these are not recommended for use in IBS patients.[3]
  - Small bowel aspirates and culture are cumbersome and expensive; these tests also are reserved for research settings.
- Endoscopy (esophagoduodenoscopy and colonoscopy) may be unnecessary in young patients presenting with classic features of IBS without any alarm symptoms.
  - These studies should be considered in all patients older than 50 years (also important part of routine colon cancer screening).[3]
  - In this setting, colonoscopy offers the following advantages:
    - Rule out inflammation or tumors (especially in patients older than 50 years).
    - Identify melanosis coli indicative of laxative abuse.
    - Allow detection of visceral hypersensitivity to visceral pain via endoscopic insufflation of the colon.

TREATMENT

General Principles

- The approach to therapy in IBS is multifaceted and should be tailored to the patient, given the individual's constellation and severity of symptoms.[8] **Two key factors that determine therapy** are as follows:
  - Dominant symptoms (diarrhea, constipation, pain, other)
  - Symptom severity (intensity, bother, effects on quality of life)
- Current management approaches include peripherally acting agents, centrally acting agents, and psychological-behavioral therapy.
- Cases with mild or intermittent symptoms can be managed with symptomatic treatment using peripherally acting agents administered on an as-needed basis.
- Patients with moderate symptoms (as designated by intermittent interference with daily activities) may benefit from regular use of peripheral agents as an initial approach, with the option of introducing centrally acting agents if this approach fails.
- Patients with severe symptoms (regular interference with daily activities and concurrent affective, personality, and psychosomatic disorders) benefit from combinations of peripherally and centrally acting agents but may also need contemporary pharmaceutical agents and cognitive-behavioral therapy (CBT) to manage their overlapping affective, personality, and psychosomatic disorders.
- Although medical therapy is available and new drugs are currently in development, IBS is a lifelong condition with exacerbations and remissions, and medications should be minimized to the extent possible.
- Clearly, **narcotics have no role in the management of IBS**.

TABLE 17-4	GENERAL APPROACH TO IRRITABLE BOWEL SYNDROME AND THE FUNCTIONAL BOWEL DISORDERS

Minimize invasive testing, targeted to exclude other disorders as appropriate
Avoid repetitive testing unless necessary
Determine patient expectations and goals
Education and reassurance with emphasis on benign nature of condition
Dietary modifications and fiber supplementation are first-line therapy
Medications for more persistent or difficult cases
Behavioral or psychological interventions for refractory and motivated patients with IBS

- Given the lack of identifiable biomarkers, trials of medications are frequently part of the IBS diagnostic process.
  - These trials should be pursued for ≥4 weeks before moving on to different therapy.
- If failure to respond to a single agent in a drug class is experienced, response to a different drug in the same class may still be observed.
- It is important to recognize the substantial (up to 50%) placebo response rates present in this patient population.
- **Patient education and reassurance** while establishing a therapeutic relationship are cornerstones in the management of this condition.
  - The strength of the physician's relationship with the patient correlates to higher rates of patient satisfaction and fewer return visits.
- Table 17-4 summarizes general management principles for patients with IBS or other functional bowel disorders.

Peripherally Acting Agents

- **Therapies for constipation-predominant IBS** (IBS-C)
  - Increasing the amount of **dietary fiber** is a simple, inexpensive option in mild IBS-C and can be instituted as an early approach.
    - Limited randomized controlled studies seem to show some benefit in global symptom relief with this approach, with a number needed to treat of 6.[3]
    - Natural fiber sources (e.g., psyllium) or synthetic fiber (e.g., methylcellulose) are available.
    - In patients who complain of bloating or gas, fiber supplementation can be associated with an increase in those symptoms and slow titration and exclusion of flatulogenic foods should be encouraged.
  - **Osmotic laxatives** such as milk of magnesia, sorbitol, lactulose, or polyethylene glycol may also be considered for patients with IBS-C.
    - Currently, there are no randomized controlled trial data to support their use.[3]
    - These agents are generally safe for long-term use and are preferable to stimulant laxatives.
    - Nonabsorbable carbohydrates such as lactulose and sorbitol can induce bloating symptoms and are probably best avoided.
  - **Lubiprostone** (Amitiza) is a chloride channel activator indicated in the treatment of IBS-C in women at a dose of 8 mcg twice daily.

- Lubiprostone has shown benefit in reducing global IBS symptom scores.[3]
- Side effects include nausea, diarrhea, and headache.
- Women of childbearing age should have a negative pregnancy test before starting lubiprostone therapy and should be capable of complying with effective contraception while on this medication.
○ Tegaserod (Zelnorm) is a partial 5-hydroxytryptamine-4 receptor agonist that exerts GI stimulatory effects and had been indicated for short-term treatment of women with constipation-predominant symptoms.
  - In 2007, tegaserod was withdrawn from the market because of a small but statistically significant increase in cardiovascular events in patients taking it.
- **Therapies for diarrhea-predominant IBS** (IBS-D)
  ○ The antidiarrheal **loperamide** (2 to 4 mg up to four times daily) is the only agent with randomized controlled data supporting its use in IBS-D.
    - On the basis of its mechanism of action, diphenoxylate 2.5 mg with atropine 0.025 mg (Lomotil, up to QID) may also be used.[3]
    - Suspension forms of these medications are available for patients who need dose titrations.
  ○ **Cholestyramine** (Questran) and **colesevelam** (WelChol) can be considered as an adjunct, or for early use when diarrheal symptoms exacerbated by cholecystectomy.
  ○ **Alosetron** (Lotronex), a selective 5-hydroxytryptamine-3 receptor antagonist, was approved for treatment of women with IBS-D.
    - Alosetron was voluntarily withdrawn from the market in 2000 because of a possible relationship with acute ischemic colitis and severe constipation induced by this medication (1.1 and 0.66 cases per 1000 patient-years, respectively).
    - It was reapproved by the U.S. Food and Drug Administration in 2002 for chronic, severe IBS-D that has failed to respond to conventional therapy; currently, its use requires a patient use agreement and prescriber registration with the manufacturer.
  ○ **Anticholinergic or "antispasmodic" agents** often are used in all classes of IBS, though probably are most useful in the setting of IBS-D.
    - Anticholinergic medications possess antidiarrheal properties via decreases in intestinal transit and modulation of bowel secretory function.
    - **Hyoscyamine** (Levsin) 0.125 to 0.25 mg orally or sublingual and **dicyclomine** (Bentyl) 10 to 20 mg orally, up to three times a day.
    - **Glycopyrrolate** (Robinul) 1 to 2 mg two to three times a day and **methscopolamine** (Pamine) 2.5 to 5 mg twice a day are also available and have decreased CNS side effect potential.
    - These agents are most useful in patients with postprandial symptoms of abdominal pain, bloating, diarrhea, or fecal urgency.
    - They should be prescribed to circumvent symptoms, such as before meals.
    - These agents often become less effective with long-term use.
  ○ Limited data also exist, supporting the use of peppermint oil as an antispasmodic agent.[3,9]
- The use of antibiotic regimens in IBS recently has generated considerable interest.
  ○ Gut-selective antibiotics such as rifaximin or neomycin have been proposed for use in patients with IBS for whom bacterial overgrowth is suspected, particularly in those with significant gas-bloat symptoms.

- ○ The results of two large, randomized, controlled studies recently demonstrated a benefit in global and individual symptom scores using rifaximin 550 mg three times daily for 2 weeks in non–IBS-C patients (the number needed to treat around 11). These benefits persisted past the period of time patients were on the drug.[10]
- Emerging data support the use of **probiotics** in the management of IBS symptoms.
  - ○ All probiotics are not equally effective, however; the most benefit has been shown with *Bifidobacteria* spp. and little to no benefit shown using *Lactobacillus* spp.[3]

Centrally Acting Agents

- **Antidepressant medications** are most useful in patients with chronic, refractory symptoms.
- They are particularly helpful with those who have concomitant psychiatric and somatic complaints, although their efficacy is independent of any direct influence on these comorbid conditions.
- It is thought that antidepressants serve to interrupt or modulate the CNS interpretation of peripheral gut signaling.
- Patient perceptions and expectations should be adequately addressed in using antidepressants in the management of IBS to optimize compliance.
- **Tricyclic antidepressants** (TCA), such as nortriptyline, amitriptyline, imipramine, and desipramine, are the best studied agents.
  - ○ They are used in doses much lower than those traditionally used in depression management (starting dose, 10 to 25 mg at bedtime).
  - ○ The anticholinergic properties of TCA may be beneficial in IBS-D but should not dissuade use in patients with IBS-C.
  - ○ Side effects can include sedation, dry mouth, urinary difficulties, sexual dysfunction, and dizziness.
  - ○ Individuals experiencing such side effects may tolerate use of agents with fewer anticholinergic effects such as desipramine.
- **Selective serotonin reuptake inhibitors** increasingly also are being used in IBS and appear to be nearly as effective as TCAs.
  - ○ Citalopram may be a good option because of its low side effect profile and its effect on colonic tone and sensitivity.
  - ○ Paroxetine may be useful in patients with IBS-D because of its anticholinergic effect.
  - ○ The SNRI venlafaxine has been shown to reduce colonic compliance and relax the colon in healthy volunteers, an effect not seen with citalopram or fluoxetine.[3]

Cognitive and Behavioral Therapy

- Psychological and behavioral therapies, such as **CBT**, may be useful in IBS management, particularly in patients who correlate an increase in severity of symptoms with life stressors.
  - ○ CBT has been demonstrated to be beneficial in IBS in randomized controlled trials, particularly in its positive influence on global well-being.[11,12]
  - ○ Although response is sporadic, factors favoring a good response include high patient motivation, diarrhea or pain as the predominant symptom, overt psychiatric symptoms, and intermittent pain exacerbated by stress.

REFERENCES

1. Drossman DA, Corazziari E, Tally NJ, et al., eds. *Rome III: The Functional Gastrointestinal Disorders. Diagnosis, Pathophysiology and Treatment: A Multinational Consensus.* 3rd ed. McLean, VA: Degnon Associates; 2006.
2. Russo MW, Gaynes BN, Drossman DA. A national survey of practice patterns of gastroenterologists with comparison to the past two decades. *J Clin Gastroenterol.* 1999;29: 339–343.
3. Brandt LJ, Chey WD, Fox-Orenstein AE, et al. An evidence based systematic review on the management of irritable bowel syndrome. *Am J Gastroenterol.* 2009;104(suppl 1):s1–s35.
4. Gralnek I, Hays RD, Kilbourne A, et al. The impact of irritable bowel syndrome on health-related quality of life. *Gastroenterology.* 2000;119:654–660.
5. Posserud I, Stotzer PO, Bjornsson ES, et al. Small intestinal bacterial overgrowth in patients with irritable bowel syndrome. *Gut.* 2007;56:802–808.
6. Gunnarson J, Simren M. Peripheral factors in the pathophysiology of irritable bowel syndrome. *Dig Liver Dis.* 2009;41:788–793.
7. Whitehead WE, Palsson O, Jones KR. Systematic review of the comorbidity of irritable bowel syndrome with other disorders: what are the causes and implications? *Gastroenterology.* 2002;122:1140–1156.
8. Drossman DA, Camilleri M, Mayer E, et al. AGA technical review on irritable bowel syndrome. *Gastroenterology.* 2002;123:2108–2131.
9. Spanier JA, Howden CW, Jones MP. A systematic review of alternative therapies in the irritable bowel syndrome. *Arch Intern Med.* 2003;163:265–724.
10. Pimentel M, Lembo A, Chey WD, et al. Rifaximin therapy for patients with irritable bowel without constipation. *N Engl J Med.* 2011;364(1):22–32.
11. Drossman DA, Toner BB, Whitehead WE, et al. Cognitive-behavioral therapy versus education and desipramine versus placebo for moderate to severe functional bowel disorders. *Gastroenterology.* 2003;125:19–31.
12. Lackner JM, Brasel AM, Quigley BM, et al. Rapid response to cognitive behavioral therapy predicts outcome in patients with irritable bowel syndrome. *Clin Gastroenterol Hepatol.* 2010;8(5):426–432.

Acute Liver Disease

18

Anil B. Seetharam and Kevin M. Korenblat

- Acute liver disease encompasses a wide range of disorders from asymptomatic aminotransferase elevations to acute liver failure (ALF).
- Viral hepatitis and drug-induced liver injury (DILI) are the most frequent causes.
- Histologic changes to the liver are typically those of acute inflammation with varying degrees of necrosis and collapse of the liver's architectural framework. These features contrast with changes of cirrhosis and development of portal hypertension that characterize the end stages of chronic liver disease.

VIRAL HEPATITIS

- Hepatotropic viruses include hepatitis A (HAV), hepatitis B (HBV), hepatitis C (HCV), hepatitis D (HDV), and hepatitis E (HEV). Nonhepatotropic viruses known to cause liver injury include Epstein-Barr virus, cytomegalovirus, herpes virus, measles, Ebola virus, and others.
- Acute viral hepatitis is defined by the sudden onset of aminotransferase elevation as a consequence of diffuse necroinflammatory liver injury.
  - ○ Clinical presentation is widely variable and often nonspecific.
  - ○ The condition may resolve or progress to ALF or chronic hepatitis.

HEPATITIS A VIRUS

GENERAL PRINCIPLES

Hepatitis A is an enterically transmitted RNA virus that in unimmunized patients often results in self-limited icteric hepatitis and rarely in fulminant hepatic failure.

Classification
- HAV is an RNA virus within the *Picornaviridae* family.

Epidemiology
- HAV is responsible for 30% of acute viral hepatitis in the United States.
- Morbidity and mortality (case-fatality rate) of infection are determined by age of onset.
  - ○ In developing countries, infection in childhood is universal and typically asymptomatic for those younger than 6 years.
  - ○ Adults are more likely to be symptomatic with infection and at greater risk for developing ALF.

Pathophysiology

- HAV infection is usually transmitted enterically.
- It is associated with unsanitary living conditions or improper food-handling techniques.
- The period of greatest infectivity is 2 weeks before onset of clinical illness; fecal shedding continues for 2 to 3 weeks after onset of symptoms.

Risk Factors

- **High-risk groups** include people living in or traveling to developing countries (food and water contamination), men having sex with men, injection drugs users, patients with clotting factor disorders, persons working with nonhuman primates, staff and attendees at daycare centers, and patients with chronic liver disease (increased risk for fulminant hepatitis A).

Prevention

- Immunization programs are available (see Treatment section under Hepatitis A Virus)

DIAGNOSIS

- Diagnosis of acute HAV infection is made by the detection of **anti-HAV IgM antibodies** in serum.
- **Aminotransferase elevations** range from 10 to 100 times the upper limits of the reference range (ULR).
- Resolution of the illness is associated with emergence of **anti-HAV IgG antibodies,** and this change provides the basis for distinguishing acute from convalescent infection.

Clinical Presentation

- HAV can be silent (subclinical), especially in children and young adults. Symptoms vary from mild illness to ALF.[1]
- Malaise, fatigue, pruritus, headache, abdominal pain, myalgias, arthralgias, nausea, vomiting, anorexia, and fever are common but nonspecific symptoms.

History

- History should include a review of symptoms, temporal course of illness, and assessment for any potential exposures from traveling to developing countries or food and water ingestion.

Physical Examination

- Physical examination may reveal jaundice, hepatomegaly, and, in rare cases, lymphadenopathy, splenomegaly, or a vascular rash.

TREATMENT

- Treatment is **supportive;** however, careful attention should be paid to identifying those at risk for ALF.
- Liver transplantation may be an option for ALF.

Medications

- **Preexposure prophylaxis**
  - ○ **Inactivated HAV vaccines** (containing the single HAV antigen) and **combination vaccines** (containing both HAV and hepatitis B antigens) are available. Vaccinations should be administered intramuscularly into the deltoid muscle in a two-dose regimen (single antigen HAV vaccine; first dose at time zero and second dose at 6 to 18 months) or in a three-dose regimen (combination vaccine; first dose at time zero, second dose at 1 month, and third dose at 6 months).
- **Postexposure prophylaxis**
  - ○ Immune globulin (GamSTAN adult dose 0.02 mL/kg/dose) given within 14 days of exposure. Efficacy beyond 2 weeks after exposure has not been established.
  - ○ Immune globulin is not needed if at least one dose of the HAV vaccine was administered >1 month prior to exposure.
  - ○ Hepatitis A vaccine is not licensed for use as postexposure prophylaxis; however, patients who have been administered one dose of vaccine at >1 month prior to exposure do not need immune globulin.
  - ○ In one study, treatment with HAV vaccine was shown to be noninferior to postexposure prophylaxis with immune globulin, though slightly higher rates of hepatitis A infection developed in those who received vaccine only.
  - ○ If HAV vaccine and immune globulin are recommended, they may be administered simultaneously at separate injection sites.

OUTCOME/PROGNOSIS

- Most symptoms of infection, including jaundice, resolve by 3 to 4 months.
- Although there is no chronic phase of HAV infection, a polyphasic form of the disease can occur associated with relapse of symptoms.
- ALF is relatively rare, but risk increases with age: 0.1% in patients younger than 15 years to >1% in patients older than 40 years.
- HAV does not induce chronic hepatitis or cirrhosis.

HEPATITIS B VIRUS

GENERAL PRINCIPLES

HBV is a parenteral or sexually transmitted virus that is rarely associated with fulminant hepatic failure but can develop into chronic infection with progression to cirrhosis, end-stage liver disease, and hepatocellular carcinoma (HCC). At-risk populations are protected by administration of recombinant vaccine that confers hepatitis B surface antibody positivity.

Classification

- HBV is a DNA virus in the *Hepadnaviridae* family.
- Eight genotypes of HBV have been identified, designated A through H.

Epidemiology

- Two billion people worldwide have serologic evidence of past or present infection, and ~400 million people are chronic carriers.
- Prevalence of HBV genotypes varies depending on the geographic location. Genotypes A, B, and C are the most prevalent in the United States.[2]
- HBV is the indication for 5% to 10% of cases of liver transplantation.

Pathophysiology

- **Modes of transmission** include
  - **parenteral or percutaneous routes** (e.g., injection drug use, hemodyalisis, transfusions, needlestick injury);
  - **sexual contact** (e.g., men who have sex with men, intercourse with HBV-infected partners); and
  - **vertical or perinatal transmission** (from mother to infant).

Risk Factors

- **High-risk groups** include individuals with a history of multiple blood transfusions, patients on hemodialysis, injection drug users, sexual promiscuity, men having sex with men, household and heterosexual contacts of hepatitis B carriers, residents and employees of residential care facilities, travelers to endemic regions, and individuals born in areas of high or intermediate prevalence.

Prevention

- Immunization programs are available (see Treatment section under Hepatitis B Virus)

Associated Conditions

- **Extrahepatic manifestations** include polyarteritis nodosa, glomerulonephritis, cryoglobulinemia, serum sickness–like illness, and aplastic anemia.

DIAGNOSIS

Clinical Presentation

- The period from exposure to symptoms ranges from 60 to 180 days.
- Presentation can be subclinical, especially in children and young adults.
- Symptoms vary from mild illness to ALF. Malaise, fatigue, pruritus, headache, abdominal pain, myalgias, arthralgias, nausea, vomiting, anorexia, and fever are common but nonspecific symptoms.
- Progression to chronicity depends on age of acquisition.
- Most acute HBV infections are self-limited in adults.

History

- History should include a thorough investigation of risk factors.

Diagnostic Testing

- Diagnosis of HBV often requires the combination of data obtained from liver chemistries, serology, and histology. With rare exceptions, the diagnosis of hepatitis B is made by the presence of hepatitis B surface antigen (HBsAg)

Laboratories

- **Liver chemistries** typically abnormal in acute hepatitis include aspartate aminotransferase (AST), alanine aminotransferase (ALT), alkaline phosphatase (AP), and total bilirubin.
- Tests that measure cholestasis [AP, γ-glutamyltransferase (GGT), and total bilirubin] or liver synthetic function [albumin and prothrombin time (PT)/international normalized ratio (INR)] may be abnormal according to the disease stage.
- HBV contains two genes (s and core) that produce antigens that elicit a corresponding antibody response.
  - HBV antigens detected in serum and used for diagnostic purposes in clinical practice include **HBsAg** and **hepatitis B e antigen (HBeAg).**
- **HBV antibodies** are specific to their corresponding antigen and include
  - Antibody against HBsAg **(anti-HBs),** antibody against HBeAg **(anti-HBe),** and IgM and IgG antibodies against HBcAg **(IgM and IgG anti-HBc).**
- **HBV viral DNA** (HBV DNA) is the **most accurate marker of viral replication.** It is detected by the polymerase chain reaction (PCR) and most commonly expressed as international units per milliliter (IU/mL).
- **Genotypic determination** is growing in clinical significance as data are emerging with respect to response to antivirals, disease progression, and risk of HCC.
- The presence of HBsAg for >6 months separates chronic from acute HBV infection.

Diagnostic Procedures

- **Liver biopsy** is useful to assess the degree of necroinflammation and fibrosis in patients with chronic hepatitis.

TREATMENT

- Most cases of symptomatic, acute HBV infection in adults resolve with the development of antibodies to the surface protein (anti-HBs), the central neutralizing antibody to HBV. Thus, generally no role exists for antiviral therapy with acute infection; however, case reports have suggested a potential role for antiviral therapy in subjects who develop signs that they may progress to ALF.

Medications

- Seven agents are currently available for the treatment of HBV infection. They are divided into three main groups:
  - **interferon-based therapy** (interferon α and pegylated interferon α),
  - **nucleoside analogues** (lamivudine, entecavir, and telbivudine), and
  - **nucleotide analogues** (adefovir and tenofovir).
- These classes of medications are indicated for the treatment of chronic HBV infection.
- Of the oral agents, **entecavir and tenofovir** are the two agents with the highest genetic barrier to resistance and therefore are **preferred if treatment of acute HBV infection is indicated.**

Other Nonoperative Therapies

- **Preexposure prophylaxis**
  - ○ **HBV vaccine** should be considered for everyone, but particularly for individuals at high risk (see risk factor section).
  - ○ HBV vaccination schedule includes three intramuscular injections at 0, 1, and 6 months in infants or healthy adults. Protective antibody response is >90% after the third dose. Response to vaccination is measured by anti-HBs ≥10 IU/mL.
- **Postexposure prophylaxis**
  - ○ **Infants born to HBsAg-positive mothers** should receive HBV vaccine and hepatitis B immune globulin (HBIG), 0.5 mL, within 12 hours of birth to prevent vertical transmission of the virus.
  - ○ **Susceptible sexual partners** of individuals with HBV and **those with needlestick injury** should receive HBIG (0.04 to 0.07 mL/kg) and the first dose of HBV vaccine at different sites preferably within 48 hours but no >7 days after exposure. A second dose of HBIG can be administered 30 days after exposure, and the vaccination schedule should be completed.

Surgical Management

- Liver transplantation is indicated for patients with ALF secondary to HBV infection.

OUTCOME/PROGNOSIS

- Depending on the age at infection, people may have spontaneous resolution or progression to chronicity.
  - ○ Children younger than 5 years: 90% will develop chronic HBV infection.
  - ○ Adults: 5% to 10% will develop chronic HBV.

HEPATITIS C VIRUS

HCV is a parentally transmitted virus that in the acute phase is not frequently recognized; however, upon establishment of chronicity, it can lead to cirrhosis, end-stage liver disease, and HCC. It is the most frequent indication for liver transplantation in the United States, but it almost always recurs.

GENERAL PRINCIPLES

Classification

- HCV is an RNA virus of the *Flaviviridae* family.
- Six HCV genotypes are recognized worldwide with >60 subtypes.

Epidemiology

- HCV is a global health problem, with ~180 million carriers worldwide.[3]

Pathophysiology

- HCV infection occurs primarily through exposure from infected blood (see risk factors section).

Pathophysiology

- HDV infection clinically presents as a coinfection (acute hepatitis B and D), superinfection (chronic hepatitis B with acute hepatitis D), or as a latent infection (e.g., in the setting of liver transplantation).

Risk Factors

- High-risk groups are similar to HBV (see HBV Epidemiology section).

Prevention

- Although there is no vaccine to prevent HDV infection in carriers of HBV, both infections can be prevented by HBV vaccination.

DIAGNOSIS

Clinical Presentation

- In patients with **coinfection,** the course is transient and self-limited. The rate of progression to chronicity is similar to that reported for acute HBV infection.
- In **superinfection,** HBV carriers may present with a severe acute hepatitis exacerbation with frequent progression to chronic HDV infection.

Diagnostic Testing

Laboratories
- Diagnosis is made by finding **HDV RNA** or **HDV antigen** in serum or liver and by detecting **antibody to the HDV antigen**.

TREATMENT

Medications

- **Interferon α–based therapy** is the treatment of choice for chronic hepatitis D.

HEPATITIS E VIRUS

GENERAL PRINCIPLES

Hepatitis E is an **enterically transmitted RNA virus** that leads to acute hepatitis in special populations including pregnant women and immunosuppressed solid-organ transplant patients.

Classification

- Hepatitis E virus (HEV) is an RNA virus belonging to the *Hepeviridae* family.

Epidemiology

- HEV is implicated in epidemics in India, Southeast Asia, Africa, and Mexico.
- Hepatitis E is considered a zoonotic disease and reservoirs include pigs and potentially other species.[5]

Pathophysiology

- Transmission is through the fecal-oral route and resembles that of HAV infection.

Prevention

- No approved pre- or postexposure prophylaxis exists.

DIAGNOSIS

Clinical Presentation

- Acute hepatitis E is clinically indistinguishable from other acute viral hepatitis.
- A **high fatality rate is seen in pregnant women** in the second and third trimesters.

TREATMENT

- Treatment is supportive.

OUTCOME/PROGNOSIS

- Although generally considered an acute illness, chronic HEV infection has been detected in immunosuppressed organ transplant patients.

HERPES SIMPLEX VIRUS HEPATITIS

GENERAL PRINCIPLES

Herpes simplex virus (HSV) rarely causes hepatitis; however, liver involvement in immunosuppressed or pregnant women can cause severe anicteric hepatitis leading to fulminant hepatic failure prompting consideration of empiric treatment while the diagnosis is being established.

Classification

- Infection with both HSV-1 and HSV-2 can lead to visceral dissemination and hepatitis.

Epidemiology

- Commonly acquired infection, with 62% of adolescents testing positive for HSV-1 and 12% for HSV-2.
- Hepatitis is an uncommon manifestation of HSV.
- Usually occurs in neonates or malnourished children; rare in adults.
- Most adult patients are immunocompromised (most often deficiency of cell-mediated immunity) or pregnant, but HSV hepatitis has been described in immunocompetent patients.

Pathophysiology

- Large HSV inoculum at the time of initial infection may result in dissemination.

- Activation of latent infection may occur.
- HSV strains have affinity to the liver ("hepatovirulent").

Risk Factors

- High-risk groups include **neonates, pregnant women** (primarily in the third trimester), and those who are **immunosuppressed.**[6]

DIAGNOSIS

- Diagnosis of acute HSV infection may be made by serologic tests; however, if index of suspicion is high, it is reasonable to initiate treatment.
- **Aminotransferase elevations** range from 10 to 100 times the ULR. These elevations may be out of proportion to the degree of jaundice; thus, HSV hepatitis is often considered anicteric hepatitis.

Clinical Presentation

- Symptoms vary from mild illness to ALF.
- Malaise, fatigue, pruritus, headache, abdominal pain, myalgias, arthralgias, nausea, vomiting, anorexia, and fever are common but nonspecific symptoms.

History

- History should include a review of symptoms, temporal course of illness, and any potential HSV exposures.

Physical Examination

- Hepatosplenomegaly. Jaundice is uncommon.
- Oral mucocutaneous lesions in HSV infection are found in 40% to 50% of cases.

TREATMENT

- Treatment is with **intravenous (IV) acyclovir,** it can be initiated presumptively if there is any degree of clinical suspicion.
- Liver transplantation may be an option for ALF.

OUTCOME/PROGNOSIS

- Cases may rapidly progress to fulminant hepatic failure; however, prompt administration of parenteral antiviral therapy may result in complete resolution of liver dysfunction.

ACETAMINOPHEN

GENERAL PRINCIPLES

When ingested at toxic levels, acetaminophen (APAP) and its metabolites may lead to hepatocellular damage and fulminant hepatic failure. Recognition of potential toxic ingestions allows for prompt administration of its antidote *N*-acetylcysteine (NAC), which may prevent progression to fulminant hepatic failure.

Epidemiology

- APAP toxicity is the most common cause of toxic medication-related ingestion in the United States.
- It is most frequently a consequence of intentional ingestion; however, unintentional overdoses do occur and can result in severe liver injury. APAP is a safe and generally well-tolerated analgesic medication.[7]

Pathophysiology

- Significant hepatic injury generally requires ingestions above a threshold value of 150 mg/kg body weight.
- APAP can be metabolized to a toxic metabolite [N-acetyl-p-benzoquinone imine (NAPQI)], which can induce toxic free radical damage to liver parenchymal cells.
- Chronic, excessive alcohol use may predispose to liver injury, although only with overdoses of APAP.

DIAGNOSIS

- Made with **measurement of APAP level** in the serum.
- **History is critical** to assess time of ingestion, as well as concurrent substances ingested, which effects treatment (see later).

TREATMENT

Medications

- Antidote to treatment, **NAC** administered within 8 hours of ingestion, is indicated in those with APAP levels above the "possible" toxicity line on the **Rumack-Matthew nomogram** (line connecting 150 μg/mL at 4 hours with 50 μg/mL at 12 hours) (Fig. 18-1)
  - NAC can be given orally (loading dose of 140 mg/kg followed by 70 mg/kg every 4 hours for a total of 17 doses) or intravenously (loading dose 150 mg/kg over 1 hour followed by 14 mg/kg/hour for 4 hours and then 7 mg/kg/hour for 16 hours).
  - For ingestions that present late (>8 hours), a longer duration of IV treatment is recommended (loading dose, 140 mg/kg IV over 1 hour followed by 14 mg/kg/hour for 44 hours).
- **Hypophosphatemia** is a frequent finding in APAP-related liver injury. Serum phosphorous levels should be monitored and treated if low.

Surgical Management

- Liver transplantation can be considered in patients with ALF secondary to APAP.

PROGNOSIS/OUTCOME

- In addition to APAP's effects on the liver, acute renal failure can occur independently of hepatic injury.
- Prognosis is excellent with timely recognition and administration of NAC; however, complications from ALF can occur (see ALF section).

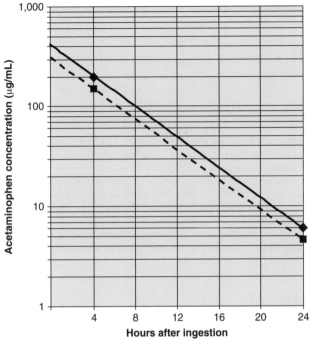

FIGURE 18-1. Acetaminophen toxicity nomogram. The area below the *dashed line* represents nontoxic ingestion. The area between the two lines is potentially toxic, and the area above the *solid line* is likely to be toxic. Treatment should be initiated for any level above the *dashed line*. (Adapted from Rumack BH, Matthews H. Acetaminophen poisoning. *Pediatrics.* 1975;55:871–866, with permission.)

DRUG-INDUCED LIVER INJURY

GENERAL PRINCIPLES

- Drug-induced liver injury (DILI) is a common cause of acute liver disease. Prognosis often depends upon the dose-dependent or idiosyncratic effect of the specific offending agent.

Classification

- **Three major patterns** of DILI occur as a result of both dose-dependent and idiosyncratic hepatotoxicity:
  ○ **Hepatocellular**
  ○ **Cholestatic**
  ○ **Mixed hepatocellular and cholestatic** injury

- Less common forms of DILI include granulomatous hepatitis and carcinogenesis.

Epidemiology

- DILI causes ~50% of the cases of ALF in the United States, with APAP the most common agent.

Pathophysiology

- **Intrinsic hepatotoxicity** results from usually predictable and dose-dependent hepatotoxic effects of the drug or its metabolite.[9]
- **Idiosyncratic hepatotoxicity** can be divided into hypersensitivity (allergic) and metabolic (nonallergic) reactions. These reactions depend on multiple variables and are not predictable.
  - ○ **Hypersensitivity responses** occur as a result of stimulation of the immune system by a metabolite of a drug alone or after haptenization (covalently binding) to a liver protein. Repeated challenge with the same agent leads to prompt recurrence of the reaction.
  - ○ **Metabolic hepatotoxicity** occurs in susceptible patients as a result of altered drug clearance or accelerated production of hepatotoxic metabolites. The latency of this reaction is variable.

DIAGNOSIS

Clinical Presentation

- Acute presentation can be clinically silent. When symptoms are present, they are nonspecific and include nausea/vomiting, general malaise, fatigue, and abdominal pain.
- In the acute setting, the majority of patients will recover after cessation of the offending drug.
- Fever, rash, and eosinophilia may also be seen in association with hypersensitivity reactions.

Diagnostic Criteria

- No diagnostic criteria are established, but diagnosis requires clinical suspicion, temporal relation of liver injury to drug usage, and resolution of liver injury after the suspected agent has been discontinued.

Diagnostic Testing

Laboratories

- Biochemical abnormalities include the following:
  - ○ **Hepatocellular injury:** AST and ALT elevation more than two times the upper limit of normal
  - ○ **Cholestatic injury:** AP and conjugated bilirubin elevation more than two times upper limit of normal
  - ○ **Mixed injury:** Increases in all of these biochemical abnormalities to more than two times upper limit of normal

Diagnostic Procedures

- Liver biopsy can be useful as part of the diagnostic workup.

TREATMENT

- Treatment includes **cessation of offending drug** and supportive measures.
- An **attempt to remove the agent from the GI tract** should be made in most cases of acute toxic ingestion, using lavage or cathartics.

Surgical Management

- Liver transplantation may be an option for patients with ALF.

Outcome/Prognosis

- Prognosis of DILI if often unique to the offending medication.
- It is important to be attuned to the development of jaundice because this sign is associated with case fatality rates of 10% to 50%.[9]

ISCHEMIC HEPATITIS

GENERAL PRINCIPLES

Ischemic hepatitis is characterized by a transient and often dramatic rise in aminotransferases that results from cardiovascular collapse.

Definition

- Ischemic hepatitis ("shock liver") results from liver hypoperfusion.

Etiology

- Clinical scenarios associated include severe blood loss, cardiac failure, heat stroke, sepsis, and sickle cell crisis.[11]

DIAGNOSIS

Clinical Presentation

History

- Ischemic hepatitis presents as acute and transient rise of liver enzymes to levels as high as >20 times the upper limit of normal range during or following a hypotensive episode.

Diagnostic Testing

Laboratories

- Laboratory studies demonstrate a rapid rise and fall in levels of serum AST, ALT (>1000 mg/dL), and lactic dehydrogenase within 1 to 3 days of the insult, with subsequent slow decline in aminotransferases if the underlying cause is corrected.
- Total bilirubin, AP, and INR may initially be normal but subsequently rise even as the levels of aminotransferases improve.

Diagnostic Procedures

- Liver biopsy is not usually needed for diagnosis.
  - Centrilobular necrosis and sinusoidal distortion with inflammatory infiltrates in zone 3 (central areas) are classic histologic features.

TREATMENT

- Correction of the underlying condition that caused circulatory collapse.

OUTCOME/PROGNOSIS

- Prognosis is determined by the rapid and effective correction of hemodynamics or treatment of the underlying cause.

BUDD-CHIARI SYNDROME

GENERAL PRINCIPLES

Budd-Chiari syndrome is characterized as hepatic venous outflow obstruction most often resulting from thrombosis, which can lead to an acute or subacute illness characterized by ascites, hepatomegaly, and jaundice. Treatment is centered on decompression of the portal system.

Definition

- **Hepatic vein thrombosis (HVT; also known as Budd-Chiari syndrome)** causes hepatic venous outflow obstruction. It has multiple etiologies and a variety of clinical consequences.

Etiology

- Thrombosis is the main factor leading to obstruction of the hepatic venous system, frequently in association with myeloproliferative disorders (polycythemia rubra vera) or hypercoagulable states (e.g., antiphospholipid antibody syndrome, paroxysmal nocturnal hemoglobinuria, factor V Leiden, protein C and S deficiency, and contraceptive use).
- HVT can occur during pregnancy and in the postpartum period.
- Less than 20% of cases are idiopathic.

DIAGNOSIS

Clinical Presentation

- Patients may present with acute, subacute, or chronic illness characterized by ascites, hepatomegaly, and right upper quadrant abdominal pain.
- Jaundice, encephalopathy, and lower extremity edema are variably present.

Diagnostic Testing

Laboratories

- Serum to ascites albumin gradient is >1.1 g/dL. Serum albumin, bilirubin, AST, ALT, and PT/INR are mildly abnormal.
- Laboratory evaluation to identify a potential hypercoagulable state or myeloproliferative disorder should be performed.

Imaging
- Doppler ultrasound can be used as a screening test and can demonstrate the absence of flow in hepatic veins.
- Definitive diagnosis is made with hepatic venography.

TREATMENT

Medications
- Nonsurgical treatment includes anticoagulation, thrombolytics, diuretics, angioplasty, stents, and transjugular intrahepatic portosystemic shunt (TIPS).[12] These agents work best in subjects without decompensated cirrhosis.

Surgical Management
- Both surgical shunts and liver transplantation have been used as therapeutic options.

WILSON'S DISEASE

GENERAL PRINCIPLES

Wilson's disease is a genetic disorder in which ineffective excretion of copper results in hepatocellular damage; its presentations include fulminant hepatic failure, and progression of disease may lead to cirrhosis and end-stage liver disease.

Definition
- Wilson's disease is an autosomal-recessive disorder (ATP7B gene on chromosome 13) that results in progressive copper overload.

Epidemiology
- Incidence is 1 in 30,000; female to male ratio of 2:1.

Pathophysiology
- Absent or reduced function of ATP7B protein leads to decreased hepatocellular excretion of copper into bile, resulting in hepatic copper accumulation and injury.

Associated Conditions
- **Extrahepatic manifestations** include **Kayser-Fleischer rings** on slit-lamp examination (gold to brown rings due to copper deposition in the Descemet membrane in the periphery of the cornea), Coombs-negative hemolytic anemia, renal tubular acidosis, arthritis, and osteopenia.[13]

DIAGNOSIS

Clinical Presentation
- Liver disease can be highly variable, ranging from asymptomatic with only biochemical abnormalities to ALF.

- The diagnosis of acute Wilson's disease should be considered in patients with unexplained liver disease with or without neuropsychiatric symptoms, first-degree relatives with Wilson's disease, or individuals with fulminant hepatic failure (with or without hemolysis).
- The average age at presentation of liver disease is 6 to 20 years, but it can manifest later in life.
- Neuropsychiatric disorders usually occur later, most of the time in association with cirrhosis. The manifestations include asymmetric tremor, dysarthria, ataxia, and psychiatric features.

Diagnostic Testing

Laboratories

- **Low serum ceruloplasmin level** (<20 mg/dL), **elevated serum free copper level** (>25 mcg/dL), and **elevated 24-hour urinary copper level** (>100 mg).
- Most patients with the ALF presentation of Wilson's disease have a characteristic pattern of findings including: Coombs-negative hemolytic anemia with features of acute intravascular hemolysis; rapid progression to renal failure; modest rise in serum aminotransferases (typically <2000 IU/L) from the beginning of clinical illness; normal or subnormal serum AP (typically <40 IU/L).

Diagnostic Procedures

- **Liver biopsy**
  - The liver histology (massive necrosis, steatosis, glycogenated nuclei, chronic hepatitis, fibrosis, cirrhosis) findings are nonspecific and depend on the presentation and stage of the disease.
  - Elevated hepatic copper levels of >250 mcg/g dry weight (normal <40 mcg/g) on biopsy are highly suggestive of Wilson's disease.

TREATMENT

Medications

- Treatment is with copper-chelating agents.
  - **Penicillamine** 1 to 2 g/day (in divided doses BID or QID) plus pyridoxine 25 mg/day. Indicated in patients with hepatic failure. Use may be limited by side effects (hypersensitivity, bone marrow suppression, and proteinuria, systemic lupus erythematosus, and Goodpasture syndrome). Penicillamine should not be given as initial treatment to patients with neurologic symptoms.
  - **Trientine** 1 to 2 g/day (in divided doses BID or QID). This has similar side effects as penicillamine but at a lower frequency. The risk of neurologic worsening with trientine is less than with penicillamine.

Surgical Management

- Liver transplantation is the only therapeutic option in ALF or in progressive dysfunction despite chelation.

OUTCOME/PROGNOSIS

- In the absence of neurologic symptoms, liver transplantation has a good prognosis and requires no further medical treatment.

ACUTE LIVER FAILURE

GENERAL PRINCIPLES

ALF is the relatively rapid development of coagulopathy and encephalopathy in the absence of preexisting liver disease; its etiologies are diverse and intensive monitoring is critical, as is timely referral for the evaluation of liver transplantation.

Definition
- ALF is a rare condition that includes evidence of coagulation abnormalities (usually an INR >1.5) and any degree of mental alteration (encephalopathy) in a patient without preexisting cirrhosis and with an illness of <26 weeks' duration.

Classification
- Terms used signifying length of illness in ALF such as hyperacute (<7 days), acute (7 to 21 days), and subacute (>21 days to <26 weeks) are generally considered unhelpful, as they do not have prognostic significance distinct from the cause of illness.[14]

Epidemiology
- Approximately 2000 cases of ALF occur in the United States yearly.

Etiology
- APAP hepatotoxicity and viral hepatitis are the most common causes of ALF.[15]
- Other causes include AIH, drug and toxin exposure, ischemia, acute fatty liver of pregnancy, Wilson's disease, and hepatitis B infection.
- In 20% of cases, no clear cause is identified.

DIAGNOSIS

Clinical Presentation
- Patients may present with mild to severe mental status changes in the setting of moderate to severe acute hepatitis and coagulopathy.
- Jaundice may or may not be initially present.
- A history of APAP overdose, toxin ingestion, or risk factors for viral hepatitis may be obtained.
- Cardiovascular collapse, acute renal failure, cerebral edema, and sepsis may be part of the clinical presentation.

Diagnostic Testing
Laboratories
- **Aminotransferases** are typically elevated and in many cases are >1000 IU/L.
- **INR is ≥1.5.**
- **Initial workup** to determine the etiology of ALF should include
  - ○ acute viral hepatitis panel;
  - ○ serum drug screen, which includes APAP;
  - ○ ceruloplasmin;

○ AIH serologies; and
○ pregnancy test.

Imaging
- **Right upper quadrant Doppler ultrasound** may be used to evaluate for obstruction of venous inflow or outflow.
- **Computed tomographic scan of the head** may be obtained to evaluate and track progression of cerebral edema; however, the radiologic findings may lag behind the development of cerebral edema.

Diagnostic Procedures
- Liver biopsy is seldom used to establish etiology or prognosis. Given the presence of coagulopathy, a transjugular biopsy is the preferred approach.

TREATMENT

- **Supportive therapy in the intensive care unit** at a center experienced with liver disease and liver transplantation is essential.
- **Precipitating factors should be identified** and treated if possible.
- **Sedation should be avoided** to allow for serial assessments of mental/neurologic status.
- Blood glucose, electrolytes, acid–base, coagulation parameters, and fluid status should be monitored serially.
- The **coagulopathy** of ALF need only to be corrected in the setting of active bleeding or when invasive procedures are required.
- **Cerebral edema and intracranial hypertension** are related to severity of encephalopathy (Table 18-1). In patients who reach grade III or IV encephalopathy, intracranial pressure monitoring should be considered (intracranial pressure should be maintained below 20 to 25 mm Hg, cerebral perfusion pressure should be maintained above 50 mm Hg). Therapies to decrease cerebral edema include mannitol (0.5 to 1 g/kg IV), hyperventilation (reduce $Paco_2$ to 25 to 30 mm Hg), hypothermia (32°C to 34°C), and barbiturates.
- **Lactulose is not indicated for encephalopathy.** Its use may result in increased bowel distention, which may complicate liver transplantation.
- **Liver transplantation is the ultimate therapy** for those with ALF (see Chapter 21). Several criteria have been proposed to identify those unlikely to recover spontaneously and in whom liver transplantation would be lifesaving. The King's College criteria are most commonly used (Table 18-2).
  ○ In the United States, patients with ALF are eligible to be listed for transplantation with the highest priority status.

TABLE 18-1	GRADES OF ENCEPHALOPATHY
I	Behavioral changes
II	Disorientation, drowsiness, inappropriate behavior
III	Confusion, somnolence but responds to painful stimuli, incoherent speech
IV	Comatose, unresponsive to noxious stimuli.

| TABLE 18-2 | KING'S COLLEGE CRITERIA |

Acetaminophen induced

Arterial pH <7.3
or
All three of the following:
  PT >100 sec (INR >6.5)
  Serum creatinine >3.4 mg/dL
  Grade III or IV encephalopathy

Nonacetaminophen induced

INR >6.5 irrespective of coma grade
or
Three of the following five criteria:
  Patient age <10 or >40
  Serum bilirubin >17.5 mg/dL
  PT >50 sec (INR ≥3.5)
  Unfavorable cause (seronegative hepatitis or DILI)
  Jaundice >7 days before encephalopathy

INR, international normalized ratio; PT, prothombin time.

OUTCOME/PROGNOSIS

- Prior to transplantation, survival was <15%; in the posttransplant era, survival is >65%.
- Death often results from progressive liver failure, GI bleeding, cerebral edema, sepsis, or arrhythmia.
- Poor prognostic indicators in APAP-induced ALF include arterial pH <7.3, INR >6.5, creatinine >2.3 mg/dL, and encephalopathy grades III to IV.

REFERENCES

1. Cuthbert JA. Hepatitis A: old and new. *Clin Microbiol Rev.* 2001;14(1):38–58.
2. Lok AS, McMahon BJ. Chronic hepatitis B. *Hepatology.* 2007;45(2):507–539.
3. Ghany MG, Strader DB, Thomas DL, et al. AASLD position paper: diagnosis, management, and treatment of hepatitis C: an update. *Hepatology.* 2009;49(4):1335–1374.
4. Hughes SA, Wedemeyer H, Harrison PM. Hepatitis delta virus. *Lancet.* 2011;378(9785): 73–85.
5. Dalton HR, Bendall R, Ijaz S, et al. Hepatitis E: an emerging infection in developed countries. *Lancet Infect Dis.* 2008;8(11):698–709.
6. Montalbano M, Slapak-Green GI, Neff GW. Fulminant hepatic failure from herpes simplex virus: post liver transplantation acyclovir therapy and literature review. *Transplant Proc.* 2005;37(10):4393–4396.
7. Rumack BH. Acetaminophen misconceptions. *Hepatology.* 2004;40:10–15.
8. Lucey MR, Mathurin P, Morgan TR. Alcoholic hepatitis. *N Engl J Med.* 2009;360(26):2758–2769.
9. Navarro VJ, Senior JR. Drug-related hepatoxicity. *N Engl J Med.* 2006;354(7):731–739.

10. Czaja AJ, Manns MP. Advances in the diagnosis, pathogenesis, and management of auto-immune hepatitis [published online ahead of print May 5, 2010]. *Gastroenterology.* 2010;139(1):58.e4–72.e4.

11. Weisberg IS, Jacobson IM. Cardiovascular diseases and the liver. *Clin Liver Dis.* 2011;15(1):1–20.

12. Plessier A, Valla DC. Budd-Chiari syndrome. *Semin Liver Dis.* 2008;28(3):259–269.

13. Roberts EA, Schilsky ML. AASLD position paper: diagnosis and treatment of Wilson disease: an update. *Hepatology.* 2008;47(6):2089–2111.

14. Polson J, Lee WM. AASLD position paper: the management of acute liver failure. *Hepatology.* 2005;41(5):1179–1197.

15. Lee WM. Etiologies of acute liver failure. *Semin Liver Dis.* 2008;28(2):142–152.

Chronic Liver Disease

19

Jennifer Shroff and Mauricio Lisker-Melman

CHRONIC VIRAL HEPATITIS

GENERAL PRINCIPLES

Definition

- Chronic viral hepatitis is defined by the persistence of viral infection for longer than 6 months, resulting in liver necroinflammatory and fibrotic changes which can lead to cirrhosis.
- Histopathologic classification of chronic liver disease is based on etiology, grade, and stage; grade represents the severity of necroinflammatory changes and stage represents the severity of fibrosis.

Classification

- The two most frequent viruses that result in chronic hepatitis are the hepatitis B (HBV) and C (HCV) viruses. The hepatitis D virus (HDV) is an infrequent etiology of chronic hepatitis in the United States. In rare occasions, and when associated with liver transplantation, the hepatitis E virus can also cause chronic hepatitis.

CHRONIC HEPATITIS B

GENERAL PRINCIPLES

Epidemiology

- There are about 2 billion people worldwide infected with HBV and about 350 to 400 million chronic carriers with measurable hepatitis B surface antigen (HBsAg).
- Acute infection can lead to chronic hepatitis B in 90% of newborns of hepatitis B e antigen (HBeAg)-positive mothers, 25% of infants/children, and 5% to 10% of adults.[1]
- Approximately 0.5% of chronic HBsAg carriers will clear this antigen yearly: 8% to 12% of chronic HBeAg-positive carriers will clear HBeAg. Spontaneous HBeAg clearance is affected by age, baseline alanine–aminotransferase (ALT) levels, and HBV genotype.
- Patients with chronic HBV have <1% per annum risk of developing hepatocellular carcinoma (HCC) with or without development of cirrhosis.

Etiology

- HBV is a DNA virus and belongs to the *Hepadnavirus* family.
- In endemic regions, such as Asia and sub-Saharan Africa, hepatitis B infection is frequently transmitted from mother to child (vertical transmission), whereas

in Western countries, where chronic hepatitis B is relatively rare, infection is transmitted from adult to adult (horizontal transmission).

- Infection is **acquired through sexual contact, parenteral routes** (e.g., needle stick, injection drug use, and blood transfusions), or **perinatal transmission**.

Natural History

- **Chronic carriers** are defined by HBsAg positivity for longer than 6 months.
- The **four clinical phases** of chronic hepatitis B infection consist of the **immune-tolerant phase, immune active** or **immune clearance phase, inactive phase,** and "**resolution phase.**" These are explained under "Interpretation of Laboratory Tests," on page 225.
- Patients with hepatitis B can have a fluctuating disease course and may progress from one stage to another.

Risk Factors

- **High-risk groups for chronic hepatitis B infection** include individuals with a history of homosexual or heterosexual promiscuity, intravenous (IV) drug users, patients on hemodialysis (HD), health care workers, children of HBeAg-positive mothers, recipients of multiple blood transfusions, residents and employees of residential care facilities, travelers to endemic areas, and natives of Alaska, Asia, or the Pacific Islands.
- **Risk factors for developing** HCC include family history of HCC, age more than 40 years, male sex, high viral replication, coinfection (i.e., HIV, HCV, HDV), aflatoxin exposure, and alcohol use.

Prevention

- **Screening** is recommended for people born in high or intermediate endemic areas, unvaccinated US-born adults whose parents are from countries with high or intermediate HBV prevalence, patients with chronically elevated liver function tests, those receiving immunosuppression or chemotherapy, men with active homosexual partners, history of sexually transmitted diseases, history of sexual promiscuity, prison inmates, IV drug users, patients on HD, HIV/HCV patients, pregnant women, and household and sexual contacts of patients with HBV infection.
- **Preexposure prophylaxis with HBV vaccine** should be considered for everyone, but particularly for individuals with a history of multiple blood transfusions, patients on HD, health care workers, injection drug users, household and heterosexual contacts of hepatitis B carriers, men with active homosexual partners, residents and employees of residential care facilities, travelers to hyperendemic areas, persons born in intermediate and high endemic areas, patients receiving long-term immunosuppression or chemotherapy, and natives of Alaska, Asia, and the Pacific Islands.
  - The Centers for Disease Control and Prevention recommends universal vaccination programs for infants and sexually active adolescents in the United States.
  - Vaccination is administered as a three-shot series at 0, 1, and 6 months. For patients who require rapid immunity, vaccination can be administered at 0, 1, and 2 months with a follow-up booster shot at 6 months for long-lasting immunity.
  - Additional doses, higher doses, and alternative vaccine routes can be considered in nonresponders and hyporesponders (antihepatitis B surface antibody

[anti-HBs] <10 IU/mL) to elicit protective anti-HBs levels and long-lasting immunity.

○ Booster doses may be needed in immunocompromised individuals in whom anti-HBs levels fall below 10 IU/mL on annual testing.

- **Postexposure prophylaxis**

  ○ It should be considered in infants born to HBsAg-positive mothers. Newborns should receive HBV vaccine and hepatitis B immune globulin (HBIG) within 12 hours of birth. This strategy has been shown to be 95% efficacious in preventing vertical transmission of HBV; efficacy may be lower in mothers with high viral load (VL).

  ○ Susceptible sexual partners of HBV-infected individuals and individuals with HBV-contaminated needle-stick injuries should receive HBIG followed by the first dose of HBV vaccine at different body sites as soon as possible. A second dose of HBIG should be administered at 30 days postexposure and the vaccine series should be completed.

  ○ Those who remain susceptible to HBV infection, including health care workers, patients on dialysis, and sexual partners of carriers should be tested for vaccination response 1 to 2 months after the last dose of the vaccine.

  ○ In HBV seronegative patients receiving antihepatitis B core antibody-positive liver transplants, lifelong antiviral therapy is indicated.

  ○ All chronic HBV patients should receive two doses of hepatitis A virus (HAV) vaccine 6 to 12 months apart if not immune to HAV.

Associated Conditions

- Patients with chronic hepatitis B (about 10% to 15% of patients) may develop **immune-mediated extrahepatic manifestations,** including polyarteritis nodosa, glomerulonephritis, cryoglobulinemia vasculitis, serum sickness-like illness, papular acrodermatitis (predominantly in children), and aplastic anemia.

DIAGNOSIS

Clinical Presentation

- Chronic hepatitis B usually progresses with nonspecific symptoms until complications develop from cirrhosis or HCC.

History

- This should include details about place of birth, family history of HBV infection and liver cancer, personal history of smoking, ETOH use, tattooing, IV drug abuse, drug transfusions, sexual habits, travel to endemic countries, and employment.

- The clinical presentation of chronic viral hepatitis varies significantly from asymptomatic to manifestations of advanced liver disease. Frequently, patients manifest vague symptoms like **malaise, fatigue and weakness, abdominal pain, myalgias, arthralgias, nausea, and anorexia.**

Physical Examination

- Physical examination findings of chronic viral hepatitis vary according to the stage of the disease at diagnosis. In early phases, the patient may not show physical examination abnormalities.

- Physical examination **findings of cirrhosis** include jaundice, parotid gland enlargement, gynecomastia, ascites, abdominal collateral circulation, peripheral edema, telangiectasia, muscle wasting, palmar erythema, and mental status abnormalities; these findings are not specific to any particular liver disease etiology.

Diagnostic Criteria

Chronic hepatitis B infection is generally defined by the following characteristics:

- HBsAg positive for more than 6 months
- Presence or absence of HBeAg
- Elevated levels of serum HBV DNA (levels vary depending on the phase of the infection)
- Persistent or intermittent elevation in ALT or aspartate aminotransferase (AST) levels
- Liver biopsy showing chronic hepatitis with different degrees of inflammation and fibrosis

Diagnostic Testing

- Diagnosis of chronic hepatitis B is based on the detection of antigens/antibodies of the HBV and HBV DNA. Additional testing includes routine liver chemistry, HBV genotype (soon to become a routine test), and liver biopsy when indicated.

Laboratory Testing

Patients with chronic HBV infection are evaluated for the presence or absence of markers of infection, as follows:

- **Hepatitis B surface antigen (HBsAg)** is detectable in serum or hepatocyte cytoplasm (immunoperoxidase staining) in acute or chronic HBV infection. This disappears if the virus is cleared. The persistence of HBsAg is the diagnostic hallmark of chronic HBV infection.
- **Antibody against HBsAg (anti-HBs)** appears after the disappearance of HBsAg and after vaccination. The presence of anti-HBs demonstrates clearance or immunity to the disease.
- **Hepatitis B core antigen (HBcAg)** is not detectable in serum but can be found in the hepatocyte nuclei by immunoperoxidase staining during active viral replication.
- **IgM antibody against HBcAg (anti-HBc IgM)** is present during acute infection and in periods of high viral replication in chronic disease (flares).
- **IgG antibody against HBcAg (anti-HBc IgG)** is usually present in patients with chronic disease and in conjunction with anti-HBs in patients who cleared the disease. In some cases, patients with isolated IgG anti-HBc can reactivate the HBV infection after immunosuppression or chemotherapy.
- **Hepatitis B e antigen (HBeAg)** appears in the serum shortly after HBsAg. This is indicative of active viral replication and high infectivity. Patients harboring HBV infection with precore or basal core promoter mutations cannot synthesize or secrete this antigen (HBeAg negative) despite high viral replication.
- **Antibody against HBeAg (anti-HBe)** usually indicates low-level replication and lower degree of infectivity. The best-known exception is the patient infected with precore or basal core promoter mutations (HBeAg negative but anti-HBe positive).
- **HBV DNA is the most accurate and sensitive marker of viral replication.** It is detected by polymerase chain reaction and reported as international units per milliliter (IU/mL).

Diagnostic Procedures
- **Liver biopsy** is useful in determining the degree of inflammation (grade) and fibrosis (stage) in patients with chronic hepatitis B.

Interpretation of Laboratory Tests (Table 19-1)
Patients with chronic HBV infection may progress through four clinical phases.

- **Immune tolerant phase.** It is generally seen in patients with perinatally acquired infection. Patients generally have subclinical or mild disease and normal ALT levels. HBV is actively replicating (>1,000,000 IU/mL). HBeAg is present. The liver biopsy is generally normal or with mild inflammatory changes. Some of these patients may develop active liver disease later in life.
- **Immune active or immune clearance phase.** It is characterized by elevated HBV DNA levels (>20,000 IU/mL), positive (wild type) or negative (precore mutation or basic core promoter mutation) HBeAg, elevated liver enzymes, and abnormal biopsy with different degrees of inflammation and fibrosis.
- **Inactive phase.** These patients have few or no symptoms. There is low replicative activity with low HBV DNA levels (<2000 IU/mL), negative HBeAg, and normal liver enzymes. The liver biopsy shows mild or no inflammation and different degrees of fibrosis. Inactive carriers may flare to active replication even after years of quiescent disease.
- **Resolution phase.** These patients have no symptoms of liver disease. It is characterized by loss of HBsAg and seroconversion to anti-HBs. HBV DNA falls and eventually disappears and liver enzymes normalize. Liver histology may return to normal. These patients develop permanent immunity (anti-HBs, anti-HBc).

TABLE 19-1	**USE OF LABORATORY TESTS IN CHRONIC HBV**				
Test	Immune Tolerant	High Replication Chronic HBV	Low Replication Chronic HBV	Precore/ BCP Mutation	Resolution of HBV
HBsAg	+	+	+	+	−
HBeAg	+	+	+	−	−
Anti-HBs	−	−	−	−	+
Anti-HBe	−	−	+	+	+
IgM anti-HBc	−	+	−	−	−
IgG anti-HBc	+	+	+	+	+
HBV DNA	>10^6 IU/mL	>10^5 IU/mL	<10^3 IU/mL	>10^4 copies /mL	Absent
ALT/AST	Normal	+++	Normal	+/++	Normal

ALT, alanine transaminase; AST, aspartate transaminase; BCP, basal core promoter; HBc, hepatitis B core antigen; HBeAg, hepatitis B e antigen; HBsAg, hepatitis B surface antigen; HBV, hepatitis B virus.

Additional Tests

- **Genotype determination** of HBV has growing clinical significance and is becoming a standard marker in clinical practice.
- Patients with genotypes A and B are more likely to have spontaneous HBeAg seroconversion at an earlier age, have slower progression to cirrhosis, have less hepatic inflammation, and are more responsive to interferon treatment.

TREATMENT

Goals

- Treatment of chronic HBV infection has the following goals: clearance/suppression of HBV DNA, HBeAg and HBsAg seroconversion, normalization of serum ALT, and normalization of liver histology.

Indication

- Treatment is indicated for patients with decompensated cirrhosis despite low HBV-DNA levels (<2000 IU/mL), compensated cirrhosis with HBV DNA VL >2000 IU/mL, HBeAg-positive and HBeAg-negative patients with high HBV DNA (VL >20,000 IU/mL and >2000 IU/mL, respectively), and ALT more than two times the upper limit of normal (ULN).[2]
- Patients with mildly elevated ALT levels (less than double the ULN) or persistently elevated DNA levels should be evaluated for possible treatment on a case-by-case basis. Liver biopsy evaluation of necroinflammatory changes and fibrosis may help determine treatment. Patients with moderate or severe inflammation or significant fibrosis may benefit from treatment.

Medications

Current treatment options include **pegylated interferon alpha therapy (pIFNα), nucleoside, and nucleotide analogs** (Table 19-2).

First-Line Treatments

- **Interferon therapy**
  ○ Interferons are glycoproteins with antiviral, immunomodulatory, and antiproliferative actions. The addition of polyethylene glycol to the standard IFN (α2a or α2b) molecule results in prolonged half-life with improved bioavailability.
  ○ pIFNα is administered as weekly subcutaneous injections. No antiviral-resistance mutations are induced by IFN.
  ○ Interferon therapy is contraindicated in patients with decompensated liver disease. Side effects include flu-like syndrome (headache, fatigue, myalgias, arthralgias, fever, and chills), neuropsychiatric symptoms (depression, irritability, and concentration impairment), reversible bone marrow suppression, and other effects (alopecia, thyroiditis, and injection-site reactions).
- **Nucleoside and nucleotide analogs**
  ○ Nucleoside or nucleotide analogs are orally administered agents that are better tolerated than IFN therapy; the major concern for long-term use of these agents is the selection of antiviral-resistant mutations.
  ○ First-line agents are tenofovir and entecavir. These analogs have robust antiviral activity and are associated with lower rates of drug resistance mutations. Both should be dose-adjusted in patients with renal disease.

TABLE 19-2 THERAPEUTIC AGENTS IN CHRONIC VIRAL HEPATITIS

	Indication	Side Effects	Contraindications
Ribavirin (*always in conjuction with pegylated-IFN*)	Chronic hepatitis C	Teratogenicity, hemolytic anemia, hyperuricemia, itching, rash, pulmonary symptoms, renal disease. Severe anemia and lactic acidosis when used with didanosine or AZT in HIV patients.	Pregnancy Renal insufficiency Inability to tolerate anemia Erythrocyte membrane enzymatic defects
Pegylated-IFN	HBeAg+ patients HBeAg– patients Chronic hepatitis C	Flu-like symptoms, neuropsychiatric symptoms, bone marrow suppression, autoimmune phenomena	Advanced liver disease with complications
Nucleotide Inhibitors (TFV, ADV)	HBeAg+ patients HBeAg– patients Cirrhotics LAM-resistant patients	Tolerable medication with few important side effects. Debate about renal failure, Fanconi's syndrome, hypophosphatemia, bone loss. Few common side effects include nausea, diarrhea, muscle pain and weakness.	Caution if concurrent nephrotonic agents. Dose adjust in patients with renal disease. Pregnancy category B (TFV) and category C (ADV).
Nucleoside Inhibitors (ETV, LAM, TBD)	HBeAg+ patients HBeAg– patients Cirrhotics	Tolerable medication with few important side effects. Lactic acidosis has been reported as a serious reaction to ETV. Common side effects include headaches, fatigue, dizziness, nausea.	Caution if concurrent nephrotoxic agents. Dose adjust in patients with renal disease. Pregnancy category B (TBD) and category C (ETV).

ADV, adefovir; AZT, azidothymidine (zidovudine); ETV, entecavir; LAM, lamuvidine; TBD, telbuvudine; TFV, tenofovir.

- **Tenofovir**
  - Tenofovir disoproxil fumarate is a nucleotide analog that effectively suppresses HBV DNA in HBeAg-positive, HBeAg-negative, cirrhotic (decompensated and compensated), and lamivudine/adefovir-resistant patients. HBV DNA suppression was defined as VL <400 copies/mL. HBV suppression occurred in 96% to 99% of HBeAg-positive patients and in 99% of HBeAg-negative patients after 192 weeks of tenofovir therapy. In lamivudine-resistant HBeAg-positive patients, the efficacy was 98% after 96 weeks of treatment. In a recent study with patients with decompensated cirrhosis, 71% of patients suppressed HBV DNA after 48 weeks of tenofovir therapy.[3] HBsAg loss in HBeAg-positive and HBeAg-negative patients was 10% (192 weeks of treatment) and 7% (96 weeks of treatment), respectively.[4]
  - The daily dose is 300 mg. Tenofovir has an excellent safety profile. Resistance mutations are not yet known through 4 years of therapy.
- **Entecavir**
  - Entecavir is a nucleoside analog that effectively suppresses HBV DNA in HBeAg-positive, HBeAg-negative, and cirrhotic (decompensated and compensated) patients, but its use is associated with high rates of failure in lamivudine-resistant patients. HBV DNA suppression was defined as VL <400 copies/mL. HBV DNA suppression occurred in 94% of HBeAg-positive patients after 5 years of therapy and 85% to 96% of HBeAg-negative patients after 96 weeks of entecavir therapy.[5] In lamivudine-refractory HBeAg-positive patients, the efficacy of entecavir after 96 weeks of treatment was about 40%. In patients with decompensated cirrhosis, HBV DNA suppression occurred in 72% of patients after 48 weeks of therapy in a recent study.[3] Loss of HBsAg occurred in 5.1% of HBeAg-positive nucleoside-naïve chronic HBV patients after 96 weeks of treatment.
  - Entecavir reduces necroinflammation and reverses fibrosis and cirrhosis in some patients after many years of treatment. The dose is 0.5 to 1 mg daily. It has an excellent safety profile. Only 1% of treatment-naïve HBeAg-positive patients developed entecavir resistance over 5 years.[5] However, in lamivudine-resistant patients, 51% developed entecavir-resistance mutations and 43% developed virologic breakthrough (≥ 1 $\log^{10}$ rise in HBV DNA).

Second-Line Agents
- **Adefovir**
  - Adefovir is a nucleotide analog. The usual dose is 10 mg daily. This should be adjusted in patients with renal disease. It is effective for treating naïve HBeAg-positive and -negative and lamivudine-resistant HBV patients. The use of adefovir and lamivudine in combination leads to a significant reduction of lamivudine and adefovir–induced resistant mutations.
- **Lamivudine**
  - Lamivudine is a nucleoside analog. The usual dose is 100 mg daily. It is safe in patients with advanced or decompensated liver disease. Treatment success is proportional to treatment duration. The high rate of antiviral-resistant mutations (15% to 20% per year of treatment) has diminished its use in patients with hepatitis B.
- **Telbivudine**
  - Telbivudine is a nucleoside analog with a few advantages over other members of the same class.

Nonpharmacologic Therapies

- **Liver transplantation** is indicated in patients with advanced cirrhosis caused by HBV. Immunoprophylaxis with HBIG combined with a nucleoside or nucleotide analog is used to diminish the possibility of post-liver transplantation recurrence.

MONITORING/FOLLOW-UP

- Patients with chronic HBV should be screened with imaging studies (abdominal ultrasound, computed tomography [CT], magnetic resonance imaging [MRI]) and α-fetoprotein every 6 to 12 months for early detection of HCC.

CHRONIC HEPATITIS C

GENERAL PRINCIPLES

Epidemiology

- About 180 million people are infected throughout the world with the HCV.[6]
- In the United States, 4 million people are positive for antibodies against HCV (anti-HCV).
- HCV infection is the main cause of liver disease–related deaths and the primary indication for liver transplantation in the United States.

Etiology

- HCV is an RNA virus that belongs to the *Flaviviridae* family.
- HCV is transmitted parenterally via transfusion, injection drug use, or needlestick injury. It is rarely acquired through sexual or vertical transmission (mother to child).
- Acute hepatitis progresses to chronicity in 60% to 80% of HCV patients and will result in cirrhosis in about 15% to 20% of patients. Cirrhotic patients are at increased risk for the development of HCC.

Natural History

- The incubation period is 15 to 150 days.
- Chronic HCV has an indolent clinical course over decades. Patients with immunosuppression, alcoholism, and obesity may have a faster progression to cirrhosis.

Risk Factors

- The highest prevalence is among hemophiliacs receiving **blood transfusion before 1987** and people with **history of IV drug use** (leading mode of transmission in the United States). There is a moderate prevalence in recipients of blood transfusions or patients with organ transplantation before 1992.
- There is a lower prevalence among **patients on HD**, those with **tattooing or body piercing, monogamous sexual partners of HCV-infected people,** and **health care workers with occupational exposure to needlesticks.**
- Risk factors for rapid development of cirrhosis include male gender, older age, alcohol consumption (more than 50 g/day), obesity with hepatic steatosis, and HIV coinfection.

Prevention

- There is no available vaccine for HCV prevention.

Associated Conditions

- **Extrahepatic manifestations** of hepatitis C include mixed cryoglobulinemia vasculitis (10% to 25% of patients with HCV), glomerulonephritis, porphyria cutanea tarda, cutaneous necrotizing vasculitis, lichen planus, and lymphoma.

DIAGNOSIS

Clinical Presentation

History and Physical Examination

- Chronic HCV symptoms and physical examination are similar to those described in other forms of chronic viral hepatitis (see Chronic Hepatitis B, Clinical Presentation).

Diagnostic Testing

Laboratories

- Diagnosis of HCV infection is suspected by the presence of anti-HCV antibodies and confirmed with the detection of HCV RNA. **Anti-HCV antibodies** may be undetectable for the first 8 to 12 weeks after infection; **acute HCV** can be diagnosed by the presence of **HCV RNA** during this time.
- A **false–positive-anti-HCV test** can be seen in the setting of hypergammaglobulinemia or autoimmune hepatitis (AIH). A **false–negative-anti-HCV test** may be seen in immunocompromised patients on HD and solid organ transplant recipients.
- **HCV RNA** is detected in serum as early as 1 to 2 weeks after infection. This test is useful both for diagnosis and for assessment of sustained virologic response (SVR) after treatment.
- **HCV genotype** determination influences the duration, dosage, and susceptibility to treatment. Genotype 1 (subtypes 1a and 1b) accounts for the majority of infections in the United States and generally has a poorer susceptibility to treatment. Genotypes 2 and 3 account for 20% of HCV infection in the United States and generally are treatment sensitive.

Diagnostic Procedures

- **Liver biopsy** is useful in determining the grade and stage of liver disease.
- Liver biopsy status may be helpful in determining when to start therapy and as a prognostic factor.

TREATMENT

Goals

- Goals of treatment are to clear the hepatitis C virus and prevent complications of chronic HCV infection, including cirrhosis and HCC.
- **Treatment response** is assessed by normalization of ALT levels, clearance of HCV RNA, and improvement in liver biopsy parameters of inflammation and

fibrosis. Treatment response is defined on the basis of the time of clearance of the HCV RNA.

○ **Rapid virologic response** is defined as undetectable HCV RNA level at 4 weeks of therapy. **Complete early virological response** is defined as negative VL at 12 weeks of therapy.

○ **End of treatment response** is defined as undetectable HCV RNA levels at the termination of treatment. **Sustained virologic response** is defined as undetectable HCV RNA levels 6 months after treatment discontinuation. Infection is considered eradicated when SVR is obtained. SVR is generally achieved in about 40% to 50% of all patients treated with antivirals.

○ **Nonresponders** are patients with no decrease in HCV RNA levels at 12 weeks of therapy. **Partial responders** ("**slow responders**") are patients whose HCV RNA levels decline by more than 2 logs after 12 weeks of treatment to become undetectable by 24 weeks. **Relapsers** are patients with negative HCV RNA levels at the end of treatment who flare after treatment discontinuation.

Medications

First Line

- Chronic HCV infection is treated with combination of subcutaneous **pegylated-interferon-α (pIFNα) and ribavirin.**
  ○ The dose for pIFN-α-2a is 180 mcg/week, whereas the dose for pIFN-α-2b is 1.5 mcg/kg/week.
  ○ The dose for oral ribavirin is 800 to 1400 mg/day (dependent on body weight).
  ○ Genotypes 1 and 4 patients are typically treated for 48 weeks with pIFN plus standard weight-based ribavirin. Patients with genotype 1 who obtain rapid virologic response (about 16%) may achieve SVR with shorter treatments.
  ○ Patients with genotypes 2 and 3 are usually treated with pIFN-α-2a and ribavirin for 24 weeks.
  ○ See Chronic Hepatitis B section for side effects of IFN.

Side effects of ribavirin include teratogenicity, hemolytic anemia, hyperuricemia, itching, rash, and pulmonary symptoms. It should be used cautiously in patients with renal disease. Severe anemia and lactic acidosis are side effects when used in conjunction with didanosine or azidothymidine (AZT, also called zidovudine) in HIV patients. Contraindications include pregnancy, chronic renal insufficiency, and inability to tolerate anemia.

Other Medications

- **Specifically targeted antiviral therapies** or **drug antiviral agents** for hepatitis C are in varying phases of clinical development.
- **Protease inhibitors** (telaprevir and boceprevir) are being evaluated by the Food and Drug Administration for use in chronic HCV. They are particularly useful for patients infected with genotype 1.
- Phase 2b and 3 studies have shown SVRs in the order of 61% to 68% in patients treated with triple therapy (pIFN, ribavirin, and a protease inhibitor) with low rates of relapse (2% to 14%).[7] These new treatments may also offer the advantage of shorter treatment courses.

Treatment Response

- Treatment outcomes are based on clinical status (acute versus chronic), HCV genotype, VL at initiation of therapy, and degree of fibrosis.

- Favorable characteristics for treatment response include female gender, non–African American race, lower body weight, and adherence to pIFN and ribavarin doses.
- Recent studies have shown that IL28B polymorphism (rs12979860) along with other single-nucleotide polymorphisms around the gene coding for IL28B are strong predictors of SVR and spontaneous clearance of HCV.[8]

Other Nonpharmacologic Therapies

- **Liver transplantation** may be indicated in patients with advanced cirrhosis.
  - Disease recurrence after transplantation is almost universal in those transplanted with viremia.
  - Posttransplantation recurrence is treated with pIFN and ribavirin; however, SVR in patients treated post–liver transplantation is lower than in nonimmunosuppressed patients.

SPECIAL CONSIDERATIONS

- Patients with cryoglobulinemia and mild/moderate proteinuria with slowly progressive renal disease can be treated with standard IFN or reduced doses of pIFN and ribavirin. Salvage therapy in those with poor response to pIFN and ribavirin includes rituximab, cyclophosphamide, methylprednisone, or plasma exchange.
- Patients with reduced creatinine clearance, HD, or decompensated cirrhosis may be treated cautiously with reduced doses of pIFN and ribavirin.

ALCOHOLIC LIVER DISEASE

GENERAL PRINCIPLES

Classification

- Liver toxicity induced by alcohol generates a spectrum of liver damage: **fatty liver, hepatitis, fibrosis, and cirrhosis**.

Epidemiology

- Fatty liver disease, the most common manifestation of alcoholic liver disease, is present in 90% of chronic alcohol users.[9]
- Progression to cirrhosis is seen in 5% to 15% of these patients despite abstinence, and in 30% to 37% if alcohol use continues.
- Despite the high prevalence of fatty liver disease in heavy drinkers, only 10% to 35% will develop alcoholic hepatitis.

Risk Factors

- Risk factors for liver disease in alcoholics include higher doses and longer duration of alcohol use (i.e., more than 60 g/day), obesity, iron overload, concomitant viral hepatitis, genetic factors, malnutrition, and female gender.
- Consumption of approximately 30 to 40 units per week of alcohol results in cirrhosis in 3% to 8% of patients with more than 12 years of alcohol use (one unit is equal to 8 g of alcohol, one glass of wine, or one 240 mL can of 3.5% to 4% beer).
- Rates of alcohol-related cirrhosis are higher among Blacks and Hispanics.

Associated Conditions

- Associated conditions induced by alcohol include **cardiomyopathy, skeletal muscle wasting, pancreatic dysfunction, and neurotoxicity**.

DIAGNOSIS

Clinical Presentation

Clinical presentation varies according to the stage of liver damage at time of presentation.

History and Physical Examination

- Physical examination findings in patients with alcoholic liver disease vary according to the stage of the disease at diagnosis.
- Patients with **fatty liver disease** are usually asymptomatic.
- **Alcoholic hepatitis** has a spectrum of clinical presentations and severity. Patients may have clinically silent disease or severe hepatitis with rapid development of hepatic failure and death.
- Patients with **alcoholic cirrhosis** may show classic signs and symptoms of advanced liver disease (see Hepatitis B section, 2.1.2.).

Diagnostic Testing

- Patients with evidence of liver disease should be screened for alcohol dependency by obtaining a thorough social history and sometimes random alcohol levels.
- The **CAGE questionnaire** has high sensitivity and specificity for identification of alcohol dependency. It consists of four questions: (1) Have you ever felt you needed to **C**ut down on your drinking? (2) Have people **A**nnoyed you by criticizing your drinking? (3) Have you ever felt **G**uilty about drinking? (4) Have you ever felt you needed a drink first thing in the morning (**E**ye-opener) to steady your nerves or to get rid of a hangover? Two "yes" responses is an indicator for further evaluation.

Laboratories

- Alcoholic hepatitis should be suspected in patients with elevated aminotransferases when the **AST to ALT ratio is >2:1.**
- A cholestatic picture characterized by **elevated alkaline phosphatase (AP), total bilirubin (predominantly conjugated)**, and **abnormal coagulation parameters** may also be found.
- Poor prognosis may be indicated by elevated creatinine, leukocytosis, marked cholestasis, and coagulopathy that does not improve with subcutaneous vitamin K administration.
- **Discriminant function** (DF) can be determined to assess in-hospital mortality. DF = 4.6 × (PT patient − PT control) + serum total bilirubin. DF >32 is associated with poor prognosis.

Imaging

- **Abdominal ultrasound** or radiologic cross-sectional studies (**MRI or CT**) are used to investigate other liver diseases including obstructive biliary pathology and infiltrative and neoplastic disease.

Diagnostic Procedures

- **Liver biopsy** is rarely indicated during the acute phase of alcoholic hepatitis. In later stages, it may be used to assess the stage and severity of liver damage.

- **Histology** includes Mallory hyaline bodies, ballooning degeneration, neutrophilic infiltrate, confluent parenchymal necrosis of hepatocytes, megamitochondria, intrasinusoidal and pericentral collagen deposition, lobular inflammation, nuclear vacuolation, bile duct proliferation, fatty change, and perivenular and perisinusoidal fibrosis.

TREATMENT

Nonpharmacologic Treatment

- **Abstinence from alcohol is the cornerstone of treatment.**
- Treatment in alcoholic liver disease also includes **nutritional support.**
  - ○ In the absence of hepatic encephalopathy or with a functioning gastrointestinal tract, enteral feeding should be considered if the patient is not eating.
  - ○ In patients with hepatic encephalopathy or with ileus, total parenteral nutrition should be considered (confers a mortality benefit).
  - ○ In patients with alcoholic cirrhosis, a regular oral diet with multiple feedings and high protein and caloric content improve survival.

Medications

- **Corticosteroids**
  - ○ Treatment of alcoholic hepatitis with corticosteroids is controversial. Evidence suggests, however, that patients with a DF >32 and hepatic encephalopathy may benefit from steroid therapy.[10]
  - ○ Prednisolone is started at 40 mg/day PO for 4 weeks and then tapered over 2 to 4 weeks.
- **Pentoxifylline**
  - ○ Treatment with pentoxifylline, a nonselective phosphodiesterase inhibitor with anti-inflammatory properties, has been shown to improve short-term survival in severe alcoholic hepatitis (DF >32), largely by reducing the development of hepatorenal syndrome.[11]
  - ○ The usual dose of pentoxifylline is 400 mg PO TID.
- **Other nonpharmacologic therapies**
  - ○ **Liver transplant** is indicated in patients with advanced liver disease from alcohol.
  - ○ A minimum of 6 months of abstinence and participation in a rehabilitation program are required to be considered a candidate for liver transplantation.

AUTOIMMUNE LIVER DISEASE

GENERAL PRINCIPLES

- Autoimmune liver disease encompasses a spectrum of illnesses, including AIH, primary sclerosing cholangitis (PSC), primary biliary cirrhosis (PBC), and overlap syndromes. These diseases have different clinical presentations and the diagnosis is often challenging to the physician (Table 19-3). Patients with autoimmune liver disease may have concurrent nonhepatic autoimmune illnesses.

TABLE 19-3 CLINICAL PROFILES IN PATIENTS WITH AUTOIMMUNE AND METABOLIC LIVER DISEASE

	Liver Test Pattern	Serologies	Liver Biopsy	"Clinical Pearls"
Autoimmune Liver Diseases				
Autoimmune Hepatitis	Hepatocellular	Type 1: Anti-SMA Type 2: Anti-LKM-1	Interface hepatitis and Plasma cell infiltrate	Responsive to steroids
PBC	Cholestatic	90% AMA positive	Destructive cholangitis affecting interlobular and septal bile ducts. Lymphocyte and mononuclear infiltrate. Several stages	Decrease morbidity and mortality in those treated with Ursodeoxycholic acid.
PSC	Mixed, predominantly, cholestatic	50%–80% pANCA positive	Ductular proliferation, obliterative fibrous cholangitis, Inflammation and fibrosis. Several stages	Associated with IBD. ERCP diagnostic method of choice.
Metabolic Liver Diseases				
Hemochromatosis	Hepatocellular	HFE-gene mutation, High transferrin sat.	Iron deposition in hepatocytes. HII 1.9>; High Iron per mcg/g dry weight	If treated appropriately mortality/morbidity equal to the general population
Wilson's Disease	Hepatocellular	Low ceruloplasmin	Fatty infiltration, glycogenic nuclei. Orcein stain positive	Chelating therapy is the cornerstone of treatment
α-1-antitrypsin deficiency	Hepatocellular	Low α-1-antitrypsin levels	PAS, diastase-positive periportal globules	No medical therapy for early stages. Liver transplantation ideal option for end stage liver disease.

AMA, antimitochondrial antibody; ERCP, endoscopic retrograde cholangiopancreatigraphy; IBD, inflammatory bowel disease; anti-LKM, anti-lower-kidney-microsomal antibody; pANCA, perinuclear antineutrophil cytoplasmic antibody; PBC, primary biliary cirrhosis; PSC, primary sclerosing cholangitis; SMA, smooth muscle antibody.

Definition

- AIH is a chronic inflammatory disease of the liver with no known cause.
  - Ongoing inflammation results in progressive hepatitis to fibrosis and eventually cirrhosis.
  - AIH is associated with circulating autoantibodies and hypergammaglobulinemia.

Classification

- There are two main types of AIH: Type 1 and Type 2.[12]
- Type 1 AIH affects predominantly females with a peak incidence in the second through fourth decades of life.
- Type 2 AIH predominantly affects children with elevated serum IgG levels.
- Both types are commonly associated with other autoimmune diseases, can progress to cirrhosis, and vary in their diagnostic markers (see "Diagnosis" section).

Epidemiology and Natural History

- AIH occurs worldwide and in all age groups; it most commonly affects women aged 10 to 30 years and older than 60 years (20% of all cases).
- Cirrhosis is more often the initial clinical presentation in African Americans than Caucasian patients.
- Older patients (older than 60 years) generally have greater degree of fibrosis, cirrhosis, and a higher frequency of portal hypertension at presentation.
- Incidence of HCC is about 1.1% per year.

Pathophysiology

- Environmental and genetic factors, along with regulatory T-cell dysfunction, cause dysregulation of immune responses to autoantigens resulting in a loss of immune-tolerance.
- Genetic studies have demonstrated different HLA antigen alleles in the AIH of adults (Type 1) compared with the AIH of children (Type 2), indicating that genetic factors may influence the presentation in different age groups.

Associated Conditions

- Extrahepatic manifestations may be found in 30% to 50% of patients. They include celiac sprue, Coombs' positive hemolytic anemia, autoimmune thyroiditis, Graves' disease, rheumatoid arthritis, ulcerative colitis (UC), type 1 diabetes, and vitiligo.
- Patients with AIH may have concurrent autoimmune liver diseases (e.g., PBC, PSC, autoimmune cholangitis).

DIAGNOSIS

Clinical Presentation

- AIH has a range of clinical presentations. In approximately 30% of cases, the presentation is acute with fever, abdominal pain, jaundice, and malaise. Some of these patients may progress to fulminant hepatic failure.
- AIH may have an indolent course with 25% to 30% of patients progressing to cirrhosis over time.

- About 40% of patients are asymptomatic (usually men with lower serum ALT levels).
- Careful history should be obtained to investigate the use of excessive alcohol, viral hepatitis risk factors, use of hepatoxins, and risk factors for metabolic disorders to rule out overlapping conditions and confounding variables.

Diagnostic Criteria

- Diagnosis is made by detection of elevated serum aminotransferases, circulating autoantibodies, elevated immunoglobulin levels, and liver biopsy.

Diagnostic Testing

Laboratories

- The most commonly elevated antibodies include **antinuclear antibody (ANA), antismooth muscle antibody (ASMA), and anti–liver-kidney microsomal antibody (LKM-1).** In type 1 AIH, ANA and ASMA are positive, whereas in type 2, anti-LKM-1 antibody is positive.
- **Other causes of liver disease should be excluded** such as Wilson's disease (WD), α_1-antitrypsin (α_1-AT) deficiency, viral hepatitis, alcohol-mediated liver disease, PBC, PSC, and other infections or medications that could cause liver disease.

Diagnostic Procedures

- **Liver biopsy** is essential for the diagnosis of AIH.
- "Piecemeal necrosis" or interface hepatitis with lobular or panacinar inflammation along with lymphocytic and plasmacytic infiltration are the histologic hallmarks. Bridging necrosis, fibrosis, or well-developed cirrhosis is found in advanced stages.

TREATMENT

Treatment Outcomes

- **Treatment is directed at achieving disease remission:** normalization of serum bilirubin, immunoglobulin levels, AST, ALT; disappearance of symptoms; and resolution of histologic changes. Remission should be achieved for 2 to 4 years to decrease likelihood of relapse.
- Other treatment outcomes include **incomplete response** (no remission after 3 years of treatment) and **relapse** (increase in serum AST to more than three times the ULN or increase in serum γ-globulin to >2 g/dL with redevelopment of interface hepatitis).

Treatment Indications

- Patients with AST levels at least ten-fold upper limit of normal range, or more than five-fold upper limit of normal with serum IgG more than two-fold the upper limit of normal, and those with bridging fibrosis or multilobular necrosis have a high mortality rate and should be treated promptly.[12]

Medications

- Therapy is initiated with **prednisone** (60 mg/day) alone or prednisone (30 mg/day) with **azathioprine** (1 to 2 mg/kg/day). Prednisone is tapered by 5 to 10 mg every week to 2 weeks when biochemical and clinical improvement is noted. Incomplete responders require lifelong low-dose prednisone and/or azathioprine therapy.

- **Relapses** should be re-treated with prednisone and azathioprine, with eventual weaning of prednisone and continuation of azathioprine at 2 mg/kg daily chronically.[13] An alternative treatment includes low-dose prednisone to maintain AST level less than three times upper limit of normal.
- **Side effects** associated with azathioprine include cholestatic hepatitis, pancreatitis, nausea, rash, worsening bone marrow suppression, malignancy, teratogenicity, and diarrhea. Side effects associated with corticosteroids include diabetes, psychosis, cataracts, glaucoma, and severe osteoporosis.
- **Refractory disease** occurs in about 20% of patients and may require "salvage" therapy with mycophenolate mofetil, cyclosporine, or tacrolimus.
- **Budesonide,** a synthetic steroid with high affinity for glucocorticoid receptors and high first-pass metabolism in the liver, is being studied as a safer alternative to prednisone. A recent study showed that budesonide, when used in conjunction with azathioprine, was effective in causing remission of disease in noncirrhotic AIH patients after 6 months of treatment with less steroid-specific side effects compared with prednisone.[14]
- AIH patients should be **vaccinated against HBV and HAV prior to treatment**.

Other Nonpharmacologic Therapies

- **Liver transplantation** is considered for patients with advanced cirrhosis and treatment failure. Five-year patient and graft survivals exceed 80%.
- Recurrent AIH posttransplant is seen in about 25% of patients and responds well to augmentation of existing immunosuppression with steroids and calcineurin inhibitors.[13]
- *De novo* AIH (AIH in patients receiving a transplant for nonautoimmune disease) should be treated with prednisone and azathioprine.[15]

PRIMARY SCLEROSING CHOLANGITIS

GENERAL PRINCIPLES

Definition

- PSC is a cholestatic liver disorder characterized by chronic inflammation and fibrosis resulting in progressive destruction of the extrahepatic and intrahepatic biliary ducts and ultimately cirrhosis.

Variant Diseases

- **Small duct PSC** is a variant in which the main bile ducts are normal on cholangiography but with cholestatic and histologic features of PSC; it has a more favorable prognosis.
- **Secondary sclerosing cholangitis** is a variant in which the destruction of bile ducts and resulting cirrhosis are a consequence of long-term biliary obstruction (i.e., cystic fibrosis), infection, ischemia of the biliary ducts, and inflammation instead of an autoimmune disorder.
- **IgG4-associated sclerosing cholangitis** is a poorly defined entity in which patients have increased levels of serum IgG4 and bile ducts infiltrated with IgG4-positive plasma cells.

Epidemiology

- The prevalence of PSC is about 10 per 100,000 in Northern European descendants.
- PSC occurs mainly in the fourth or fifth decade of life in adults and affects males more than females.
- Approximately 75% of patients have involvement of both large and small ducts, 15% have small duct disease (affecting ducts too small to evaluate with endoscopic retrograde cholangiopancreatography [ERCP]), and 10% have large duct disease only.
- The lifetime risk of cholangiocarcinoma in patients with PSC is from 7% to 15%.
- PSC median survival without liver transplantation fluctuates from 7 to 12 years depending on the stage at diagnosis.

Risk Factors

- Genetic associations in PSC and complex family inheritance patterns have been demonstrated. A significant increased risk of PSC exists among siblings.

Associated Conditions

- PSC is frequently associated with **UC** although their clinical courses have no correlation. In the United States, 70% of patients with PSC have UC and approximately 2% to 4% of patients with UC have PSC.
- **Other autoimmune diseases,** such as autoimmune pancreatitis and AIH, can coexist with PSC.

DIAGNOSIS

Clinical Presentation

- Physical examination findings of PSC vary according to the stage of the disease at diagnosis.
- Many patients are initially asymptomatic with normal physical examinations and isolated elevation of liver enzymes. Presentation with a cholestatic syndrome with jaundice and pruritus is also common.
- **Acute cholangitis** manifested by fever or rigors, right upper quadrant pain, and jaundice may be a clinical emergency. Usually, these patients have bacteremia and require IV antibiotics.
- Patients may present to the physician for the first time in late stages with cirrhosis.

Diagnostic Criteria

- Diagnosis is supported by liver chemistry, biliary tree imaging, and sometimes a liver biopsy.

Differential Diagnosis

- The differential diagnosis for PSC includes postoperative biliary strictures, choledocholithiais, chronic bacterial cholangitis, HIV-related cholangiopathy, biliary neoplasms, ischemic and medication-induced biliary injuries, metabolic liver diseases, viral hepatitis, and PBC.

Diagnostic Testing

Laboratories

- **AP** is the most commonly elevated liver test. **ALT and AST** are often elevated up to 2 to 3 times the ULN. **Serum IgG levels** are elevated to 1.5 times the ULN in about 60% of patients.
- **ANA** is often positive and **perinuclear antineutrophil cytoplasmic antibody (p-ANCA)** is positive in about 50% to 80% of the cases.

Imaging

- **Abdominal ultrasound** may be normal or may show bile duct wall thickening and focal bile duct dilation. Gallbladder pathology including gallbladder dilation or wall thickening, gallstones, cholecystitis, and mass lesions can also be present.
- **Abdominal CT** may show thickening and enhancement of biliary ducts, intrahepatic duct dilation, evidence of portal hypertension, and significant lymphadenopathy.
- PSC is confirmed by demonstration of multiple strictures and segmental dilations or irregularities of the intrahepatic and/or extrahepatic bile ducts ("beaded" pattern) by **ERCP or magnetic resonance cholangiopancreatography**.
- The finding of a "dominant stricture" (stenosis <1.5 mm in the common bile duct or <1 mm in the hepatic duct) should raise concern for cholangiocarcinoma. Stricture brush cytology and biopsies should be obtained to rule out malignancy. Digital image analysis and fluorescent in situ hybridization enhance the sensitivity of obtained brush cytologies.

Other Diagnostic Procedures

- **Liver biopsy** is usually unnecessary in the setting of positive ERCP for diagnosis of large-duct PSC, but it can be helpful in the diagnosis of small duct PSC, in excluding other diagnoses, and when overlap syndromes (i.e., PSC–AIH overlap syndrome) are suspected.
- Characteristic findings of PSC include concentric periductal fibrosis ("onion-skinning") that progresses to narrowing and obliteration of small bile ducts.
- PSC patients should also obtain a **screening colonoscopy with biopsies** to rule out inflammatory bowel disease.

TREATMENT

Medications

- **Pruritis** associated with PSC can be treated with **cholestyramine** followed by rifampin and opiate antagonists. Serotonin antagonists can also be used. In refractory states, plasmapheresis and liver transplantation should be considered.[16,17]
- **IgG4-associated sclerosing cholangitis is steroid responsive.**
- **Ursodeoxycholic acid (UDCA) has not been proven to have a survival benefit** in PSC patients despite improving liver biochemistries; it may cause adverse effects at higher doses.[18]

Nonpharmacologic Therapies

- **Dominant biliary duct strictures** can be treated with **balloon dilation and stenting;** prophylactic antibiotics should be administered before these endoscopic procedures. Endoscopic treatment of dominant strictures is associated with improved 3- and 5-year survival rates.
- **Episodes of cholangitis require antibiotics** and may require endoscopic therapy to treat biliary duct strictures. Rarely, surgical management of biliary strictures (biliary diversion) is indicated.
- **Liver transplantation** is a treatment option for PSC patients with advanced disease. Unique indications include intractable pruritis, recurrent cholangitis, and limited-stage cholangiocarcinoma.
  - 5-year survival rates post-liver transplantation is about 85%.
  - Recurrent PSC after liver transplantation has been documented. Other causes of posttransplant biliary strictures should be ruled out before establishing the diagnosis of posttransplant PSC recurrence.
- **PSC patients with cholangiocarcinoma can undergo surgical resection** in the absence of cirrhosis and in particular cases be considered for adjuvant chemotherapy and liver transplantation.

MONITORING/FOLLOW-UP

- Patients are monitored for chronic complications of cholestasis and for fat-soluble vitamin deficiencies.
- Surveillance for cholangiocarcinoma is conducted every 6 to 12 months with abdominal MRI/magnetic resonance cholangiopancreatography, CA19-9, and ERCP.

PRIMARY BILIARY CIRRHOSIS

GENERAL PRINCIPLES

Definition

- PBC is a cholestatic liver disorder of unknown etiology with autoimmune features.
- In patients with PBC, granulomatous destruction of interlobular and septal bile ducts results in progressive ductopenia, cholestasis, fibrosis, and cirrhosis.

Epidemiology and Natural History

- PBC is seen worldwide but is more commonly described in North America and Northern Europe. It has a worldwide prevalence of <1:2000.[19]
- PBC most commonly affects women in the fourth and fifth decades of life. It has a progressive course which may extend over many decades.

Associated Conditions

- **Extrahepatic manifestations** associated with PBC include keratoconjunctivitis sicca, renal tubular acidosis, gallstones, thyroid disease, scleroderma, Raynaud's phenomenon, and CREST syndrome (Calcinosis, Raynaud's phenomenon, Esophageal hypomotility, Sclerodactyly, and Telangiectasia).

DIAGNOSIS

Clinical Presentation

- Many patients are asymptomatic at the time of diagnosis.
- As the disease progresses, the most common clinical features of PBC include **fatigue** and **pruritus**. Patients with PBC develop features of portal hypertension.
- Patients with PBC frequently develop clinical **complications from chronic cholestasis**.
  - ○ Jaundice and pruritis are the most common clinical manifestations associated with chronic cholestasis and are often the first symptoms of PBC.
  - ○ Decreased secretion of bile acids and bile salts into the small bowel results in **malabsorption of fat and fat-soluble vitamins,** including vitamins A, D, E, and K.
- Clinical consequences of vitamin malabsorption include the development of osteoporosis and rarely osteomalacia. Increased risk of bleeding with abnormal prothrombin time/INR is common.
  - ○ Chronic cholestasis results in **hypercholesterolemia** and the associated development of **xanthomas and xanthelasma.** Xanthomas and xanthelasma are more commonly seen in PBC than in other diseases with chronic cholestasis.
  - ○ Cholestasis increases the production of melanin in the skin resulting in hyperpigmentation.
- **Sicca syndrome** can occur with PBC; it presents with dry eyes, dental caries, dry mouth, dysphagia, vaginal dryness, and dry skin.
- Patients with PBC may develop cirrhosis after 10 to 15 years of disease progression.
  - ○ Portal hypertension develops as a result of fibrosis or portal venule obliteration causing nodular regenerative hyperplasia (portal hypertension without cirrhosis).

Diagnostic Criteria

- Diagnosis of PBC is based on laboratory tests and liver biopsy showing cholestasis, positive autoimmune markers, and histology with nonsuppurative cholangitis and destruction of small and medium-sized bile ducts.

Differential Diagnosis

- The differential diagnosis for PBC includes cholestasis due to drug reaction, biliary obstruction, sarcoidosis, AIH, and PSC.

Diagnostic Testing

Laboratories

- Elevated **AP** is the most common abnormality seen in PBC. Hyperbilirubinemia, high cholesterol, elevated IgM, and bile acids are also frequently found. AST and ALT are mildly elevated.
- **Antimitochondrial antibody** is present in more than 90% of PBC patients and is the serologic hallmark for diagnosis.

Diagnostic Procedures

- **Liver biopsy** is helpful for both diagnosis and staging.
  - ○ Stages 1 to 3 disease is characterized by portal or periportal hepatitis with granulomatous destruction of bile ducts, bile duct proliferation, and bridging necrosis and fibrosis. Stage 4 disease is characterized by cirrhosis.

TREATMENT

Medications

- **UDCA** at a dose of 13 to 15 mg/kg/day may improve liver test abnormalities and delays progression of disease with improvement in survival when given long term (>4 years).[19] UDCA can be an effective treatment for any histologic stage of PBC. Side effects of UDCA include minimal weight gain, loose stools, and hair thinning.
- Symptom-specific therapy for pruritus, steatorrhea, and malabsorption can be added to treatment with UDCA.
- Pruritis can be treated with cholestyramine, rifampin, sertraline, and naltrexone.

Other Nonpharmacologic Therapies

- Liver transplantation is indicated in PBC patients with advanced cirrhosis. Recurrent PBC has been documented after transplantation.

NONALCOHOLIC FATTY LIVER DISEASE

GENERAL PRINCIPLES

Definition

- Nonalcoholic fatty liver disease (NAFLD) is a clinicopathologic syndrome that encompasses several clinical entities, including simple steatosis, steatohepatitis, fibrosis, and end-stage liver disease in the absence of significant alcohol consumption.

Classification

- **Nonalcoholic steatohepatitis (NASH)**, which is part of the spectrum of NAFLD, is defined by the presence of steatosis, hepatocellular ballooning, lobular inflammation, and pericellular or perisinusoidal fibrosis. It accounts for about one-fifth of NAFLD and has the risk for progression to cirrhosis.
- **Non–NASH fatty liver** consists of "simple" steatosis lacking significant inflammation and is characterized by more stable disease with lesser risks for progression to cirrhosis.

Epidemiology

- A worldwide condition, NAFLD is a common liver disease in the United States affecting 20% to 30% of the adult population. The prevalence of NASH is about 2% to 3% with a higher prevalence among Mexican-Americans.
- NAFLD affects both children and adults; its incidence increases with age.
- Approximately 30% of patients with NASH will progress to fibrosis over 5 years and 15% to 20% progress to cirrhosis over time.[20] About 37% of patients with fibrosis will progress to cirrhosis, 34% will have stable disease, and about 29% will have histologic improvement. Three percent to four percent of NASH patients progress to end-stage disease each year.
- Mortality among NASH patients is more often from cardiovascular disease than cirrhosis.

Etiology and Pathophysiology

- The mechanism by which NAFLD progresses to NASH is not completely clear.
- Decreased lipid output from the liver, increased peripheral lipolysis, and increased hepatic uptake of fatty acids lead to the development of macrovesicular

steatosis which is worsened by insulin resistance. In addition, hyperinsulinemia induces mitochondrial dysfunction which causes increased hepatic oxidative stress and development of steatohepatitis.[20]

- Secondary causes of NASH include hepatotoxic drugs (amiodarone, nifedipine, estrogens), surgical procedures (jejunoileal bypass, extensive small bowel resection, pancreatic and biliary diversions), and miscellaneous conditions (total parenteral nutrition, hypobetalipoproteinemia, environmental toxins).

Risk Factors

- Risk factors for NAFLD include female gender, insulin resistance, type II diabetes, central obesity, hypertension, and dyslipidemia.[21]

DIAGNOSIS

Clinical Presentation

- Disease presentation can vary from asymptomatic to advanced disease and HCC.

History

- Significant ETOH use (defined as more than two drinks per day for males and more than one drink per day for females) must be ruled out by history.
- A thorough review of patients' medications is essential, including over-the-counter medications, herbal remedies, and vitamin supplements.

Diagnostic Criteria

- Diagnosis is suspected clinically and confirmed by imaging and liver biopsy.

Diagnostic Testing

Laboratories

- **Liver enzyme elevations are generally mild.** Up to 80% of patients have normal liver enzymes.

Imaging

- Imaging studies, such as ultrasonography, CT, and MRI may detect steatosis.
- Magnetic resonance spectroscopy offers a quantitative measurement of liver fat content but is not commonly available in US medical centers.

Diagnostic Procedures

- **Liver biopsy remains the gold standard of diagnosis.**
  - Histologic lesions necessary for diagnosis include macrosteatosis, hepatocyte ballooning, and mixed lobular inflammation. More severe injury on initial biopsy is found in patients who are older, have elevated body mass index, and have diabetes.

TREATMENT

Medications

- **No specific established therapy** for NAFLD exists. However, multiple agents have been shown to improve liver histology and liver function tests in NAFLD.

- ○ **Vitamin E** has been shown to improve steatohepatitis, lobular inflammation, and aminotransferases in a portion of patients but does not significantly improve fibrosis scores.[22]
- ○ **Gemfibrozil, pravastatin, and atorvastatin** have been shown to improve aminotransferases and lipid profiles of NAFLD patients.
- ○ **Metformin** has been shown to decrease aminotransferase levels, insulin, and c-peptide levels significantly. Thiazolidinediones have been found to improve aminotransferases and liver histology in NAFLD patients.[22]
- ○ **Correction of associated conditions** such as hyperlipidemia, diabetes, and insulin resistance is warranted. It is imperative to discontinue possible offending agents (hepatotoxins).
- ○ **Agents under research** include TNF-α inhibitors (reduction of hepatic inflammation) and angiotensin receptor blockers (stellate cell inhibitor for prevention of hepatic fibrosis).

Nonpharmacologic Therapies

- **Weight loss and exercise** should be recommended to improve insulin resistance and other parameters of the metabolic syndrome.
- **Liver transplantation** should be considered in patients with advanced cirrhosis. Recurrence of NAFLD may occur after transplantation.

MONITORING/FOLLOW-UP

- Since NASH is associated with increased risk of HCC, annual screening with abdominal imaging studies and α-fetoprotein is warranted.

METABOLIC LIVER DISEASES

The most frequently encountered metabolic liver diseases include hereditary hemochromatosis (HH), α_1-AT deficiency, and WD (Table 19-3). These diseases generate different degrees of liver damage or progression to cirrhosis through different mechanisms.

HEREDITARY HEMOCHROMATOSIS

GENERAL PRINCIPLES

Definition
- HH is an autosomal recessive disorder of iron overload resulting in oxidative damage of hepatocytes.

Epidemiology
- HH is the most common inherited form of iron overload affecting Caucasians. HH is most common in middle-aged, Caucasian males.
- The degree of iron overload has a direct impact on life expectancy in individuals with HH; thus, diagnosis is targeted at identifying individuals before they become symptomatic. Thirty-eight percent to 50% of patients homozygous for HFE C282Y develop iron overload and 10% to 33% develop hemochromatosis-associated morbidity.[23]

Etiology/Pathophysiology

- HH is primarily caused by a missense mutation (C282Y) in the HFE gene located on chromosome 6.
- **HFE gene mutation** causes deficient synthesis of the hormone hepcidin, causing increased iron entry into the bloodstream which exceeds the storage capacity of ferritin and the binding capacity of transferrin; this promotes increased iron accumulation in liver parenchymal cells. Iron overload leads to production of highly reactive oxygen species which damage intercellular structures. Furthermore, abnormal iron absorption in the duodenum as well as increased release of iron from reticuloendothelial macrophages leads to excessive and damaging iron deposition in the heart, pancreas, skin, and endocrine system (in addition to the liver).[24]
- Approximately, 80% of patients with HH who are of Northern European descent are homozygotes for the C282Y mutation.

Risk Factors

- The major risk factor for development of HH is **family history** of HH.
- Alcohol abuse is the main modifiable risk factor associated with disease progression to cirrhosis.
- Patients with cirrhosis caused by HH are at increased risk of HCC despite adequate iron depletion therapy.

Prevention

- Family members of patients with HH should be screened with fasting transferritin saturation and ferritin levels. Genetic testing may be performed if needed.
- Screening should also be considered in patients with liver disease of unknown etiology, porphyria cutanea tarda, and chondrocalcinosis.

Associated Conditions

- Cardiomyopathies, hypogonadism, and diabetes are frequently associated with HH.

DIAGNOSIS

- Diagnosis is based on laboratory testing, imaging, and liver biopsy.

Clinical Presentation

- Some patients are asymptomatic at presentation.
- Clinical manifestations include slate-colored skin, diabetes, cardiomyopathy, arthritis, and hypogonadism. More common symptoms include fatigue, malaise, arthralgias, and hepatomegaly.
- Patients with progressive liver iron overload will develop fibrosis and clinical manifestations of cirrhosis.

Diagnostic Testing

Laboratories

- **High fasting transferrin saturation** (>45%) is suggestive of the diagnosis.
- Other nonspecific laboratory tests include **elevated serum iron** and **ferritin** levels.
- The diagnosis is confirmed by the presence of **specific mutations in the HFE gene.**

Imaging

- **MRI is the imaging of choice** for noninvasive assessment of iron storage in the liver.

Diagnostic Procedures
- **Liver biopsy is not required to establish the diagnosis** of HH; however, it is helpful in staging the disease, especially in individuals at increased risk of advanced fibrosis or cirrhosis and in those with iron overload without typical HFE gene mutations.

TREATMENT

First-Line Treatment
- Therapy consists of weekly **phlebotomy** until iron depletion is achieved (ferritin level <50 mcg/L and transferrin saturation <30%).
- Maintenance phlebotomy of 2 to 4 units of blood yearly is continued for life, with goal ferritin levels between 50 and 100 mcg/L.
- Treatment with phlebotomy before the onset of cirrhosis or diabetes significantly reduces the morbidity and mortality of HH.
- Phlebotomy can improve ALT/AST levels, skin pigmentation, hepatic fibrosis, daily insulin requirements, and symptoms of weakness, lethargy, and abdominal pain.[24]
- HH-related hypogonadism, cirrhosis, destructive arthritis, and diabetes are usually irreversible.
- Asymptomatic individuals homozygous for the HFE gene mutation with iron overload should be treated. Symptomatic individuals should also be treated to minimize extent of end-organ damage.

Medications
- **Deferoxamine** is an iron-chelating agent used in the setting of HH if phlebotomy is contraindicated secondary to severe anemia, cardiac failure, poor venous access, or poor tolerance. Deferoxamine binds free iron and facilitates its urinary excretion.
- **Deferasirox** is a new oral iron-chelating agent which has been shown to be effective in lowering serum ferritin levels in patients with HH in a recent phase 1/2, dose-escalation trial.[25]
- The usual starting dose is 10 mg/kg/day. Higher doses may cause creatinine and aminotransferases elevations.

Other Nonpharmacologic Therapies
- Liver transplantation may be considered in cases of HH with cirrhosis.
- Patients who undergo liver transplantation for HH tend to have poorer 1- and 5-year survival rates when compared with other liver transplant recipients.

Prognosis
- Patients with appropriately treated HH without cirrhosis have survival rates identical to that of the general population.

α_1-ANTITRYPSIN DEFICIENCY

GENERAL PRINCIPLES

Definition
- α_1-AT deficiency is an autosomal recessive disorder with codominant expression in which a mutant α_1-AT protein is formed. Retention of mutant α_1-AT

protein in hepatocytes and decreased serum α_1-AT levels causes cirrhosis and early-onset panlobular emphysema.

Epidemiology

- PiZZ genotype has an incidence of about 1:3500 and occurs mostly in people of Northern European ancestry. More than 30% of patients with PiZZ genotype develop cirrhosis (more common in older males).
- The disease onset has a bimodal distribution from neonatal hepatitis and cholestatic jaundice in infants to chronic liver disease in adults (fifth decade of life).
- There is an increased incidence of cholangiocarcinoma and HCC in PiZZ patients.

Pathophysiology

- α_1-AT is a serine protease inhibitor (prime inhibitor of neutrophil elastase). Accumulation of misfolded α_1-AT in the endoplasmic reticulum of the hepatocytes produces hepatic injury. Deficiency of serum α_1-AT causes lung injury because of uninhibited proteolytic damage to the lung connective tissue from unopposed action of elastase.
- The gene associated with this disorder is located on chromosome 14. The most common allele is M which gives rise to the normal protein protease inhibitor (Pi) M.
- The most common deficiency alleles are S (expresses 50% to 60% of α_1-AT) and Z (expresses 10% to 20% of α_1-AT), with S being slightly more prevalent. Deficiency genotypes associated with liver disease include PiSZ, PiZZ, and possibly PiMZ. PiZZ genotype is associated with more severe disease manifestations.[26]

Associated Conditions

- Associated conditions include panniculitis, systemic vasculitis, interstitial fibrosis (in patients with rheumatoid arthritis), peripheral neuropathy, multiple sclerosis, intracranial aneurysms, and membranoproliferative glomerulonephritis.

DIAGNOSIS

Clinical Presentation

- Patients may present with clinical features of cholestasis or cirrhosis. Asymptomatic patients present with isolated abnormal aminotransferases.
- α_1-AT deficiency can present as emphysema in early adulthood.

Diagnostic Criteria

- It includes quantification of the protease inhibitor and genotyping.

Diagnostic Testing

Laboratories

- **Low serum α_1-AT level** (<10% to 15% of normal) is suggestive of the disease.
- Other suggestive tests include decreased α_1-globulin level (protein electrophoresis). Patients with proven enzyme deficiency should be tested for their α_1-AT genotype.

Diagnostic Procedures

- **Liver biopsy is essential for diagnosis.** It shows characteristic periodic acid–Schiff–positive, diastase-resistant intracellular globules in the periportal hepatocytes.

TREATMENT

Medications

- Currently, **no specific medical treatment** exists for the liver disease associated with α_1-AT deficiency. Gene therapy for α_1-AT is a potential future alternative for these patients. For patients with emphysema, "augmentation therapy" (IV purified pooled human plasma α_1-AT) raises serum α_1-AT levels but does not necessarily improve the rate of FEV1 decline.[26]

Other Nonpharmacologic Therapies

- Liver transplantation is indicated in patients with α_1-AT deficiency and decompensated cirrhosis.
- Liver transplantation corrects the underlying disorder by normalizing α_1-AT production. It is unclear whether liver transplantation slows the onset of emphysema.

WILSON'S DISEASE

GENERAL PRINCIPLES

Definition

- Wilson's disease is an autosomal recessive disorder that results in progressive copper overload in the liver, kidney, brain, and cornea.

Epidemiology

- The incidence of Wilson's disease is 1:30,000.[27]
- This disease usually presents primarily as hepatic disease in younger patients and with neurologic or psychiatric symptoms in the second decade of life.

Pathophysiology

- Wilson's disease is caused by a mutation in the ATP7B gene located on chromosome 13.
- Absence or reduced function of the ATP7B gene results in decreased hepatocyte excretion of copper, precipitating copper accumulation within the liver.
- Progressive copper buildup results in hepatocyte injury, fibrosis, and cirrhosis.
- Copper is subsequently released into the bloodstream and deposited into the brain, kidneys, and cornea.

Prevention

- DNA testing for family members of affected individuals is becoming commercially available.
  - The analysis requires identification of the patient's ATP7B gene mutation or haplotype; this same haplotype is screened for in first-degree relatives.
  - Many patients are compound heterozygotes, making identification of mutations more difficult.
  - To date, more than 200 mutations of the ATP7B gene have been identified.

DIAGNOSIS

Clinical Presentation

- Wilson's disease can present as chronic hepatitis, cirrhosis, or rarely as fulminant hepatic failure.
- The diagnosis should be considered in patients with unexplained liver disease with or without neuropsychiatric symptoms, first-degree relatives with Wilson's disease, or individuals with fulminant hepatic failure.
- Cirrhosis is frequently identified in patients with Wilson's disease between the age of 10 and 20 years.
- **Neuropsychiatric manifestations** include asymmetric tremor, dysarthria, ataxia, and psychiatric features.
- **Other extrahepatic manifestations** include **Kayser-Fleischer rings** on slit lamp examination (gold to brown rings caused by copper deposition in Descemet's membrane in the periphery of the cornea), **hemolytic anemia, renal tubular acidosis, arthritis,** and **osteopenia.**

Diagnostic Testing

- Diagnosis is based on laboratory studies, imaging, and liver biopsy.

Laboratories

- Laboratory findings include **low ceruloplasmin levels** (<20 mg/dL), although normal values do not rule out the diagnosis.
- **Elevated serum copper level** (>200 mcg/dL) and **elevated 24-hour urinary copper level** (>100 mg/24 hours) may also be detected. These laboratory tests are better used for monitoring treatment in patients with Wilson's disease than for diagnostic purposes.
- Laboratory results may also show an AP to bilirubin ratio of <4 and an AST to ALT ratio of >2.2.

Imaging

- **Brain imaging** can demonstrate basal ganglia changes due to copper accumulation.

Diagnostic Procedures

- Liver biopsy findings are nonspecific and depend on the presentation and stage of the disease.
- Liver histology can include steatosis, glycogenated nuclei, chronic hepatitis, fibrosis, and cirrhosis.
- Elevated hepatic copper levels >250 mcg/g dry weight (normal <40 mcg/g dry weight) on biopsy are highly suggestive of Wilson's disease.

TREATMENT

Medications

- Treatment is with copper chelating agents or zinc salts. Chelating agents like trientine and penicillamine are used for initial and maintenance therapy, whereas zinc salts are used for maintenance therapy.[28]
- Patients require lifelong therapy.

Chelating Agents

Penicillamine

- Penicillamine 1 to 2 g/day PO in divided doses BID or QID plus pyridoxine 2.5 mg/day can be used in patients with hepatic failure.
- Side effects include hypersensitivity, bone marrow suppression, proteinuria, systemic lupus erythematosus, or Goodpasture's syndrome.
- Penicillamine should never be given as initial treatment to patients with neurologic symptoms.

Trientine

- Trientine 1 to 2 g/day PO in divided doses BID or QID is also used.
- Side effects are similar to those of penicillamine but occur in lower frequency. The risk of neurologic decompensation with trientine is less than with penicillamine.

Tetrathiomolybdate

- Tetrathiomolybdate is both a chelating agent and inhibitor of copper absorption; the normal dose is 120 mg/day divided as 20 mg TID with meals and 60 mg at bedtime (without food). It can be given with zinc therapy.
- Tetrathiomolybdate is the treatment of choice for patients presenting with neurologic symptoms. It has a good safety profile; possible side effects include anemia, leukopenia, and mild elevations of aminotransferases.
- Dietary restriction of copper-containing food should be used in conjunction with drug treatment.

Zinc Salts

- **Zinc salts** at a dose of 50 mg PO TID are indicated for treatment of WD in patients with chronic hepatitis and cirrhosis in the absence of hepatic failure.
- It can be used in association with penicillamine and trientine.
- Other than gastric irritation, zinc has a very good safety profile.

Other Nonpharmacologic Therapies

- Liver transplantation is the therapy of choice for fulminant hepatic failure and for progressive liver dysfunction despite chelation therapy.
- Plasmapheresis and hemofiltration may help bridge patients to transplant by markedly reducing serum copper levels, thereby reducing hemolysis and second organ damage.
- In the absence of neurologic symptoms, liver transplantation has a good prognosis and requires no further medical treatment.

REFERENCES

1. Lok AS, McMahon B. AASLD practice guidelines. Chronic hepatitis B: update 2009. *Hepatology.* 2009;50:1–36.
2. Lai M, Liaw YF. Chronic hepatitis B: past, present, and future. *Clin Liver Dis.* 2010;14:531–546.
3. Liaw Y, Sheen I, Lee C, et al. Tenofovir disoproxil fumarate (TDF), emtricitabine/TDF, and entecavir in patients with decompensated chronic hepatitis B liver disease. *Hepatology.* 2011;53:62–72.
4. Yuen MF, Lai C. Treatment of chronic hepatitis B: Evolution over two decades. *J Gastroenterol Hepatol.* 2011;26:138–143.
5. Chang TT, Lai CL, Kew Yoon S, et al. Entecavir treatment for up to 5 years in patients with hepatitis B e antigen-positive chronic hepatitis B. *Hepatology.* 2010;51:422–430.

6. Ghany MG, Strader DB, Thomas DL, et al. Diagnosis, management, and treatment of hepatitis C: an update. *Hepatology.* 2009;49:1335–1374.

7. Jang JY, Chung RT. New treatments for chronic hepatitis C. *Korean J Hepatol.* 2010;16(3):263–277.

8. Clark PJ, Thompson AJ, McHutchinson JG. IL28B genomic-based treatment paradigms for patients with chronic hepatitis C infection: the future of personalized HCV therapies. *Am J Gastroenterol.* 2010;370:1–7.

9. O'Shea Robert, Dasarathy S, McCullough AJ, et al. AASLD Practice Guidelines. Alcoholic liver disease. *Hepatology.* 2010;51:307–328.

10. Rambaldi A, Saconato HH, Christensen E, et al. Systematic review: glucocorticoids for alcoholic hepatitis-a Cochrane Hepato-Biliary Group systematic review with meta-analyses and trial sequential analysis of randomized clinical trials. *Aliment Pharmacol Ther.* 2008;27:1167–1178.

11. Akriviadis E, Botla R, Briggs W, et al. Pentoxifylline improves short-term survival in severe acute alcoholic hepatitis: a double-blind, placebo-controlled trial. *Gastroenterology.* 2000;119:1637–1648.

12. Mann MP, Czaja AJ, Gorham JD, et al. AASLD Practice Guidelines. Diagnosis and management of autoimmune hepatitis. *Hepatology.* 2010;51:2193–2213.

13. Yeoman AD, Longhi MS, Heneghan MA. Review article: the modern management of autoimmune hepatitis. *Aliment Pharmacol Ther.* 2010;31:771–787.

14. Manns M, Woynarowski M, Kreisel W, et al. Budesonide induces remission more effectively than prednisone in a controlled trial of patients with autoimmune hepatitis. *Gastroenterology.* 2010;139:1198–1206.

15. Muratori L, Muratori P, Granito A, et al. Current topics in autoimmune hepatitis. *Dig Liver Dis.* 2010;42:757–764.

16. Chapman R, Fevery J, Kalloo A, et al. Diagnosis and management of primary sclerosing cholangitis. *Hepatology.* 2010;51:660–678.

17. Mendes F, Lindor K. Primary sclerosing cholangitis: overview and update [published online ahead of print 2010]. *Nat Rev Gastroenterol Hepatol.* doi:10.1111/j.1365-2036.2011.04753.x.

18. Lindor KD, Kowdley KV, Luketic VA, et al. High-dose ursodeoxycholic acid for the treatment of primary sclerosing cholangitis. *Hepatology.* 2009;50:808–814.

19. Poupon R. Primary biliary cirrhosis: a 2010 update. *J Hepatol.* 2010;52(5):745–758.

20. Pasumarthy L, Srour J. Nonalcoholic steatohepatitis: a review of the literature and updates in management. *South Med J.* 2010;103:547–550.

21. Neuschwander-Tetri B, Clark J, Bass N, et al. Clinical, laboratory and histological associations in adults with nonalcoholic fatty liver disease. *Hepatology.* 2010;52:913–924.

22. Sanyal AJ, Chalasani N, Kowdley KV, et al. Pioglitazone, vitamin E, or placebo for nonalcoholic steatohepatitis. *N Engl J Med.* 2010;362:1675–1685.

23. Whitlock EP, Garlitz BA, Harris EL, et al. Screening for hereditary hemochromatosis: a systematic review for the U.S. Preventive Services Task Force. *Ann Intern Med.* 2006;145:209–223.

24. Pietrangelo A. Hereditary hemochromatosis: pathogenesis, diagnosis, and treatment. *Gastroenterology.* 2010;139:393–408.

25. Phatak P, Brissot P, Wurster M, et al. A phase 1/2, dose-escalation trial of deferasirox for the treatment of iron overload in HFE-related hereditary hemochromatosis. *Hepatology.* 2010;52:1671–1679.

26. Fairbanks K, Tavill A. Liver disease in alpha 1-antitrypsin deficiency: a review. *Am J Gastroenterol.* 2008;103:2136–2141.

27. Ala A, Walker AP, Ashkan K, et al. Wilson's disease. *Lancet.* 2007;369:397–408.

28. Roberts EA, Schilsky ML. Diagnosis and treatment of Wilson disease: an update. *Hepatology.* 2008;47:2089–2111.

Cirrhosis

20

Anupam Aditi and Jeffrey S. Crippin

GENERAL PRINCIPLES

- Cirrhosis is the common endpoint of a multitude of insults to the liver, with myriad complications caused by progressive liver dysfunction and portal hypertension.
- Ascites, hepatic encephalopathy, gastrointestinal (GI) bleeding, and renal dysfunction are the major sources of morbidity and mortality.
- Treatment of the underlying cause of cirrhosis as well as prevention of complications are the mainstays of treatment.
- Screening for hepatocellular carcinoma (HCC) and evaluation for liver transplantation are important steps in management.

Definition

- Cirrhosis is a pathologic diagnosis.
- The World Health Organization defines cirrhosis as a "diffuse process characterized by fibrosis and conversion of normal liver architecture into structurally abnormal nodules which lack normal lobular organization."[1]

Classification

- Classified by morphology, histology, and etiologic agent[1]
  - Morphology may be classified as micronodular, macronodular, or mixed.
  - Histology may be classified as portal, postnecrotic, posthepatitic, biliary, or congestive.
  - Etiology corresponds to specific morphologic and histologic findings.
- Clinical classification using **Child-Turcotte-Pugh score** (Table 20-1)[2]
  - This scoring system incorporates ascites, presence of encephalopathy, serum albumin, total bilirubin, and prothrombin time.
  - It can be used to determine 1-year mortality.

Epidemiology

- According to the summary health statistics from the 2007 National Health Interview Survey, ~2.6 million adults suffer from chronic liver disease and cirrhosis. However, this may be an underestimation, as 2.7 to 3.9 million are thought to have chronic hepatitis C in the United States alone.[3,4]
- Cirrhosis is the twelfth leading cause of death in the United States, with 29,963 deaths per year.[5]
- Cirrhosis is the fourth leading cause of death in the 45 to 54 age group amongst both men and women.[5]

TABLE 20-1 CHILD-TURCOTTE-PUGH SCORING SYSTEM

Criteria	1	2	3
Ascites	None	Slight	Moderate-severe
Encephalopathy	None	Mild	Moderate-severe
Bilirubin, mg/dL	<2	2–3	>3
Albumin, g/dL	>3.5	2.8–3.5	<2.8
Prothrombin time (seconds above normal prothrombin time)	1–3	4–6	>6

Child's class determined by adding scores from each of the five criteria together: class A, 5–6 points; class B, 7–9 points; class C, 10–15 points.

Etiology

- Cirrhosis is a common endpoint for many causes of liver disease (Table 20-2), with alcoholic liver disease and hepatitis C accounting for the majority of cases.[6]
- Other causes include autoimmune hepatitis, Wilson's disease, hemochromatosis, nonalcoholic fatty liver disease, drug hepatotoxicity, veno-occlusive disease, and cryptogenic cirrhosis.[6]

Pathophysiology

- The pathway to cirrhosis begins with hepatocellular damage.
  - Fenestrated sinusoids with absent intercellular junctions and basement membranes ensure close interactions between the sinusoidal blood and hepatocytes; therefore, hepatocytes are sensitive to blood-borne toxins.[7]
- Hepatocellular injury leads to the initiation of an inflammatory cascade with the release of cytokines, which amplify and sustain the overall response.
- Cytokines activate effector cells, especially hepatic stellate cells, initiating an autocrine loop of inflammation and fibrosis.[7–9]
  - Stellate cells are transformed into cells with fibrinogenic, contractile, and proliferative properties. Because of increased stellate cell contractility, there is increased intrahepatic resistance and decreased sinusoidal blood flow.
  - Stellate cell transformation also leads to "capillarization" of the hepatic sinusoids with a shift from a fenestrated sinusoid to a "nonfenestrated" capillary.
  - Capillarization induces a shift toward vasoconstriction, with increased production of endothelin and decreased production of nitric oxide.
  - Thrombosis of the microvasculature occurs with formation of intrahepatic arterial shunts.[9]
  - An erratic proliferation of hepatocytes takes place in hypoperfused areas, leading to a nodular pattern of regeneration within areas of fibrosis.

Risk Factors

- Cirrhosis is a common endpoint of chronic diseases that cause hepatic injury.
- These include chronic viral hepatitis, alcohol liver disease, iron overload, and chronic inflammatory conditions, such as nonalcoholic steatohepatitis.

TABLE 20-2 EVALUATION OF CIRRHOSIS

Historical Factors	Laboratory Evaluation	Suspected Cause
Excessive alcohol use	Increased AST to ALT ratio	Alcoholic liver disease
Intravenous drug abuse, tattoos, multiple sexual partners, sharing of needles, transfusions before 1992	Positive hepatitis B or C serologies	Chronic viral hepatitis
Fatigue, jaundice, pruritus	Antimitochondrial antibody, elevated alkaline phosphatase	Primary biliary cirrhosis
Ulcerative colitis, bacterial cholangitis, or cholangiocarcinoma	Elevated alkaline phosphatase	Primary sclerosing cholangitis
Neuropsychiatric symptoms	Kaiser-Fleisher rings, low serum ceruloplasmin, high urinary copper	Wilson's disease
Skin changes, arthritis, diabetes mellitus, hypogonadism	Ferritin, iron studies, hemochromatosis gene (HFE) mutations	Hemochromatosis
Autoimmune disease	ANA, increased serum quantitative immunoglobulins, smooth muscle antibody	Autoimmune hepatitis
Diabetes mellitus, obesity, dyslipidemia	Dyslipidemia, elevated levels of sugars	Nonalcoholic fatty liver disease
Emphysema without smoking history, positive family history	Emphysema, phenotype testing (PiZZ phenotype), α_1-antitrypsin level	α_1-Antitrypsin deficiency
Methotrexate or amiodarone use		Drug hepatotoxicity
History of anasarca, venous thromboembolism, or malignancy	Hypercoagulable state, nephrotic syndrome, paroxysmal nocturnal hemoglobinuria	Budd-Chiari syndrome
Stem-cell transplant		Veno-occlusive disease
Unknown factors		Cryptogenic cirrhosis

ALT, alanine aminotransferase; ANA, antinuclear antibody; AST, aspartate aminotransferase.

- ○ **Alcohol:** men with intake of >168 g/week; women with intake of >112 g/week.[10]
- ○ **Hepatitis C:** intravenous drug use, transplant or transfusion prior to 1992, and HIV infection.[11]

DIAGNOSIS

- Many patients present with overt complications of cirrhosis; however, one must have a high clinical suspicion in patients with subtle symptoms. Manifestations of cirrhosis in different organ systems is presented in Table 20-3.

Clinical Presentation

- **Subtle symptoms**
  - ○ Anorexia, nausea/vomiting, hyperirritability, pruritis, change in sleep pattern, decreased libido, shortness of breath, jaundice
- **Overt complications** of cirrhosis
  - ○ Hematemesis/melena, abdominal distention, ascites, confusion, edema/fluid overload
  - ○ Complications can also include a myriad of infections, coagulopathy, acute on chronic liver failure, hepatopulmonary syndrome, and HCC.

History

- The history should focus on common causes of liver disease and cirrhosis.
- Duration and quantity of alcohol intake, intravenous/intranasal drug use, sexual activity, family history of liver disease, prescription medications, and over-the-counter drug use.

TABLE 20-3	MANIFESTATIONS AND PRESENTATION OF CIRRHOSIS
Constitutional	Fatigue, weight loss, anorexia, malaise, muscle wasting
Gastrointestinal	Hematemesis, melena, esophageal or gastric varices, portal hypertensive gastropathy, gastritis, ascites
Pulmonary	Shortness of breath, dyspnea on exertion, hypoxia, hepatopulmonary syndrome, respiratory alkalosis, hepatic hydrothorax, portopulmonary syndrome
Cardiovascular	Hypotension, hyperdynamic circulation
Renal	Hepatorenal syndrome, hyponatremia
Endocrine	Decreased libido, impotence, testicular atrophy, dysmenorrhea, gynecomastia
Neurologic	Confusion, short-term memory loss, hyperirritability, insomnia encephalopathy
Dermatologic	Jaundice, spider angioma, palmar erythema, Dupuytren's contracture, caput medusa
Hematologic	Splenomegaly, thrombocytopenia, anemia, leukopenia, coagulopathy
Infectious	Spontaneous bacterial peritonitis, sepsis

- Personal history of ulcerative colitis, metabolic syndrome, premature emphysema, and history of autoimmune disease places patients at risk for primary sclerosing cholangitis, nonalcoholic fatty liver disease, α_1-antitrypsin deficiency, and autoimmune hepatitis, respectively.
- A history of a hypercoagulable state or prior malignancy may lead to hepatic venous thrombosis (Budd-Chiari syndrome). A stem cell or bone marrow transplant increases the risk of veno-occlusive disease.
- A constellation of skin changes, arthritis, diabetes mellitus, and hypogonadism is seen in individuals with hereditary hemochromatosis.

Physical Examination
- The physical examination can reveal **signs of cirrhosis**.
  - Muscle wasting, jaundice, spider angiomata, gynecomastia, caput medusa, prominent venous collaterals, palmar erythema, Dupuytren's contracture, testicular atrophy, and ecchymoses.
  - Splenomegaly, a coarse liver edge, and evidence of ascites (fluid wave, dullness in flanks, and/or shifting dullness) may be present on abdominal examination.
  - Rectal examination may reveal hemorrhoids, guaiac-positive stools, or melena.
  - Confusion, agitation, asterixis, and hyporeflexia are signs of hepatic encephalopathy.

Diagnostic Testing
- Etiology-specific testing for the cause of cirrhosis should be performed as outlined in Table 20-2; however, evaluation should begin with basic laboratory studies.

Laboratories
- Complete blood cell count, basic metabolic panel, and hepatic function panel
  - **Complete blood cell count** may reveal megaloblastic anemia due to liver disease or microcytic/normocytic anemia due to GI blood loss. Leukocytosis can be an indicator for underlying infection, especially spontaneous bacterial peritonitis (SBP) in the setting of ascites. Leukopenia and thrombocytopenia are markers for hypersplenism due to portal hypertension.
  - **Basic metabolic panel** may reveal hyponatremia in the setting of fluid overload or intravascular volume depletion. Blood urea nitrogen and serum creatinine may be acutely elevated because of the hepatorenal syndrome (HRS). Hypoglycemia may be present due to dysregulation of hepatic compensatory mechanisms.
  - **Hepatic function panel** may show hypoalbuminemia, indicating impaired hepatic synthetic function. Serum bilirubin may be elevated indicating an acute insult superimposed on chronic disease versus poor hepatic function. Transaminase elevations may indicate acute on chronic liver disease; however, the aspartate aminotransferase and alanine aminotransferase will often be normal to mildly elevated.
- Coagulation studies, ammonia, and blood culture
- **Clotting factors** are synthesized in the liver. Therefore, clotting is often abnormal, with elevated prothrombin time (PT)/international normalized ratio (INR). PT/INR can be used as a marker for evaluating synthetic function.

- **Ammonia level** is often used in the diagnosis and treatment of hepatic encephalopathy. However, ammonia levels have very poor specificity and are not particularly useful in the diagnosis of hepatic encephalopathy; some use ammonia levels to monitor treatment response, but no convincing data exist for reliability in monitoring patient course.

Imaging

- Imaging studies of the liver are useful in assessing the size and echotexture of the liver, the presence of ascites, biliary ductal dilation, and splenomegaly. They also help screen for liver masses and HCC.
- Ultrasonography, computed tomography, and magnetic resonance imaging are commonly used.
  - ○ **Ultrasonography** has the added benefit of evaluating hepatic vasculature and grading the severity of portal hypertension using color Doppler.
  - ○ **Magnetic resonance imaging** may be used to further characterize hepatic masses and vasculature.
  - ○ **Endoscopic retrograde cholangiopancreatography** allows direct imaging and intervention of the biliary tree.

Diagnostic Procedures

- **Paracentesis**
  - ○ A diagnostic paracentesis should be performed on all patients admitted to the hospital with ascites, given the high incidence of SBP. There is no need to correct coagulopathy prior to paracentesis unless the platelet count is <15,000/mm^3 or INR is >2.5.[12]
  - ○ Fluid sample should be obtained for cell count with differential, albumin level, and protein level.
    - An absolute ascites neutrophil count of >250 cells/mm^3 suggests SBP. A bedside blood culture bottle inoculation with ascitic fluid should be performed if SBP is suspected.
    - Serum ascites albumin gradient (SAAG) >1.1 suggests portal hypertension or heart failure while a SAAG <1.1 suggests peritoneal carcinomatosis or tuberculous peritonitis: See Chapter 10 for explanation of SAAG.
    - An ascitic fluid total protein level of >2.5 g/dL may suggest alternate etiologies such as heart failure, whereas a protein level of <2.5 g/dL is consistent with portal hypertension.
- **Liver biopsy**
  - ○ This is not necessary if imaging, laboratory, and clinical findings are consistent with cirrhosis. It can be very useful if the specific etiology of cirrhosis needs to be determined.

TREATMENT

- Management focuses on treatment of the underlying cause of cirrhosis and management of complications.
- Complications of cirrhosis include GI hemorrhage, encephalopathy, ascites, SBP, and HRS.

Gastrointestinal Hemorrhage

- Upper GI bleeding in cirrhotic patients is usually caused by variceal rupture, gastritis, portal hypertensive gastropathy, or peptic ulcer disease. Varices are present in 30% to 40% of patients with compensated cirrhosis and 60% of patients with ascites. The annual incidence of new varices is 5% to 10%.[13]

- In addition to fluid resuscitation, octreotide infusion[13] (to lower portal pressure) and antibiotic therapy[14] with a third-generation cephalosporin (to reduce SBP and mortality) are indicated early in the presentation. Endoscopic variceal ligation (EVL) is currently the mainstay of endoscopic therapy in acute variceal bleeding. See Chapter 6 for further details regarding treatment of GI hemorrhage.

Prevention and Follow-up
- **Periodic endoscopic evaluation** is essential to identify varices and prevent progression to variceal bleeding.
  - In patients with compensated cirrhosis with no varices on screening endoscopy, EGD should be performed every 2 to 3 years. In those with small varices (<5 mm), EGD should be repeated in 1 to 2 years.[13]
  - Patients with decompensated cirrhosis, defined as the development of complications of liver dysfunction with reduced hepatic synthetic function and portal hypertension, should undergo yearly EGD.[13]
  - Patients who survive an episode of active bleeding should have repeat EVL until obliteration of varices. The first surveillance EGD is performed 1 to 3 months after obliteration and is repeated every 6 to 12 months to check for recurrence.[13]
- **Nonselective β-blockers** such as nadolol, propranolol, or timolol are also used for prevention of variceal bleeding. β-blockers decrease cardiac output and produce splanchnic vasoconstriction.
  - American Association for the Study of Liver Diseases (AASLD) does not recommend nonselective β-blocker use in patients with cirrhosis without varices.[13]
    - A trial comprising 200 patients followed for 55 months without evidence of prior varices showed no difference in the development of varices (39% vs. 40%) in patients on β-blockers versus placebo.
  - AASLD recommends use of a nonselective β-blocker in patients with small and large varices.[13]
    - Two separate meta-analyses comparing β-blockers with placebo showed a 40% to 50% reduction in the risk of bleeding.
    - For secondary prophylaxis after a sentinel bleeding event, a combination of β-blockers and EVL versus endoscopic therapy alone was associated with a significantly lower rate of recurrent variceal bleeding with combination therapy (14% vs. 38% at 16 months), though the mortality rate was similar.
- **Proton pump inhibitors** should be considered in patients with peptic ulcer disease or other erosive findings on endoscopy; however, there is no recommendation for the use of a proton pump inhibitor in portal hypertensive gastropathy and esophageal varices.

Hepatic Encephalopathy

- Hepatic encephalopathy (HE) is a neuropsychiatric disorder associated with severe liver disease and is graded according to the West Haven criteria (Table 20-4).
- Excess ammonia is central to the pathogenesis of this process due to the acceleration of astrocyte swelling and cerebral edema; however, the precise molecular mechanism is unclear.[15]

TABLE 20-4	GRADES OF ENCEPHALOPATHY
Grade	Characteristics
1	Sleep reversal pattern, mild confusion, irritability, tremor
2	Lethargy, disorientation, inappropriate behavior, asterixis
3	Somnolence, severe confusion, aggressive behavior, asterixis
4	Coma

- Despite its role in encephalopathy, ammonia levels have very poor specificity in diagnosis and monitoring of HE.
- HE is a **diagnosis of exclusion** and other causes of altered mental status *must* be ruled out.
- The diagnosis is made on clinical grounds with altered mental status, asterixis, and hypo- or hyperreflexia. A precipitating cause for encephalopathy, such as sepsis, GI bleeding, constipation, dehydration, or electrolyte abnormality, should be identified and treated once the diagnosis of HE is made (Table 20-5).
- Patients with grade 3 and 4 encephalopathy may require close monitoring in an intensive care unit setting with endotracheal intubation for airway protection. The risk of cerebral edema increases with progression of encephalopathy. Advanced cerebral edema can lead to uncal herniation and death. This is much more common in patients with acute liver failure; however, it can be seen in patients with chronic liver disease.

Medications

- **Lactulose,** a disaccharide broken down by gut bacteria, is the mainstay of treatment due to its ability to reduce intraluminal pH, converting ammonia to ammonium, decreasing its absorption, and allowing it to be purged from the colon.[15]

TABLE 20-5	COMMON PRECIPITANTS OF HEPATIC ENCEPHALOPATHY
Gastrointestinal bleeding	
Post-TIPS	
Constipation	
Spontaneous bacterial peritonitis and other infections	
Narcotics or benzodiazepine use	
Hepatocellular carcinoma	
Worsening liver function	
Diuretic use	
Alkalosis	
Hypokalemia	

TIPS, transjugular intrahepatic portosystemic shunt.

○ Lactulose can be administered orally, rectally, or through a nasogastric tube, with a typical dose of 60 to 90 g/day, titrated to three to five loose bowel movements daily.

○ Abdominal bloating and diarrhea are the major side effects of lactulose; however, overtreatment with lactulose may lead to severe dehydration and hypernatremia.

• **Rifaximin** is a minimally absorbed oral antibiotic with FDA approval for the treatment of HE. Its precise role in the treatment of acute HE continues to be explored. A study published in 2010 demonstrated that remission of HE was prolonged in patients treated with rifaximin.[15]

• Rifaximin is administered orally at a dose of 550 mg twice daily.

Prevention and Follow-up

• After resolution of HE, patients with cirrhosis tend to remain on empiric therapy with lactulose and rifaximin for an indefinite period of time or until they undergo transplantation.

• Patients should be educated on possible precipitants of HE such as dehydration, sedatives, narcotics, poor compliance with lactulose therapy, and constipation.

Ascites

• Ascites is the most common complication seen in cirrhotic patients, with ~50% of patients with compensated cirrhosis developing ascites during 10 years of follow-up.

• Approximately 85% of patients with ascites in the United States have cirrhosis.[12]

• Ascites is caused by the activation of the renin-angiotensin-aldosterone system and sympathetic nervous system in response to splanchnic vasodilatation and arterial underfilling in the setting of portal hypertension. The activation of the renin-angiotensin-aldosterone system causes fluid retention and elevated hydrostatic pressure in the splanchnic microcirculation. Elevated hydrostatic pressure and low oncotic pressure cause increased lymph production, and once lymph production surpasses lymph return, ascites develops.

• Patients present with increased abdominal girth, shortness of breath, and lower extremity edema. Common physical findings include dullness to percussion in the flanks, shifting dullness, pleural effusion, a fluid wave, and umbilical and inguinal hernias.

• A paracentesis allows analysis of ascitic fluid (see Chapter 10).

Medications

• **Spironolactone,** an aldosterone antagonist, is first-line therapy for ascites due to cirrhosis. Hyperkalemia and breast tenderness are common side effects.[12]

• **Furosemide,** a loop diuretic, is usually given with spironolactone.

○ Spironolactone and furosemide are prescribed at a ratio of 2.5:1, usually at a starting dose of 100 and 40 mg daily, respectively.[12]

   ▪ This ratio often prevents hyperkalemia.

   ▪ Dosage of each medication can be increased every 1 to 2 weeks to a maximum daily dose of 400 mg of spironolactone and 160 mg of furosemide.[12]

○ Spironolactone can be substituted with amiloride in the setting of tender gynecomastia.

- Triamterene, metolazone, and hydrochlorothiazide may also be used in the treatment of ascites.
- The goal of diuretic therapy is the loss of 0.5 and 1 kg/day if peripheral edema is present.[12]
- Diuretic-resistant or -refractory ascites can be treated with bimonthly outpatient large-volume paracentesis or transjugular intrahepatic portosystemic shunt (TIPS).
  - In a meta-analysis, TIPS was more effective at decreasing ascites without a significant difference in mortality, GI bleeding, infection, and acute renal failure but with a significantly higher rate of hepatic encephalopathy.[16]

Dietary Changes

- **Sodium restriction** to 2 to 4 g/day is an important component of the treatment of ascites. Salt restriction and diuretic therapy are effective in 90% of patients with ascites.
  - Two grams of sodium is equivalent to 88 mmol/day. The body loses ~10 mmol/day of sodium chloride (NaCl) via sweat. Therefore, the kidney must excrete NaCl at a rate of 78 mmol/day to maintain homeostasis.[12]
  - A spot urine study can determine which patient may respond to sodium restriction without diuretic therapy.
    - If the urine sodium is greater than urine potassium, the patient is excreting >78 mmol/day of NaCl and will respond to salt restriction alone.[12]
- **Hyponatremia** is often seen in the setting of ascites. A **daily oral fluid restriction** of 800 to 1200 mL/day is first-line treatment. Vasopressin receptor antagonists, such as tolvaptan, show promise in the treatment of hypervolemic hyponatremia according to the Study of Ascending Levels of Tolvaptan in Hyponatremia trial (SALT1 and SALT2).[17]

Spontaneous Bacterial Peritonitis

- SBP is a common complication of cirrhosis and contributes to 25% of all bacterial infections seen in this population. It is caused by translocation of gut bacteria into the blood, causing transient bacteremia and seeding of ascitic fluid.
- Presentation may be subtle, with abdominal pain, fever, chills, jaundice, or worsening encephalopathy. Up to half of patients with SBP are asymptomatic, and a diagnostic paracentesis with a 22- to 25-gauge needle is imperative, regardless of the reason for hospital admission.
- A **diagnostic paracentesis is the gold standard diagnostic test.** Ascitic fluid should be sent for cell count with differential, Gram's stain, and aerobic and anaerobic blood cultures. The presence of >250 polymorphonuclear cells/mm^3 strongly suggests SBP and should be aggressively treated. A positive culture, regardless of the number of polymorphonuclear cells, should also be treated.

Medications

- A **third-generation cephalosporin administered for at least 5 days** is the standard of care.[12]
  - **Cefotaxime** 1 to 2 g IV every 8 to 12 hours and **ceftriaxone** 1 to 2 g every 24 hours are effective therapies.
  - If clinical deterioration is confirmed, coverage should be broadened to cover *Enterococcus,* methicillin-resistant *Staphylococcus aureus,* and anaerobic organisms.

- Following repeated episodes of SBP, patients can be given **prophylactic antibiotic therapy,** such as norfloxacin 400 mg daily, ciprofloxacin 250 mg daily, or trimethoprim/sulfamethoxazole 800/160 five times per week.[12]
- HRS is a feared complication of SBP and efforts to maintain adequate volume expansion are a necessity.
  - ○ Diuretics and large-volume paracentesis should be avoided in the setting of SBP.
  - ○ Albumin administration should be given to reduce the risk of HRS.
    - ■ In SBP patients treated with a third-generation cephalosporin, albumin administration at 1.5 g/kg on day 1 and 1 g/kg on day 3 is associated with a lower rate of renal failure (10% vs. 33%) and a lower hospital mortality rate (10% vs. 29%).[18]

Hepatorenal Syndrome
- The HRS is an ominous sign. It affects 5% of patients hospitalized for GI bleeding, 10% of patients with ascites treated by paracentesis, and 30% of patients with SBP. HRS is classified on the basis of rapidity of onset and severity of renal failure. **Type I HRS** is progressive over a period of <2 weeks and is often associated with a precipitating factor. Median survival is relatively short at 12 days, with >90% mortality rate at 10 weeks. **Type 2 HRS** is characterized by a steady and progressive reduction in glomerular filtration rate and recurrent, diuretic-resistant ascites. An identifiable precipitant may be difficult to find. Type 2 HRS is associated with a median survival of 3 to 6 months.
- Diagnosis is based on four major criteria that must be met and five additional criteria that provide supportive evidence for the diagnosis of HRS.
  - ○ The *major* **criteria** are (1) presence of low glomerular filtration rate as indicated by creatinine level of >1.5 mg/dL, (2) absence of shock or ongoing bacterial infection, (3) no sustained improvement in renal function following administration of 1.5 L of intravenous fluid, and (4) absence of proteinuria >500 mg/day.
  - ○ **Additional criteria** include (1) urine volume <500 mL/day, (2) urine sodium concentration <10 mEq/L, (3) urine osmolality > plasma osmolality, (4) urine red blood cells <50/high powered field, and (5) serum sodium concentration <130 mEq/L.
- It is necessary to **rule out reversible causes of renal failure,** including hypovolemia (owing to aggressive diuresis, GI bleeding, or poor nutrition), sepsis, nephrotoxins, obstruction, and acute tubular necrosis.

SPECIAL CONSIDERATIONS

- HCC is the third leading cause of death from cancer worldwide and the ninth leading cause of cancer deaths in the United States. Chronic hepatitis B virus and hepatitis C virus infections account for an estimated 78% of HCC cases globally.
  - ○ The relative risk for the development of HCC is 100 for chronic hepatitis B and 20 for cirrhosis secondary to chronic hepatitis C
- Surveillance with a liver ultrasonography is recommended in specific populations. The low sensitivity and specificity of α-fetoprotein make it less useful as a screening tool.[19]

- Surveillance should be performed for the following populations:
  - Asian descendant carrier of hepatitis B (men >40 years, women >50 years)
  - Cirrhosis secondary to hepatitis B or C
  - Hepatitis B carrier with family history of HCC
  - African/North American blacks with chronic hepatitis B
  - Stage 4 primary biliary cirrhosis
  - Cirrhosis due to hemochromatosis, α_1-antitrypsin deficiency, and other causes
- Surveillance must be performed every 6 to 12 months.
- **Hepatopulmonary syndrome** is seen in 8% of cirrhotic patients and is defined by the triad of hypoxia, liver disease, and intrapulmonary shunting.
  - Platypnea (shortness of breath with upright posture) and orthodeoxia (fall in arterial blood oxygen with upright posture) are often present.
  - Treatment options are limited to supplemental oxygen. Somatostatin analogues and inhaled nitric oxide inhibitors are possible strategies with uncertain efficacy.
  - Hepatopulmonary syndrome usually resolves following liver transplantation.
  - Portopulmonary hypertension occurs in 2% to 5% of all cirrhotic patients and presents with dyspnea on exertion (most common), syncope, chest pain, fatigue, hemoptysis, or orthopnea. Poor prognosis without treatment with mean survival of 15 months.
    - It is defined as precapillary pulmonary hypertension [mean pulmonary artery pressure >25 mm Hg] in the setting of portal hypertension.
    - Treatment is similar to primary pulmonary hypertension and consists of prostaglandin analogues, phosphodiesterase inhibitors, inhaled nitric oxide, and endothelin receptor antagonists.
- **Transplantation** is considered after the first episode of decompensation or worsening of liver function.
  - The **Model for End-Stage Liver Disease (MELD) score** objectively evaluates liver function for patients listed for transplantation.[20]
    - It generates a number using serum creatinine, total bilirubin, and INR in a complicated mathematical formula.
    - It enables physicians to allocate donor livers to "sicker" patients.

REFERENCES

1. Anthony PP, Ishak NG, Nayak NC. The morphology of cirrhosis: recommendations on definition, nomenclature, and classification by a working group sponsored by the World Health Organization. *J Clin Pathol.* 1978;31:395–414.
2. Child CG, Turcotte JG. Surgery and portal hypertension. In: Child CG, ed. *The Liver and Portal Hypertension.* Philadelphia, PA: Saunders; 1964:50–64.
3. Pleis JR, Lethbridge-Cejki M. Summary health statistics for U.S. adults: National Health Interview Survey, 2005. *Vital Health Stat.* 2006;(232):1–153.
4. Wise M. Changing trends in hepatitis C-related mortality in the United States, 1995–2004. *Hepatology.* 2008;47:1–8.
5. Miniño AM, Xu J, Kochanek KD. Deaths: preliminary data from 2008. *Natl Vital Stat Rep.* 2010;59(2):1-52.
6. Chung RT, Podolsky DK. Cirrhosis and its complications. In: Kasper DL, Fauci AS, Longo DL, et al., eds. *Harrison's Principle of Internal Medicine.* 16th ed. New York, NY: McGraw-Hill; 2005:1858–1868.

7. Crawford JM. Liver and biliary tract. In: Vinay KV, Abbas AA, Fausto N, eds. *Robbins and Cotran Pathologic Basis of Disease.* 7th ed. Philadelphia, PA: Elsevier Saunders; 2005: 877–927.

8. Rockey DC. Cell and molecular mechanisms of increased intrahepatic resistance and hemo-dynamic correlates. In: Sanyal AJ, Shah VH, eds. *Portal Hypertension: Pathobiology, Evaluation, and Treatment.* Totowa, NJ: Humana Press; 2005:37–50.

9. Pinzani M, Vizzutti F. Anatomy and vascular biology of the cells in the portal circulation. In: Sanyal AJ, Shah VH, eds. *Portal Hypertension: Pathobiology, Evaluation, and Treatment.* Totowa, NJ: Humana Press; 2005:15–36.

10. O'Shea RS, Dasarthy S, McCullough AJ. Alcoholic liver disease. *Hepatology.* 2010;51: 307–328.

11. Ghany MG, Strader DB, Thomas DL, et al. Diagnosis, management and treatment of hepatitis C: an update. *Hepatology.* 2009;49:1335–1374.

12. Runyon BA. Management of adult patients with ascites due to cirrhosis: an update. *Hepatology.* 2009;49:2087–2107.

13. Garcia-Tsao G, Sanyal AJ, Grace ND, et al. Prevention and management of gastroesopha-geal varices and variceal hemorrhage in cirrhosis. *Hepatology.* 2007;46:922–938.

14. Bernard B, Grange JD, Khac EN, et al. Antibiotic prophylaxis for the prevention of bacte-rial infections in cirrhotic patients with gastrointestinal bleeding: a meta-analysis. *Hepatology.* 1999;29:1655–1661.

15. Prakash R, Mullen KD. Mechanisms, diagnosis and management of hepatic encephalopa-thy. *Nat Rev Gastroenterol Hepatol.* 2010;7:515–525.

16. Saab S, Nieto JM, Lewis SK, et al. TIPS versus paracentesis for cirrhotic patients with refractory ascites. *Cochrane Database Syst Rev.* 2006;(4):CD004889. doi:10.1002/14651858. CD004889.pub2

17. Schrier RW, Gross P, Gheorghiade M, et al. Tolvaptan, a selective oral vasopressin V2-receptor antagonist, for hyponatremia. *N Engl J Med.* 2006;355(20):2099–2112.

18. Gines P, Tito L, Arroyo V, et al. Randomized comparative study of therapeutic paracentesis with and without intravenous albumin in cirrhosis. *Gastroenterology.* 1988;94:1493–1502.

19. Bruix J, Sherman M; Practice Guidelines Committee, American Association for the Study of Liver Diseases. Management of hepatocellular carcinoma. *Hepatology.* 2005;42: 1208–1236.

20. Malinchoc M, Kamath PS, Gordon FD, et al. A model to predict poor survival in patients undergoing transjugular intrahepatic portosystemic shunts. *Hepatology.* 2000;31(4): 864–871.

Liver Transplantation

Anil B. Seetharam and Thomas A. Kerr

GENERAL PRINCIPLES

- Dr. Thomas Starzl performed the first human liver transplant in 1963. Since then, dramatic advances in surgical and medical management in peritransplant and posttransplant care have improved liver transplant outcomes.
  - Advances in immunosuppression have allowed prolonged graft survival.
  - Conditions that previously were regarded as relative or absolute contraindications to liver transplantation (hepatitis B, HIV, etc.) are now medically managed in liver transplant candidates and recipients.
  - Recurrence of the disease leading to transplantation is increasingly a cause of graft loss.
- Approximately 5% of liver transplantations involve a living donor, and about 10% of liver transplant recipients are children.
- Between 2004 and 2009, a total of ~6000 to 7000 liver transplantations were performed annually in the United States, up from ~1700 in 1988.
  - Changes in organ allocation with the advent of the **Model for End-Stage Liver Disease (MELD)** have decreased wait-list mortality but have substantially increased wait-list time.
  - Limited donor supply remains a significant challenge to liver transplantation.
- Current 1-, 3-, and 5-year survival rates after liver transplantation in the United States are 88%, 80%, and 75%, respectively.[1]

INDICATIONS

- Orthotopic liver transplantation (OLT) is indicated for acute or chronic liver failure from a variety of causes (Table 21-1).
- Patients with cirrhosis should be considered for OLT referral when they develop evidence of hepatic dysfunction or when they experience major complications of end-stage liver disease (ascites, variceal bleeding, or encephalopathy).[2]
- The natural history of the patient's disease must be carefully compared with anticipated survival after OLT.
- Conditions associated with liver disease [hepatopulmonary syndrome, type I hepatorenal syndrome, hepatocellular carcinoma (HCC)] can prompt an expedited OLT evaluation regardless of hepatic synthetic dysfunction.

Disease-specific Indications

- In general, indications for liver transplantation include irreversible hepatic failure and liver cancer.[2]
- Indications for liver transplant mirror the most common forms of chronic liver disease including viral, alcohol, autoimmune, and metabolic causes (see Table 21-1).

TABLE 21-1	INDICATIONS FOR LIVER TRANSPLANTATION				
Chronic Noncholestatic Disorders	Chronic Cholestatic Disorders	Metabolic	Systemic	Malignancies	Other
Alcohol	Primary biliary cirrhosis	Nonalcoholic steatohepatitis	Amyloidosis	Hepatocellular carcinoma	Acute liver failure
Autoimmune hepatitis	Primary sclerosing cholangitis	Wilson's disease	Hyperoxaluria	Hepatoblastoma	Budd-Chiari syndrome
Hepatitis B	Alagille syndrome	Hereditary hemochromatosis	Urea cycle defects	Hemangioendothelioma	Polycystic disease
Hepatitis C	Biliary atresia	α_1-Antitrypsin deficiency		Metastatic neuroendocrine tumor	
	Cystic fibrosis	Tyrosinemia			
	Progressive familial intrahepatic cholestasis				

Hepatitis C

- Hepatitis C virus (HCV) infects 3 to 5 million individuals in the United States.
- The rate of development of cirrhosis in HCV-infected individuals is ~20% after 20 years of infection. Once cirrhosis has developed, the rate of hepatic decompensation is ~4% per year, and cancer develops at a rate of 1% to 4% per year.[3]
- Decompensated hepatitis C–related cirrhosis carries a 5-year mortality rate of >50%.
- Hepatitis C accounts for 30% to 40% of liver transplants, making it the leading indication for liver transplantation in the United States.
- Recurrent hepatitis C is nearly universal and contributes significantly to graft injury and failure with ~20% of HCV-infected recipients developing cirrhosis within 5 years.
- Histologic fibrosis 1 year posttransplant is predictive of more rapid progression to advanced fibrosis and, at many centers, prompts posttransplant hepatitis C treatment.
- Progression of recurrence with cirrhosis in a transplanted allograft can be accelerated compared with natural history in native liver infection.[4]
- Retransplantation in cases of early graft loss from hepatitis C may result in accelerated allograft failure making retransplantation for hepatitis C–related graft loss controversial.

Alcohol-related Liver Disease

- Alcohol-related liver disease is the **most common cause of cirrhosis** and accounts for 40% of deaths from cirrhosis in the United States.
- Alcohol-related liver disease is the **second most common indication for liver transplantation in the United States.**
- Abstinence is the only effective treatment but can be associated with dramatic survival improvement, even in patients with decompensated cirrhosis.[5]
- A **period of abstinence before providing transplantation may have salutary effects on liver function that obviate the need for OLT**. Most US transplant centers require 6 months of abstinence prior to OLT listing.
- Routine follow-up and alcohol abuse counseling should be undertaken in the preoperative and postoperative period to reduce rates of recidivism.
- Excellent long-term outcomes are common for patients transplanted for alcohol-related liver disease.

Nonalcoholic Fatty Liver Disease/Cryptogenic Cirrhosis

- The term nonalcoholic steatohepatitis (NASH) was first used in 1980 to describe biochemical and histologic changes consistent with alcoholic hepatitis but without a history of alcohol use.
- Nonalcoholic fatty liver disease (NAFLD) encompasses simple steatosis, NASH, and NASH-related cirrhosis. **NAFLD is strongly associated with obesity and the metabolic syndrome** and is increasing in incidence in the Unites States. Many cases of chronic liver failure previously reported as cryptogenic are likely a consequence of NAFLD.
- As NAFLD progresses to cirrhosis, fat may decrease or disappear, making it difficult to establish with certainty that NAFLD led to cirrhosis.
- NAFLD is a growing indication for liver transplantation and together with cryptogenic cirrhosis accounts for ~7% of liver transplants annually in the United States.[2]

- Patients with NAFLD-related cirrhosis often have coexisting cardiometabolic conditions (i.e., coronary artery disease) that increase peritransplant morbidity and risk of death.
- NAFLD can reoccur in an allograft liver, though this rarely leads to graft loss.[6]

Hepatitis B

- Prior to routine use of hepatitis B immune globulin (HBIG), hepatitis B infection in liver transplant patients was associated with poor outcomes and considered a contraindication to liver transplantation.
- Peri- and posttransplant HBIG has dramatically decreased the rate of allograft hepatitis B infection and permitted transplantation of hepatitis B virus (HCB)-infected patients.[7]
- Five-year survival rate is ~15% in decompensated HBV-related cirrhosis.
- The duration of posttransplant hepatitis B antiviral treatment remains a topic of controversy.

Autoimmune Hepatitis

- Corticosteroid and immunosuppressive therapy is largely effective in maintaining clinical and biochemical remission of autoimmune hepatitis (AIH). However, patients with AIH may present after years of infection when already cirrhotic or in a fulminant fashion. Both of these conditions may require transplantation.
- A fraction of patients with cryptogenic cirrhosis may have had long-standing unrecognized AIH.
- Outcome after liver transplantation for AIH is excellent, with 5- and 10-year survival rates of >75%.[8]
- Recurrent disease can occur but is usually mild and managed with conventional immunosuppression.
- Patients transplanted for any indication may develop histologic findings of AIH in their allograft. This generally responds to immunosuppression.

Primary Biliary Cirrhosis

- Patients with primary biliary cirrhosis (PBC) who present late in the course of their disease or respond inadequately to ursodeoxycholic acid may progress to cirrhosis requiring transplantation.
- Occasional patients with PBC and stable liver function may be considered for OLT if they have severe pruritus, leading to sleep deprivation and emotional disturbances.
- Seventy percent of patients receiving OLT for PBC are alive after 10 years.
- Recurrence of PBC after transplantation has been documented but has not had major impact on long-term postoperative survival.[9]

Primary Sclerosing Cholangitis

- No specific medical therapy has been shown to improve survival in patients with primary sclerosing cholangitis (PSC).
- Survival of patients with PSC after liver transplantation has been shown to be superior to that predicted for conservatively managed patients.[10]
- Recurrent disease is common (15% to 20%) after transplantation but generally does not impact posttransplant survival.
- The development of colorectal cancer can adversely influence postoperative survival if regular screening is not performed in patients with coexistent ulcerative colitis.

Metabolic Liver Diseases

- The most common metabolic diseases causing progressive liver failure in adults (excluding NASH) are α_1-**antitrypsin deficiency, Wilson disease,** and **hereditary hemochromatosis.**
- Although these conditions account for <5% of the liver transplants performed in the United States, the outcome after transplantation in adults is excellent (1 year survival rate, 88%).
- Liver transplantation is the only effective treatment of decompensated cirrhosis secondary to α_1-antitrypsin deficiency.
- After transplantation, donor α_1-antitrypsin phenotype is expressed and serum levels of α_1-antitrypsin return to normal ranges within weeks. Its impact on pulmonary disease is unknown.
- Careful assessment of lung disease should be performed in cirrhosis secondary to α_1-antitrypsin deficiency, although coexistent disease is uncommon.
- Urgent liver transplantation is the only effective option for patients with FHF resulting from Wilson disease.
- In patients receiving liver transplantation for chronic Wilson's disease, copper chelation and zinc therapy are not needed after transplantation.
- Survival of transplanted patients with hereditary hemochromatosis is lower than in those transplanted for other causes of liver disease.[11]
- Because of increased risk of cardiac complications, pretransplant cardiac evaluation is of paramount importance.

Hepatocellular Carcinoma

- Patients with chronic HBV infection and cirrhosis of any kind are at risk for HCC.
- Patient prognosis in HCC is dependent upon the stage of the tumor and the degree of liver function impairment.[12]
- Timely liver transplantation is often the most effective treatment of HCC.
- The **Milan criteria** are used to identify patients with HCC who are expected to benefit with liver transplantation. Transplantation can be considered in patients with
  ○ a single lesion 2 cm or larger but smaller than 5 cm *or*
  ○ no more than three lesions, the largest of which is smaller than 3 cm, *and*
  ○ no evidence of extrahepatic malignancy.
- In many transplant centers, patients with HCC that extend beyond Milan criteria can be considered for downstaging procedures such as transarterial chemoembolization or radiofrequency embolization to decrease tumor size to within Milan criteria and allow listing for liver transplantation.
- Enhanced priority or exception points in the MELD can be awarded to patients with HCC within Milan criteria.

Fulminant Hepatic Failure

- There are ~2000 cases of fulminant hepatic failure (FHF) in the United States annually, most commonly resulting from acetaminophen toxicity (39%).
- FHF accounts for ~5% of liver transplants annually in the United States.
- More than 60% of patients survive acetaminophen overdose without transplantation if appropriate therapy (*N*-acetyl cysteine) is given in a timely fashion.

- Nonacetaminophen-related FHF may result from drug-induced liver injury, hepatitis A and B, acute fatty liver of pregnancy, Wilson disease, immune-mediated liver disease, Budd-Chiari syndrome, and other causes.
- Given the subacute changes in physiology, as opposed to the chronic changes with most indications, critical care in the perioperative period is most intensive.[13]
- In FHF, early effort must be made to identify patients likely to require transplantation for survival and to determine whether the patient is an acceptable candidate for transplantation.
- Several scoring systems, including the King's College criteria, have been developed to identify patients who are likely to require transplantation to survive acetaminophen- and nonacetaminophen-related FHF.
- Patients with FHF should be **promptly transferred to a transplant center and cared for in an intensive care unit setting** until clinical improvement or transplantation. Brain edema, infection, and renal failure may occur and require intensive management while awaiting transplant.
- To address the urgency of FHF, a special category (status 1) was created. This gives high priority to patients with FHF.

ORGAN ALLOCATION

- The growing need for liver transplantation with a limited donor supply has generated a waiting list of >16,000 patients in the United States. The growing disparity between organ supply and demand mandates allocation policies to prioritize scarce donor organs to patients most in need.
- The outcome of all patients who receive liver transplants and candidates who are listed for OLT in the United States is continuously tracked in a comprehensive database: the **United Network for Organ Sharing** (UNOS).
- A modification of the **MELD score** is used to prioritize patients for allocation:
  - The MELD score incorporates serum bilirubin (Tbil), international normalized ratio of prothrombin time (INR), and serum creatinine [MELD = $9.57 \times$ ln(serum creatinine) + $3.78 \times$ ln(Tbil) + $11.2 \times$ ln(INR) + 6.43], where ln is the natural logarithm.
    - Patients are assigned a score in a continuous scale from 6 to 40, which equates to estimated 3-month survival rates from 80% to 7%, respectively.[14]
    - Serum creatinine is always entered as ≤4 g/dL—if dialysis has occurred twice in the past week, the maximum value should be entered.
    - The MELD score can be modified to gain priority listing through granting of "exception points" in certain instances including HCC (see Disease-specific Indications section).
    - Patients with acute liver failure needing transplantation receive UNOS priority 1A listing.

DIAGNOSIS

Patient Evaluation

- Every option for disease-specific treatment should be considered for patients with chronic liver disease. When no effective alternative therapy exits, or when treatment has been ineffective, transplantation should be considered.

- In critically ill patients in whom the outcome of medical therapy is uncertain or in whom disease is expected to advance, it is appropriate to simultaneously begin treatment and transplantation evaluation.
- Liver transplant evaluation includes a comprehensive physical, physiologic, and psychosocial patient assessment. This involves a multidisciplinary approach including transplant hepatologists, surgeons, radiologists, psychiatrists, pharmacists, social workers, and case coordinators.
- **Important considerations for candidate evaluation:**
  - Can the patient survive the operation and the immediate postoperative period?
  - Can the patient comply with a complex medical regimen and follow-up after the transplant?
  - Does the patient have comorbid conditions that require modification prior to transplant or that preclude transplant?

Components of the Transplant Evaluation

- A thorough history and physical examination.
- Cardiopulmonary assessment including evaluation for structural and ischemic heart disease with pharmacologically induced stress echocardiography and pulmonary function testing.
- Abnormalities identified on noninvasive cardiopulmonary pulmonary testing warrant further evaluation with left or right cardiac catheterization.[15]
  - Laboratory studies to confirm the etiology of liver disease and to evaluate for previously undetected medical conditions.
  - Assessment of creatinine clearance.
  - Serologic evaluation to determine the status of viral infections including hepatitis B and C virus, cytomegalovirus, Epstein-Barr virus, and HIV.
  - Cross-sectional abdominal imaging to determine the presence of HCC as well as patency of hepatic inflow (portal vein and hepatic artery) and outflow (hepatic veins).

Special Considerations

- **Age.** There is no specific age limitation to successful OLT, and candidacy is determined on an individual basis.
- **Pulmonary hypertension.** This condition is often identified on echocardiography and requires more precise measurement with right heart catheterization. Pulmonary hypertension may preclude liver transplantation and should, at a minimum, be optimally controlled with medical therapy prior to transplantation.
- **Morbid obesity.** This is generally considered a contraindication to transplantation. Attention should be directed to improving body mass index prior to transplantation.
- **Renal insufficiency:** The etiology of the renal insufficiency should be investigated prior to transplantation and, in some cases, consideration given to combined liver–kidney transplantation.
- **Previous malignancy.** Given the increased risk for recurrence of cancer with systemic immunosuppression, consultation from the treating oncologist regarding the risk of posttransplant recurrence should be obtained.
- **HIV.** Although previously regarded as a contraindication to transplantation, improved medical therapies have allowed HIV-positive individuals to be

successfully transplanted. There are numerous interactions between highly active antiretroviral therapy (HAART) and immunosuppressant medications requiring monitoring of serum drug levels.

- **Surgical issues.** Thrombosis of the main portal vein may be bypassed; however, more extensive thrombosis of the mesenteric vasculature or cavernomatous transformation of the portal vein may preclude adequate graft venous inflow.
- **Psychosocial issues.** Issues related to depression and previous alcohol or illicit substance abuses need to be explored and counseling offered.

TREATMENT

Surgical Considerations

- During transplantation, the liver is placed in the natural position in the right upper quadrant.
- Most OLTs are performed using a **whole donor liver.**
- **Split liver transplantation** involves utilizing a portion of the left lobe of the donor liver for transplantation into a child and utilizing the remaining donor organ for transplantation into an adult.
- **Living donor transplantation** is performed at some centers, though donor safety remains a significant concern.
- Complex vascular reconstruction of the hepatic artery, portal vein, and hepatic venous drainage system to the inferior vena cava is undertaken to provide adequate vascular inflow and outflow to the allograft.
- Biliary reconstruction is accomplished using an end-to-end anastamosis of the proximal donor common bile duct to the distal recipient common bile duct.
- In transplant recipients with diseased ducts (i.e., primary sclerosing cholangitis), a Roux-en-Y hepaticojejunostomy is performed. This ensures removal of the entire native biliary tree and, in the case of PSC, decreases the risk of future biliary strictures and neoplasia.

IMMUNOSUPPRESSIVE AGENTS

- Advances in posttransplant immunosuppression have allowed long-term allograft survival.
- The goal of posttransplant immunosuppression is to prevent allograft rejection while allowing physiologic defenses against infection.
- Although mechanisms are incompletely understood, the liver appears to be less susceptible to rejection than other transplanted organs.
- In general, currently used immunosuppressants deplete T cells or inhibit T-cell activation.
- **Calcineurin inhibitors (CNIs)** (cyclosporine and tacrolimus) are the most commonly used maintenance immunosuppressive medicines.[16]
  - ○ CNI bind to cyclophilin, and inhibit T-cell activation and proliferation.
  - ○ CNI require monitoring of 12-hour trough levels.
  - ○ Because CNIs are metabolized by the cytochrome P450 system, drug levels can be significantly affected by commonly prescribed medications, requiring close monitoring of drug levels.
  - ○ Side effects of CNI include nephrotoxicity, which commonly leads to chronic renal insufficiency, neurotoxicity, hypertension, and hyperlipidemia.

TABLE 21-2	EARLY AND LATE COMPLICATIONS AFTER LIVER TRANSPLANTATION

Early Complications After Liver Transplantation
Acute cellular rejection
Biliary disease (e.g., anastomotic stricture)
Hepatic artery thrombosis
Infection

Late Complications After Liver Transplantation
Chronic rejection
Malignancy (e.g., skin and cervical cancer)
Infection
Cardiometabolic complications (hypertension and hyperlipidemia)

- **Antimetabolites** include mycophenolate mofetil and mycophenolate sodium.
  - Mycophenolate mofetil and mycophenolate sodium are metabolized to mycophenolic acid (MPA), which inhibits guanosine synthesis and lymphocyte proliferation.
  - MPAs are generally not used as monotherapy but as supplements to CNIs.
  - The side effects of MPA include gastrointestinal disorders (primarily diarrhea) and bone marrow suppression.
  - MPAs carry an increased risk of spontaneous abortions and birth defects.
- **mTOR inhibitors** include sirolimus (SRL) and everolimus.
  - mTOR inhibitors bind to FK506 binding protein inhibiting T-cell proliferation.
  - SRL has been associated with hepatic artery thrombosis and delayed wound healing and generally is not used in the immediate posttransplant period.
  - SRL use in place of CNI may delay progression of chronic renal insufficiency in posttransplant patients.
- **Corticosteroids** reduce cytokine release and lymphocyte activation.
  - Corticosteroids are used in the immediate posttransplant period, though efforts are made to wean steroids by 3 to 6 months posttransplantation to avoid side effects cause by prolonged corticosteroid use (diabetes, hypertension, osteoporosis, etc.).
  - Intravenous and oral steroids are commonly used to treat episodes of acute cellular rejection.

POSTTRANSPLANT COMPLICATIONS

- **Early posttransplant complications** may relate to allograft function, surgical anatomic issues, infections, and other causes (Table 21-2).
  - Early allograft dysfunction usually prompts liver biopsy, an assessment of the hepatic vasculature, and biliary system.
  - Early rejection may be treated with steroids and other immunosuppressants.
  - Biliary tract disease leading to graft dysfunction (i.e., biliary anastomotic stricture) may require radiographic or endoscopic intervention. Extrahepatic

biliary strictures not responding to surgical intervention may require revision to Roux-en-Y anatomy.

○ Early hepatic artery thrombosis often requires retransplantation. If this occurs within 7 days of transplantation, the patient is relisted for transplantation as status 1.

• **Late posttransplant complications** include allograft rejection, recurrence of hepatic disease in the allograft, anatomic complications (i.e., hepatic artery thrombosis), infections, and malignancy.

○ Evidence of worsening hepatic function generally prompts biopsy of the allograft.

○ If no clear hepatic parenchymal cause is found on biopsy (i.e., rejection), a prompt evaluation of the allograft vasculature and biliary system is necessary.

• Posttransplant immunosuppression leads to **increased risk for a variety of malignancies** (skin cancer, cervical cancer, etc.) as well as adverse cardiometabolic risk factors (serum lipids, hypertension).

REFERENCES

1. OPTN Organ Procurement and Transplantation Network. http://optn.transplant.hrsa.gov. Accessed January 3, 2012.
2. O'Leary JG, Lepe R, Davis GL. Indications for liver transplantation. *Gastroenterology.* 2008;134:1764–1776.
3. El-Serag HB. Hepatocellular carcinoma: recent trends in the United States. *Gastroenterology.* 2004;127(suppl 1):S27–S34.
4. Berenguer M. Natural history of recurrent hepatitis C. *Liver Transpl.* 2002;8:S14–S18.
5. Veldt BJ, Laine F, Guillygomarc'h A, et al. Indication of liver transplantation in severe alcoholic liver cirrhosis: quantitative evaluation and optimal timing. *J Hepatol.* 2002; 36:93–98.
6. Contos MJ, Cales W, Sterling RK, et al. Development of nonalcoholic fatty liver disease after orthotopic liver transplantation for cryptogenic cirrhosis. *Liver Transpl.* 2001; 7:363–373.
7. Lok AS. Prevention of recurrent hepatitis B post-liver transplantation. *Liver Transpl.* 2002;8:S67–S73.
8. Vogel A, Heinrich E, Bahr MJ, et al. Long-term outcome of liver transplantation for autoimmune hepatitis. *Clin Transplant.* 2004;18:62–69.
9. Heathcote EJ. Management of primary biliary cirrhosis. The American Association for the Study of Liver Diseases practice guidelines. *Hepatology.* 2000;31:1005–1013.
10. Roberts MS, Angus DC, Bryce CL, et al. Survival after liver transplantation in the United States: a disease-specific analysis of the UNOS database. *Liver Transpl.* 2004; 10:886–897.
11. Brandhagen DJ, Alvarez W, Therneau TM, et al. Iron overload in cirrhosis-HFE genotypes and outcome after liver transplantation. *Hepatology.* 2000;31:456–460.
12. Llovet JM, Bruix J. Systematic review of randomized trials for unresectable hepatocellular carcinoma: chemoembolization improves survival. *Hepatology.* 2003;37:429–442.
13. Ellis A, Wendon J. Circulatory, respiratory, cerebral, and renal derangements in acute liver failure: pathophysiology and management. *Semin Liver Dis.* 1996;16:379–388.
14. Malinchoch M, Kamath PS, Gordon FD, et al. A model to predict poor survival in patients undergoing transjugularintrahepatic portosystemic shunts. *Hepatology.* 2000; 31:864–871.
15. Cotton CL, Gandhi S, Vaitkus PT, et al. Role of echocardiography in detecting portopulmonary hypertension in liver transplant candidates. *Liver Transpl.* 2002;8(11):1051–1054.
16. Pillai AA, Levitsky J. Overview of immunosuppression in liver transplantation. *World J Gastroenterol.* 2009;15:4225–4233.

Pancreatic Disorders

Alexander Lee and Sreenivasa Jonnalagadda

22

GENERAL PRINCIPLES

- The pancreas is a mixed endocrine and exocrine gland consisting of lobular subunits composed of acini.[1,2]
- The exocrine pancreas consists of acinar, centroacinar, and ductal cells.
  - The acinar cells secrete ~20 digestive enzymes (in zymogen granules) into the central ductule of the acinus.[1,2]
  - The central ductule of the acinus connects with the intralobular ducts to form the interlobular ducts, which join to form the main pancreatic duct.[1,2]
  - The main pancreatic duct empties into the duodenum through the ampulla of Vater.[1,2]
- The pancreas lies in the retroperitoneal space of the upper abdomen. Because of its central location, diseases of the pancreas are generally more difficult to manage than those of other abdominal viscera.
  - Lymphatic drainage of the pancreas occurs along several major routes. These include the splenic, hepatic, and superior mesenteric nodal systems, as well as the aortocaval and other posterior abdominal wall lymphatic vessels.[2]
  - Blood vessels in close proximity to the pancreas include major vessels of the epigastrum, such as the superior mesenteric vein, the portal vein, and the celiac axis. Thus, local invasion of malignant pancreatic tumors often involves these vessels, making such tumors unresectable and/or incurable.[2]
  - If the pancreas is resected, the need to excise the vessels and lymph nodes associated with it often necessitates resection of the duodenum, gallbladder, distal bile duct, spleen, upper jejunum, and part of the stomach.[2]
  - The vascular nature of the pancreas and the adjacent organs makes hemorrhage the most common postoperative complication of pancreatic resection.

ACUTE PANCREATITIS

GENERAL PRINCIPLES

Definition

- Acute pancreatitis is an autodigestive process that occurs when the proteolytic enzymes are prematurely activated within the pancreas rather than in the intestinal lumen. The active enzymes digest membranes within the pancreas, which leads to inflammation, edema, vascular damage, cellular injury, and possibly death.[3]

Classification

- Acute pancreatitis can be classified either by its clinical course or by its histologic appearance.

○ **Clinical classification**
- **Nonnecrotizing (mild) acute pancreatitis** comprises most cases. Recovery usually occurs within 7 days. Death is unusual.[4,5]
- **Necrotizing (severe) acute pancreatitis** is associated with a high rate of complications and mortality.[4,5]

○ **Histologic classification**
- **Interstitial type.** The pancreas is edematous, but its gross architecture is preserved, and hemorrhage is absent.[4,5]
- **Hemorrhagic type.** Marked pancreatic tissue necrosis and hemorrhage are apparent. Surrounding areas of fat necrosis are also prominent. Large hematomas often occur in the retroperitoneal space, and vascular inflammation or thrombosis is common. Mortality is higher in hemorrhagic than in interstitial type.[4,5]

Epidemiology

- Acute pancreatitis accounts for >220,000 hospital admissions in the United States each year.[3]
- The yearly incidence of acute pancreatitis ranges from 1 to 5 per 10,000.[6]
- Acute pancreatitis occurs at similar frequencies among all age groups, but the cause and likelihood of death vary by demographics and other clinical factors.
  ○ Gallstone pancreatitis is prevalent among white women older than 60 years.[4]
  ○ In children, trauma and systemic disease are the most common etiologies.[4]

Etiology

- **Gallstones**
  ○ Gallstone disease and excessive alcohol use account for 70% to 80% of cases of acute pancreatitis in Western countries. It is important to note, however, that pancreatitis develops in only a small percentage of patients with gallstones.[3,4]
  ○ While the precise pathogenesis is unclear, gallstones are thought to cause pancreatitis by one of two mechanisms:
    - By mechanically obstructing the pancreatic duct where it joins the common bile duct[4]
    - By allowing the reflux of bile or duodenal contents into the pancreatic duct after passage across the sphincter of Oddi[5]
  ○ Both mechanisms cause pancreatic ductal hypertension and subsequent pancreatitis.
- **Alcohol**
  ○ Alcohol-induced pancreatitis occurs in persons with long-standing alcohol use.[4]
  ○ A single binge use of alcohol rarely, if ever, causes pancreatitis.[5]
  ○ Because only ~5% of chronic heavy alcohol users develop pancreatitis, other hereditary or environmental risk factors (including smoking) likely play a role.[5]
- **Drugs**
  ○ Commonly implicated agents include azathioprine, 6-mercaptopurine, l-asparaginase, pentamidine, didanosine, valproic acid, furosemide, sulfonamides, tetracyclines, estrogens, metronidazole, and erythromycin.[6]
- **Trauma**
  ○ Acute pancreatitis can be seen after blunt or penetrating abdominal trauma.[6]

- **Iatrogenic**
  - Acute pancreatitis may occur as a complication of endoscopic retrograde cholangiopancreatography (ERCP), pancreaticobiliary surgery, or cardiopulmonary bypass.[3–5]
- **Hypertriglyceridemia**
  - The breakdown products of triglycerides can induce pancreatitis in patients with hypertriglyceridemia.[6,7]
  - When lipase in the pancreatic capillary bed acts on the high levels of triglycerides in the serum, toxic free fatty acids are generated. Although triglyceride levels of >2000 to 3000 mg/dL are usually required for pancreatitis to develop, pancreatitis can also occur when serum levels are only 500 mg/dL.[3,6,7]
  - In general, a serum triglyceride level of 1000 mg/dL suggests hypertriglyceridemia as a cause of pancreatitis.[5]
  - Importantly, acute pancreatitis itself can elevate triglycerides.
  - The typical hypocaloric regimen (nothing by mouth) recommended during acute pancreatitis results in rapid decline in triglyceride levels.
  - Fasting triglyceride levels should be measured after discharge from the hospital to ascertain whether hypertriglyceridemia was the cause of acute pancreatitis.
- **Infection**
  - Infection is thought to be a rare cause of acute pancreatitis.
  - The most common viral infections that involve the pancreas are mumps, cytomegalovirus, and coxsackie B virus.[5]
  - Viral hepatitis, especially hepatitis B, has also been associated with pancreatitis.[8]
  - Patients with HIV infection develop pancreatitis at a higher rate than the general population.
    - The virus itself appears to be the cause in some cases, but other factors (antiretroviral medications, alcohol abuse, dyslipidemia) may also play a role.[8]
    - Asymptomatic hyperamylasemia and hyperlipasemia have been reported in up to 40% of patients with acquired immunodeficiency syndrome (AIDS).[8]
  - Bacteria associated with acute pancreatitis include *Salmonella, Shigella, Campylobacter,* hemorrhagic *Escherichia coli, Legionella, Leptospira,* and *Brucella* species. Pancreatitis associated with these infections is most likely toxin mediated and improves with clearance of the organisms.[8]
- **Miscellaneous causes**
  - Other less common causes of pancreatitis include tumors (both benign and malignant), autoimmune disorders, hypercalcemia, hereditary pancreatitis, pancreas divisum, and papillary stenosis (sphincter of Oddi dysfunction).[4,5,7]
- **Idiopathic**
  - Despite an extensive workup, the cause will not be identifiable in 30% of cases of acute pancreatitis.[4]

Pathophysiology

- Processes that contribute to the initiation of pancreatitis include pancreatic duct obstruction, pancreatic ischemia, and the premature activation of zymogens within the pancreatic acinar cells.[4]
- Subsequent digestion of pancreatic membranes causes tissue injury. This leads to release of inflammatory cytokines (tumor necrosis factor, interleukin-1, platelet-activating factor) that recruit inflammatory cells and increase vascular permeability.[4]
- This cascade of events leads to the development of acute pancreatitis and its systemic manifestations. If the resulting inflammation and tissue injury causes

areas of the pancreas to become devitalized, necrotizing pancreatitis occurs and predisposes the patient to septic complications.[4]

DIAGNOSIS

Clinical Presentation

History
- The hallmark of acute pancreatitis is abdominal pain located in the epigastric and periumbilical areas, radiating to the back.[5]
- The abdominal pain typically is more intense when the patient is supine and may be relieved if the patient leans forward or assumes a fetal position.
- The abdominal pain worsens with food and alcohol ingestion.
- Nausea, emesis, and abdominal distention are also frequently reported.
- Hematemesis, melena, and diarrhea are infrequent.

Physical Examination
- Systemic features may include fever and tachycardia, depending on the severity of disease. Patients may present with shock and/or in coma.[3–5]
- Abdominal tenderness ranges from mild epigastric tenderness and distension to rigidity with rebound tenderness.
- Scleral icterus may be seen because of biliary obstruction or accompanying liver disease.
- A faint bluish discoloration around the umbilicus (Cullen's sign) or flank (Turner's sign), secondary to hemorrhage, is rarely seen.
- An epigastric mass due to pseudocyst formation may become palpable over the course of the disease.
- Less common features include polyarthritis, thrombophlebitis of the lower extremities, and panniculitis (subcutaneous nodular fat necrosis).[3–5]

Diagnostic Testing

Laboratories
- **Amylase and lipase**
  - These are enzymes that are released from the pancreas during acute pancreatitis.
  - Amylase and lipase elevations at least twice the upper limit of normal are required to establish a conclusive diagnosis of pancreatitis.[5]
  - Compared with amylase, lipase has slightly superior sensitivity and specificity.[5]
  - Plasma levels of both enzymes peak at 24 hours of symptoms, but amylase has a shorter half-life.[4,5]
- **Predictors of severity**
  - Because the severity of pancreatitis correlates with prognosis, stratifying patients early during the hospital course is important.
  - Several approaches have been used to differentiate between patients who will have a mild versus severe course. These rating schemes include **Ranson's criteria, modified Glasgow criteria**, and **Acute Physiologic and Chronic Health Evaluation (APACHE) II score** (Table 22-1). Another rating scheme, the CT Severity Index, employs imaging data (see later).[3–5,7]
  - When compared at 48 hours after admission, all of the classification systems are similar.[9]
    - The disadvantage of Ranson's criteria is that patients must be scored on admission and at 48 hours to obtain a completed score.
    - The modified Glasgow criteria and the APACHE II scoring system can be calculated anytime during the hospital stay.

| TABLE 22-1 | COMPARISON OF SEVERITY SCORING SYSTEMS FOR ACUTE PANCREATITIS |

Ranson's Criteria[a]		Glasgow Criteria	CT Scoring Criteria	
On Admission	Within 48 hr		Score	CT Findings
WBC >16,000/mm^3	Hematocrit decrease by 10%	WBC >15,000/mm^3	0	Normal pancreas
Age >55 yr	BUN increase by >5 mg/dL	BUN >45 mg/dL without response to fluids	1	Focal or diffuse pancreatic enlargement
	Calcium <8 mg/dL	Calcium <8 mg/dL	2	Peripancreatic inflammation with intrinsic pancreatic abnormalities
	Arterial po$_2$ <60 mm Hg	Arterial po$_2$ <60 mm Hg	3	Presence of single fluid collection
AST >250 IU/L	Base deficit >4 mEq/L	AST >200 U/L	4	Presence of ≥2 fluid collections or gas in the pancreas and/or retroperitoneum
LDH >350 IU/L	Fluid sequestration >6 L	LDH >600 U/L	**Score**	**Necrosis (%)**
Glucose >200 mg/dL		Glucose >180 mg/dL without diabetes	0	0
		Albumin <3.2 g/dL	2	<33
			4	33–50
			6	≥50
Mortality rate of ≤4 criteria is <15% and considered mild disease. Mortality rate rises greatly with more than four criteria.		Severe pancreatitis is defined as the presence of three or more of the above criteria within 48 hr of evaluation.	CT severity index is defined as the sum of the CT findings score and the pancreatic necrosis score. The maximum is 10 and >6 predicts severe disease. A severity score of 7–10 has a 92% complication rate and a 17% mortality rate, whereas a score of 0 or 1 has zero morbidity or mortality.	

AST, aspartate aminotransferase; BUN, blood urea nitrogen; CT, computed tomography; LDH, lactate dehydrogenase; WBC, white blood cell count.

[a]Applies to nonbiliary causes of pancreatitis. Criteria are adjusted with biliary pancreatitis. Adapted from Ranson JHC, Rifkind KM, Roses DF, et al. Surg Gynecol Obstet. 1974;139:69; Corfield AP, Williamson RCN, McMahon MJ, et al. Prediction of severity in acute pancreatitis: prospective comparison of three prognostic indices. Lancet. 1985;24:403–407; and Balthazar EJ, Robinson DL, Megibow AJ, et al. Radiology. 1990;174:331, with permission.

Imaging

- **Abdominal ultrasonography**
  - ○ Limited utility in visualizing the pancreas but very useful in establishing gall-stones as the cause.[4]
  - ○ **Should be the initial imaging modality in patients presenting with acute pancreatitis.**
- **Computed tomography**
  - ○ Not necessarily required for the initial diagnosis of pancreatitis in patients with typical symptoms and corresponding elevations of pancreatic enzymes.
  - ○ May be normal in up to 30% of patients with mild pancreatitis, but almost always abnormal in patients with moderate or severe pancreatitis.[4,5]
  - ○ Should be obtained if (1) the diagnosis is in doubt, (2) patients do not improve within a few days, or (3) initial favorable clinical response was followed by sudden clinical deterioration.[4,5]
  - ○ Should be performed using a pancreatic protocol, which involves thin cross-sectional images ("slices") through the pancreas during several contrast phases. Disruption of the pancreatic microcirculation results in necrosis of the pancreatic tissue, which can be identified on computed tomography (CT).[5]
  - ○ Severity of pancreatitis can also be staged on the basis of CT findings such as pancreatic edema, peripancreatic infiltrates, peripancreatic fluid collections, vascular thrombosis, and areas of nonenhancement due to necrosis (Fig. 22-1).
  - ○ The CT Severity Index does not use any clinical or laboratory parameters and only uses imaging findings (Table 22-1).
- **Magnetic resonance cholangiopancreatography**
  - ○ Useful when renal insufficiency or dye allergies preclude the use of CT but not routinely performed.

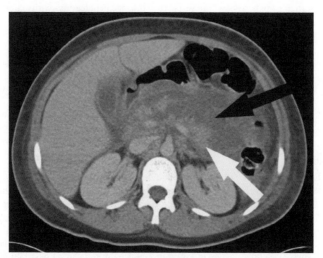

FIGURE 22-1 Computed tomography scan demonstrating pancreatic edema and necrosis in an 18-year-old man with gallstone pancreatitis. Note the large areas of low-attenuation (*dark gray*) within the pancreatic bed (*black arrow*) compared with the areas with relatively preserved blood flow (*white arrow*). Normally, the pancreas has similar attenuation as the adjacent liver.

Diagnostic Procedures

- **Endoscopic retrograde cholangiopancreatography**
  - This has both diagnostic and therapeutic utility in biliary causes of pancreatitis.[5]
  - Once identified, impacted gallstones can be extracted and infected bile can be drained via endoscopic sphincterotomy during ERCP (see later).

TREATMENT

- **Mild acute pancreatitis**
  - Treatment is supportive with bed rest, no oral intake, intravenous hydration, electrolyte replacement, antiemetics, and analgesics (meperidine or morphine).
  - Nasogastric suction may be useful to alleviate the symptoms of nausea, emesis, and abdominal distention.
  - The patient can be cautiously fed once the abdominal pain resolves.[3,4]
- **Severe acute pancreatitis**
  - The treatment of severe pancreatitis, like milder forms, is primarily supportive, but these patients typically require more vigorous fluid resuscitation and closer monitoring in an intensive care unit.
  - A patient-controlled analgesic pump is often required to achieve adequate levels of pain control.
  - Patients should be monitored closely for signs of clinical deterioration from multisystem organ failure (renal, respiratory, cardiovascular, or sepsis).[4,6,7]

Medications

- **Antibiotics**
  - The issue of prophylactic antibiotics in pancreatitis is controversial.[3–7]
  - In general, prophylactic antibiotics are recommended in cases of severe necrotizing pancreatitis or suspected biliary pancreatitis with cholangitis, whereas antibiotics are not recommended for mild pancreatitis.[4,5]
  - Appropriate antibiotics should be active against a wide variety of organisms—in particular, gram-negative bacilli.[4,5]
  - The **most commonly used regimens** include imipenem, meropenem, or a combination of a fluoroquinolone and metronidazole.[3]
  - The optimal length of treatment is not known, but antibiotics are usually continued for 10 to 14 days or until clinical improvement is seen.[4,5]
  - Caution should be exercised because prolonged use of broad-spectrum antibiotics is associated with resistant bacterial infections as well as disseminated fungal infections.[4,5]

Procedures

- **Endoscopic retrograde cholangiopancreatography**
  - Should be performed in **patients with presumed gallstone pancreatitis with suspected residual common bile duct stones,** as suggested by persistently elevated liver enzymes or bilirubin, dilated common bile duct, or obvious choledocholithiasis seen during ultrasonography or other imaging.[4,5]
  - Should also be performed in those with findings suggestive of **cholangitis** such as right upper quadrant abdominal pain and tenderness, temperature >39°C, leukocyte count >20,000.[4,5]
  - ERCP with sphincterotomy has been shown to reduce length of hospital stay and mortality in patients with suspected residual bile duct stones when performed 24 to 72 hours after presentation.[4]

Other Nonpharmacologic Therapies

- **Nutrition**
  - **Withholding oral intake is a mainstay of initial therapy for acute pancreatitis.** This serves to minimize stimulation of the exocrine pancreas, thereby minimizing abdominal pain, nausea, and vomiting.[3,4]
    - Withholding oral intake also serves to mitigate pancreatic inflammation.
    - If the pancreatitis is severe, it may require weeks or months before oral feedings are reintroduced. If symptoms do not resolve and an oral diet cannot be resumed in 5 to 7 days, other avenues for nutritional support must be considered.[4,5]
  - **Enteral tube feeding delivered to the jejunum** (beyond the ligament of Treitz) is the safest manner in which to deliver nutrition. By bypassing the stomach and duodenum, jejunal feedings theoretically avoid the meal-driven pancreatic stimulation that can lead to symptoms or recurrent attacks of pancreatitis.[10]
    - Enteral feedings are thought to maintain the health and barrier function of the bowel wall, reducing the probability of bacterial translocation and subsequent superinfection of pancreatic fluid collections.[5,10]
  - **Total parental nutrition** (TPN) is effective in delivering calories, minerals, and micronutrients. However, because it bypasses the gastrointestinal (GI) tract, TPN does not maintain bowel wall integrity. TPN should therefore be considered a second option in feeding patients with moderate to severe pancreatitis.[10]
    - TPN requires central venous access, imparting a significant risk of infection. Also, TPN is financially costly and requires monitoring of key metabolic parameters.

COMPLICATIONS

- **Fluid collection (pseudocyst)**
  - Pseudocysts develop in 15% of patients with acute pancreatitis.[3]
  - Previously, any pseudocyst larger than 6 cm persisting for 6 weeks was managed with a drainage procedure. It is now clear, however, that some of these pseudocysts that are not enlarging or causing symptoms will resolve without intervention and can be monitored with serial CT.[4,11]
  - In patients with enlarging or symptomatic noninfected pseudocysts, endoscopic or radiological drainage is an attractive option. Radiologic placement of drainage catheters is often successful but can result in pancreatocutaneous fistulas.[6,11]
  - In recent years, transluminal endoscopic approaches have been increasingly adopted to treat symptomatic fluid collections.
  - For endoscopic drainage to be successful, the fluid collection should not be multiloculated and should not contain excessive amounts of debris or necrotic material.[5]
  - The absence of pseudoaneurysms in the wall of the cyst should be confirmed with CT before attempting endoscopic drainage.[5–7]
  - During endoscopic drainage, initially the planned puncture site in the stomach or duodenum is identified with or without endoscopic ultrasonography (EUS) guidance to locate an area devoid of blood vessels. Next, a guidewire is passed into the cavity, the tract is dilated with a balloon, and "pigtail" stents or nasocystic drains are placed within.[4–6]
    - This allows for decompression and drainage of the pseudocyst contents directly into the bowel through the cystenterostomy (Fig. 22-2).

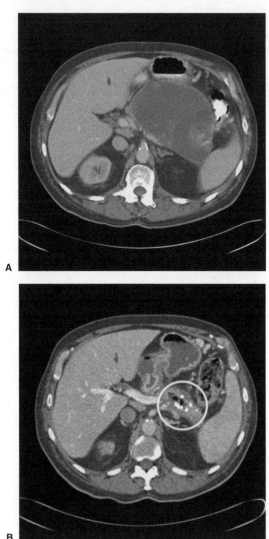

FIGURE 22-2 Demonstration of efficacy of endoscopic pancreatic pseudocyst drainage in a 58-year-old man with severe pancreatitis who developed a large pseudocyst as seen on computed tomography (**A**). He was symptomatic with abdominal pain, early satiety, and nausea. Therefore, multiple "pigtail" stents were endoscopically placed from the stomach into the cavity, and the cyst resolved over a period of 4 months (*white circle*) (**B**).

○ **Following drainage, patients are followed with serial imaging studies to document resolution of the pseudocyst.**[11]

○ Once the pseudocyst has resolved, the stents or drains may be removed.

• **Pancreatic abscess**

○ Occasionally, bacterial colonization of a pseudocyst or inflammatory mass occurs, resulting in infected pancreatic necrosis or an abscess.[3]

○ Clinical manifestations include worsening pain, fever, septic physiology, and an elevated white blood cell count.[5,6]

○ Aspiration of any low-density areas or fluid collections under CT or ultrasound guidance can guide further interventions.[5]

○ If organisms or polymorphonuclear neutrophils are seen on the aspirate, the patient should undergo **percutaneous drainage or surgical debridement.**[7]

○ The typically viscous and loculated nature of infected fluid collections tends to render endoscopic drainage ineffective. However, direct endoscopic debridement through a cystenterostomy and irrigation of the cyst for several days via a nasocystic drain may be pursued in poor surgical candidates with solitary infected fluid collections.[5,11]

• **Pancreatic necrosis**

○ May occur as diffuse or focal areas of nonviable pancreatic parenchyma.[3]

○ Can develop during the first few days of pancreatitis.[3]

○ Onset of necrosis is associated with pancreatic inflammation, hemoconcentration, and pancreatic hypoperfusion, whether due to hypovolemia or hypotension from shunting of blood to other organs.[4,5]

○ Subsequent infection of necrotic pancreatic tissue is associated with late complications and death.

○ Clinical indicators of necrosis, usually apparent after the first week of illness, include fever, leukocytosis, failure to improve, or unexpected deterioration.[5]

○ Gas bubbles may be visualized within necrotic tissue on CT.

○ Definitive diagnosis may be made by fine-needle aspiration (FNA) of the necrotic area guided by CT or ultrasonography, followed by Gram stain and culture of the aspirate.[4]

○ Treatment includes **aggressive supportive care and surgical debridement.**

▪ It has been suggested that survival is improved by delaying surgical intervention for at least 2 weeks if possible, to allow the patient's medical condition to be optimized and to allow the viability of pancreatic tissue to become more evident.[3,4]

OUTCOME/PROGNOSIS

• Most cases of mild, acute pancreatitis are self-limited, with a mortality rate of 1%.[6,7]

• Overall, about 20% of cases have a severe course, of which 10% to 30% die.[3]

• Despite numerous advances in intensive care unit medicine over the last few decades, mortality in acute pancreatitis has not declined.[3]

CHRONIC PANCREATITIS

GENERAL PRINCIPLES

Definition

• Chronic pancreatitis is characterized by progressive inflammatory changes in the pancreas leading to irreversible damage of the pancreatic architecture. This leads to impairment of exocrine and endocrine function.[12–14]

- Acute pancreatitis differs from chronic pancreatitis in that the former is the result of injury and is nonprogressive. Recurrent flares of acute pancreatitis may lead to chronic pancreatitis, however.[13]

Epidemiology

- The incidence of chronic pancreatitis is ~4 of 100,000 per year; the prevalence is ~13 of 100,000.[13]

Etiology

- **Alcohol**
  - In Western societies, alcohol consumption is the most common etiology, accounting for 70% to 80% of cases. Of note, however, only 5% to 10% of alcoholics develop chronic pancreatitis.[13]
  - In general, prolonged alcohol intake (6 to 12 years) is required to produce symptomatic chronic pancreatitis.[14]
- **Genetic syndromes**
  - Patients with **cystic fibrosis** (mutations in the CFTR gene) develop progressive pancreatic damage due to defective secretion from pancreatic ductules and acinar cells, resulting in chronic pancreatitis.[13,14]
  - Hereditary chronic pancreatitis has been described.[15]
- **Ductal obstruction**
  - May result from trauma, stones, neoplasms, or sphincter of Oddi dysfunction.[13]
- **Autoimmune disease**
  - Includes systemic lupus erythematosus, inflammatory bowel disease, and autoimmune pancreatitis.[13]
- **Idiopathic**
  - Accounts for 30% to 40% of cases.[14]
- The comprehensive TIGAR-O classification system for etiologic risk factors for chronic pancreatitis is shown in Table 22-2.

TABLE 22-2	TIGAR-O CLASSIFICATION SYSTEM OF CHRONIC PANCREATITIS
Toxic-metabolic	Alcohol, tobacco, hypercalcemia, hyperlipidemia, chronic renal failure, medications (phenacetin abuse)
Idiopathic	Early onset, late onset, tropical
Genetic	Cationic trypsinogen, CFTR mutations
Autoimmune	Sjögren's syndrome, inflammatory bowel disease, primary biliary cirrhosis
Recurrent and severe acute pancreatitis	Postnecrotic, recurrent acute pancreatitis, vascular disease, postirradiation
Obstructive	Pancreas divisum, duct obstruction (tumor), posttraumatic pancreatic duct scars, preampullary duodenal wall cysts

CFTR, cystic fibrosis transmembrane conductance regulator.
Adapted from Etemad B, Whitcomb DC. Chronic pancreatitis: diagnosis, classification, and new genetic developments. *Gastroenterology.* 2001;120:682–707.

Pathophysiology

- Pancreatic acinar cell loss, islet cell loss, calcifications, and patchy mononuclear infiltrates and fibrosis are observed in chronic pancreatitis. Protein hypersecretion and impaired ductal bicarbonate secretion occur as well.[13]
- The pathogenesis of these chronic inflammatory changes is not entirely clear.
- Intraductal plugging, chronic ischemia, excess free radical formation, and autoimmune mechanisms have been proposed as factors contributing to the development of chronic pancreatitis.[13]
- When <10% of the normal exocrine secretion of pancreatic enzymes remains in a patient with chronic pancreatitis, fat and/or protein malabsorption can occur.[13]
- Symptoms tend to occur relatively late in the course of chronic pancreatitis.

DIAGNOSIS

- The diagnosis of chronic pancreatitis often can be made on the basis of the history and relatively simple radiographic tests. Routine blood studies usually are not helpful in making the diagnosis of chronic pancreatitis, and imaging may be normal.[12]
- The classic triad of pancreatic calcifications, steatorrhea, and diabetes mellitus usually occurs only in very advanced disease.[12]

Clinical Presentation

History

- The most common presenting symptom is dull, constant epigastric/periumbilical abdominal pain that may radiate to the back. Pain could occur periodically, lasting several days, or occasionally be constant.[16]
  - Exacerbation of pain by eating is common in chronic pancreatitis, but other medical conditions (e.g., mesenteric ischemia and irritable bowel syndrome) can also have a similar presentation.[16]
  - In advanced stages, chronic pancreatitis can be painless (15% of patients). Idiopathic pancreatitis is more likely to be painless than alcoholic pancreatitis.[16]
- Nausea, vomiting, and anorexia are common.
- If chronic pancreatitis is complicated by malabsorption, the patient may present with diarrhea, steatorrhea, or azotorrhea. Compared with other malabsorptive conditions, which tend to cause frank watery diarrhea, pancreatic malabsorption causes diarrhea that is more bulky and formed, with lower fecal weights.[12,13]
- Weight loss may be multifactorial and due to anorexia, malabsorption, or complications of chronic pancreatitis such as malignancy or uncontrolled diabetes mellitus.[14]

Physical Examination

- Usually is of limited assistance in the diagnosis of chronic pancreatitis because the intensity of the patient's complaint tends to be out of proportion to the physical signs.[16]
- Epigastric tenderness may be present during the painful episodes as well as during periods of remission.
- Less common manifestations of chronic pancreatitis include jaundice (extrinsic bile duct obstruction or stricture), ascites, pleural effusion, painful subcutaneous nodules (pancreatic panniculitis), and polyarthritis of the small joints of the hands.[13]

Diagnostic Testing

Laboratories

- Leukocytosis may be observed during acute exacerbations.[12,13]
- Anemia and fat-soluble vitamin deficiency states (hypocalcemia, hypoprothrombinemia) are seldom seen in association with the steatorrhea of chronic pancreatitis.[13]
- Varying degrees of cholestasis can be seen, secondary to pancreatic fibrosis with involvement of the common bile duct. This can cause elevations in serum alkaline phosphatase and direct bilirubin fraction.[13]
- In contrast to attacks of acute pancreatitis, in which the serum levels of amylase and lipase are usually elevated, these enzymes may be elevated, normal, or low in chronic pancreatitis.[5]

Imaging

- **Plain X-ray of the abdomen**
  - This should be the **initial imaging study.**
  - Demonstration of diffuse, speckled calcification of the pancreas on a plain X-ray film is diagnostic of chronic pancreatitis.[13]
  - Although often seen in patients with advanced pancreatitis, the presence of pancreatic calcifications does not correlate with disease severity.[13]
- **Abdominal ultrasonography**
  - Findings include calcifications as well as dilation of the main pancreatic duct to >4 mm. These findings may correlate to marked pancreatic changes on ERCP.[17]
  - When a satisfactory examination is obtained, the reported sensitivity of this test for chronic pancreatitis is ~70% and the specificity is 90%.[17]
- **Computed tomography**
  - More sensitive than ultrasonography for the diagnosis of chronic pancreatitis.[18]
  - The most common diagnostic findings of chronic pancreatitis on CT include duct dilation, calcifications, and cystic lesions.[18]
  - Less common diagnostic findings include enlargement or atrophy of the pancreas and heterogeneous density of the parenchyma.[18]
  - Besides being significantly more expensive, CT carries the additional risks of contrast reactions and radiation exposure.
- **Magnetic resonance cholangiopancreatography**
  - Allows for accurate delineation of the pancreatic duct (presence of dilation, stones, or strictures), evaluation of pancreatic parenchyma, and the detection of subtle solid and cystic lesions.
  - May be more desirable than CT because it avoids exposure to ionizing radiation and iodinated intravenous contrast.

Diagnostic Procedures

- **Endoscopic ultrasound (EUS)**
  - Provides more detailed structural information of the pancreas than ultrasonography and CT, without the risk of complications of ERCP.
  - Allows for evaluation of ductal and parenchymal changes, such as echotexture of the gland, calcifications, lobulations, and bands of fibrosis.
  - Allows for direct tissue sampling by FNA if indicated.
- **Endoscopic retrograde cholangiopancreatography**
  - As in acute pancreatitis, ERCP is both a diagnostic and therapeutic tool.
  - ERCP is both sensitive and specific for the diagnosis of chronic pancreatitis.
  - Mild chronic pancreatitis is characterized by dilatation and irregularity of the side branch ducts.[13,19]

- ○ Moderate chronic pancreatitis is characterized by the additional findings of dilation and tortuosity of the main pancreatic duct.[13,19]
- ○ Advanced disease has the additional findings of ductal stenosis, stone formation, cyst formation, or atrophy of the pancreas.[13,19]
- ○ The widespread availability of EUS and magnetic resonance cholangiopancreatography (MRCP) has largely supplanted the use of ERCP for diagnostic pancreatography. ERCP is typically performed with intent to deliver therapy as directed by other imaging modalities rather than purely as a diagnostic procedure.

Tests of Pancreatic Exocrine Function
- Exocrine function can be **tested directly.**
  - ○ Testing may be performed by stimulation with secretin, cholecystokinin, or both, followed by measurement of bicarbonate concentrations or enzyme activity. Subnormal measured levels are suggestive of chronic pancreatitis.[13]
  - ○ Another method is the measurement of pancreatic polypeptide. A subnormal rise in plasma pancreatic polypeptide levels after stimulation with a protein-rich meal or secretin infusion is an indication of chronic pancreatitis.
- Exocrine function can also be **tested indirectly.**
  - ○ Testing may be performed by measuring pancreatic enzyme levels or by assessing the absorption of a compound that requires initial digestion by pancreatic enzymes.[13]
  - ○ The bentiromide test involves ingestion of *N*-benzoyl-l-tyrosyl-*p*-aminobenzoic acid (NBT-PABA), a tripeptide that is digested by chymotrypsin with the release of *p*-aminobenzoic acid (PABA). Free PABA is absorbed in the small bowel and excreted by the kidney. The quantity excreted in urine is used as a measure of pancreatic exocrine function.[13]
  - ○ Measurement of fecal chymotrypsin activity or fecal elastase levels is also an available testing modality.
    - ■ Fecal chymotrypsin activity measurement is rapid and simple, but its sensitivity is considered too low to be recommended in clinical practice.[13]
    - ■ In contrast, fecal elastase measurement is much more sensitive and specific in the diagnosis of moderate to severe pancreatic insufficiency.[20]
  - ○ Alternatively, exocrine function can be assessed by measuring the absorption of a compound that requires initial digestion by pancreatic enzymes. However, because clinically detectable nutrient malabsorption does not occur until pancreatic enzyme secretion has diminished to <10% of normal, this approach cannot detect early chronic pancreatitis.

TREATMENT

Medication for Pain

- **Analgesics**
  - ○ Initially, nonopioid analgesics such as salicylates or acetaminophen should be used. The dose or frequency of these nonopioid analgesics should be titrated and maximized before adding on or switching to an opioid.[21]
  - ○ For severe or uncontrolled pain, opioid analgesics are required.
  - ○ Because of the recurrent nature of chronic pancreatitis with the frequent use of opioid analgesics, many of these patients demonstrate opioid dependence and drug-seeking behaviors, making evaluation and treatment of pain quite complex.
  - ○ Consultation from a pain management specialist may be helpful.

- **Pancreatic enzyme replacement therapy**
  - Several groups of investigators have confirmed that intestinal administration of trypsin or chymotrypsin inhibits pancreatic enzyme secretion.[21]
  - In normal persons, intraduodenal cholecystokinin (CCK) stimulates the pancreas to secrete digestive enzymes that, in turn, degrade CCK, thus establishing a feedback loop.[21]
  - The reduction in pancreatic enzyme secretion in chronic pancreatitis causes elevated CCK levels, leading to stimulation-associated pancreatic pain.
  - Effective enzyme replacement therapy should reduce pancreatic stimulation, decrease intraductal pressure, and diminish pain.[21]
  - In most patients, a trial of high-dose, nonenteric-coated pancreatic enzymes is prescribed with meals for several weeks in any patient with painful chronic pancreatitis. Typically, a starting dose of at least 48,000 units of lipase, 90,000 units of amylase, and 90,000 units of protease is taken with each meal.[21]
  - Patients should also take a histamine-2 receptor antagonist or proton pump inhibitor to diminish enzyme degradation by gastric acid.
  - The best results are seen in pancreatitis of nonalcoholic etiology, which manifests with symptoms of constant (rather than recurrent) pain and only mild to moderate pancreatic insufficiency.[21]
- **Octreotide**
  - Synthetic long-acting analogue of somatostatin, an endogenous hormone that inhibits pancreatic secretion.
  - Octreotide has been shown to inhibit both CCK release and pancreatic enzyme secretion.
  - Randomized studies of patients with advanced chronic pancreatitis and severe pain suggest that 200 mcg of octreotide administered subcutaneously three times per day produced the greatest pain relief (65% vs. 35% of patients with placebo), especially in patients with constant, as opposed to intermittent, pain. However, this result did not reach statistical significance.[21]
  - Additional studies are needed to further clarify the role of octreotide in the management of pain in chronic pancreatitis.

Medication for Exocrine Insufficiency

- **Pancreatic enzyme replacement therapy**
  - The cornerstone of therapy for malabsorption in patients with chronic pancreatitis.
  - It is critical that sufficient amounts of enzyme are delivered to the small bowel to abolish azotorrhea and significantly reduce steatorrhea.
  - Generally, 30,000 units of **lipase** taken with each meal is adequate to reduce steatorrhea and prevent further weight loss.[13,21]
  - As with enzyme replacement therapy for pain control, the use of acid-suppressive agents reduces degradation in the stomach and increases the amount of pancreatic enzymes available in the small bowel to assist in fat digestion. The dosage of the pancreatic enzyme supplements can be titrated to treat the symptoms and malabsorption adequately.[21]
  - Although it is not common to see complete correction of steatorrhea in patients with chronic pancreatitis, it is possible to bring the steatorrhea under control.

Procedures

- **Endoscopic retrograde cholangiopancreatography**
  - ○ This has been used for control of pain in chronic pancreatitis, with the aim of alleviating obstruction of flow caused by ductal strictures, stones, or papillary stenosis.[21]
  - ○ Ductal strictures are sometimes treated by **balloon dilation,** usually followed by **stent placement** across the stricture.[21]
  - ○ Endoscopic techniques also have been used for the removal of pancreatic stones in chronic pancreatitis.[21]
  - ○ In the cases of large stones, **extracorporeal shockwave lithotripsy** is used in conjunction with ERCP to fragment and then remove stones.[21]
  - ○ Papillary stenosis is treated with **pancreatic sphincterotomy** during ERCP.[13,21]
- **Celiac plexus block**
  - ○ Injections into the celiac ganglion have been used for control of pancreatic pain.
  - ○ This can be performed either by radiologists using fluoroscopy or gastroenterologists using endoscopic ultrasound guidance. Typically, absolute alcohol is injected into the area where the celiac plexus lies.[13,21]
  - ○ In small, uncontrolled series of patients with chronic pancreatitis and debilitating pain, celiac plexus block has produced mixed results.[21]
  - ○ The pain relief usually does not last for more than a few months, and repeated treatment may not be as effective.[21]

Other Nonpharmacologic Therapies

- **Avoidance of alcohol**
  - ○ Avoiding alcohol decreases the frequency and severity of abdominal pain in chronic alcoholic pancreatitis.[13,21]
  - ○ All patients with excessive alcohol consumption should be referred to an appropriate treatment program.
  - ○ In patients who maintain significant exocrine secretory function, pain may be provoked by alcohol, which acts as a pancreatic secretagogue.[16]
  - ○ In patients whose exocrine secretion is drastically reduced, alcohol may play a lesser role in the mechanism of pain.
  - ○ Further studies are needed to clarify the role of alcohol in pain production in chronic pancreatitis.

Surgical Management

- A growing body of evidence suggests that surgical therapies for chronic pancreatitis are superior to endoscopic management in the ability to provide long-lasting pain relief.[13,21]
- The type of surgery is selected according to the perceived mechanism for the pain, the severity of pain, ductal morphology, and the extent of parenchymal disease.
- Patients who have ductal dilation have a 70% to 80% chance of obtaining pain relief with either a partial resection with pancreaticojejunostomy or lateral pancreaticojejunostomy.[13,21]
- Other options include partial pancreatectomy or near total pancreatectomy with islet cell transplantation.
- Distal pancreatectomy can also be considered in those with focal changes limited to the tail of the pancreas.[21]

COMPLICATIONS

- **Diabetes mellitus**
  - Clinically evident diabetes, which occurs relatively late in the disease, is seen in up to 60% of patients with chronic pancreatitis.[13]
  - Diabetic ketoacidosis and diabetic nephropathy are relatively uncommon in this form of diabetes.
- **Pseudocyst**
  - Develops in 10% of patients with chronic pancreatitis, which is less frequent than in acute pancreatitis.[13]
  - In chronic pancreatitis, pseudocysts are the result of ductal disruptions; in contrast, pseudocysts of acute pancreatitis are the result of peripancreatic fluid collections.
  - Pseudocysts are usually asymptomatic.
  - Additional complications of pseudocyst formation include enlargement of the pseudocyst, which may cause abdominal pain, duodenal or biliary obstruction, vascular occlusion, or fistula formation.[11]
  - Pseudoaneurysms may form as a result of pancreatic enzyme digestion of an adjacent vessel wall.[11]
  - Infection of the pseudocyst leads to abscess formation.
  - Pseudocysts are diagnosed by ultrasonography or CT.
  - Endoscopic drainage is indicated in cases of rapid enlargement, compression of surrounding structures, pain, or signs of infection.[13]
- **Bile duct obstruction or duodenal obstruction**
  - Develops in 5% to 10% of cases.[13]
  - Causes include inflammation and fibrosis in the head of the pancreas, or a pseudocyst.
  - Bile duct obstruction characteristically causes pain as well as elevated levels of transaminases and bilirubin.
    - Diagnosis is made by ERCP or MRCP.
  - Dudoental obstruction characteristically causes postprandial pain and early satiety.
    - Diagnosis is made by upper GI series, upper endoscopy, or CT.
  - If obstruction is due pseudocyst, then drainage is indicated. Otherwise, gastrojejunostomy or choledochoenterostomy is indicated.
  - For biliary stricture, endoscopic stenting can be considered.[21]
- **Pancreatic ascites**
  - May develop due to disruption of the pancreatic duct, which leads to fistulization to the abdomen or rupture of a pseudocyst. Pancreatic juice then tracks into the peritoneal cavity, causing ascites. Pleural effusions may develop in a similar manner as well.
  - Fluid obtained by paracentesis (or thoracentesis in the setting of pleural effusion) has a characteristically high amylase concentration, usually exceeding 1000 IU/L.
  - Treatment may be nonoperative, consisting of repeated aspiration, diuretics, or octreotide. Parenteral nutrition to decrease pancreatic secretion and endoscopic stenting of the pancreatic duct may be employed as well.[13,21]
  - Surgical drainage involves anastomosis of a Roux-en-Y loop of jejunum to the pancreatic duct and pseudocyst.[13]
- **Splenic vein thrombosis**
  - Because of its location along the posterior pancreas, the splenic vein may thrombose due to adjacent inflammation.
  - Gastric varices may develop due to subsequent portal hypertension.
    - Splenectomy is a curative option for patients who develop bleeding from varices.

- **Pancreatic cancer**
  ○ Chronic pancreatitis has been associated with pancreatic adenocarcinoma.
  ○ Pancreatic cancer develops in ~4% of patients within 20 years of a diagnosis of chronic pancreatitis.[22]

OUTCOME/PROGNOSIS

- Chronic pancreatitis characteristically has a prolonged, recurrent course with progressive loss of pancreatic endocrine and exocrine function.
- The "burnout" phenomenon has been observed in some patients, in whom progressive loss of exocrine function is associated with resolution of abdominal pain.[13]
- Chronic pancreatitis is associated with a 50% mortality rate within 20 to 25 years. Approximately 15% to 20% of these deaths are due to associated attacks of pancreatitis, whereas the remaining deaths are due to associated factors such as malnutrition, infection, or complications of alcohol or tobacco use.[13,14]

PANCREATIC CANCER

GENERAL PRINCIPLES

Definition
- Ductal adenocarcinoma and its variants account for >90% of all malignant exocrine pancreatic tumors.[15]

Epidemiology
- Approximately 30,000 new cases of pancreatic cancer occur every year in the United States, and nearly all of these patients eventually die from the disease.[23]
- The peak incidence of pancreatic carcinoma occurs in the seventh decade of life, and there is a slight male predominance.[23]
- The overall incidence of the disease is 30% to 40% higher in blacks than in whites.[23]

Pathophysiology
- Approximately two-thirds of ductal adenocarcinomas occur in the head of the gland, with the rest in the body or tail.[15]
- At the time of diagnosis, tumors of the head of the pancreas are usually ≥2 cm in diameter.[15,24]
- Seventy percent to 80% of malignant pancreatic tumors have metastasized to regional lymph nodes by the time they are discovered.[15,24]
- Tumors of the body and tail commonly are more advanced and larger (5 to 7 cm) when discovered, because they do not produce symptoms as early as pancreatic head tumors.
  ○ The symptoms from tumors in the body and tail are usually caused by malignant infiltration of the retroperitoneal structures, which produces pain.
- Less than 20% of patients present with localized, potentially curable tumors.
- By the time of diagnosis, almost all pancreatic cancers are unresectable.[15,24]
  ○ Because pancreatic cancer has usually spread to lymph nodes or vascular structures at the time of diagnosis, most patients have at least stage III disease.
  ○ Patients with stage IV disease (distant metastases) cannot be cured and their tumors are considered unresectable.

○ The best outcomes are seen in patients who have well-differentiated neoplasms, without retroperitoneal invasion or lymph node metastases, but such cases are unfortunately uncommon.

Risk Factors

- **Smoking**
  - ○ The risk factor most strongly linked to pancreatic cancer is cigarette smoking.
  - ○ Smoking approximately doubles the chance of developing the disease.[15,24]
  - ○ The risk of pancreatic cancer rapidly decreases when individuals discontinue cigarette use. Approximately 10 to 15 years after quitting smoking, the relative risk falls to ~1.[15]
- **Chronic pancreatitis**
  - ○ Epidemiologic studies suggest that the relative risk of developing pancreatic cancer in patients with chronic pancreatitis is increased by up to 15 times when compared with control populations.[22]
  - ○ This suggests that changes associated with chronic inflammation and fibrosis in the pancreas are important in the development of cancer.
  - ○ Chronic pancreatitis accounts for only a small fraction of patients who have pancreatic cancer.
- **Surgery**
  - ○ Patients who have had a partial gastrectomy have a three- to sevenfold greater risk of developing pancreatic cancer.[24]
  - ○ The apparent increase in incidence may be related to postsurgical altered metabolism of ingested carcinogens by the remaining stomach and small intestine.
- **Diet**
  - ○ Meats and foods of animal origin increase the risk of pancreatic cancer, whereas foods of plant origin and dietary fiber appear to be protective.[23,24]
- **Obesity**
  - ○ A body mass index of >30 kg/m^2 is also reported to be associated with increased cancer risk.[25]
- **Other factors**
  - ○ Increased risk of pancreatic cancer is seen in tropical chronic pancreatitis, hereditary chronic pancreatitis, kindreds with multiple tumor suppressor-1 gene mutations, and other familial cancer syndromes such as Peutz-Jeghers syndrome.[15]

DIAGNOSIS

- There are two main goals in the workup of a patient with suspected pancreatic cancer:
  - ○ To establish the diagnosis with certainty
  - ○ To determine whether the patient should undergo a surgical procedure to resect or palliate the disease

Clinical Presentation

History

- **Jaundice**
  - ○ Presenting symptom in 80% to 90% of patients with cancer of the head of the pancreas.[15,24]
  - ○ Light-colored stools and dark urine are seen if obstructive jaundice exists.
  - ○ Usually accompanied by abdominal pain.

- **Abdominal pain**
  - Epigastric pain or right upper quadrant pain can occur due to biliary tree obstruction.
  - Similar pain or discomfort in the left upper quadrant, back, or periumbilical areas could also result from pancreatic duct distention associated with pancreatic duct obstruction, or invasion of retroperitoneal or somatic nerves.
- **Weight loss**
  - By the time of diagnosis, weight loss of >10% of ideal body weight is common.
  - Anorexia due to tumor-associated pain and decreased food intake contribute to weight loss.
  - Proinflammatory cytokines, especially tumor necrosis factor-α, play a prominent role in the pathogenesis of cachexia of pancreatic cancer.[15,24]
  - Malabsorption from pancreatic insufficiency can also contribute to weight loss.
- **Diabetes mellitus**
  - Diabetes mellitus sometimes appears as an early manifestation of pancreatic cancer, occurring many months before the tumor becomes evident.
- Other symptoms
  - Emesis may be caused by duodenal or gastric outlet obstruction from tumor invasion.
  - GI bleeding can occur from direct invasion of the tumor into the duodenum, stomach, or colon.
  - Migratory thrombophlebitis (Trousseau's sign) is reported in ~10% of patients and may be the earliest presenting sign.[24]
  - There is also a poorly understood association between pancreatic malignancy and major depressive disorder.

Physical Examination
- May be nonspecific.
- Examination may reveal jaundice, temporal wasting, peripheral lymphadenopathy, hepatomegaly, and ascites.
- Physical findings typically reflect the anatomical consequences of the enlarging tumor.

Diagnostic Testing

Laboratories
- **Serum carbohydrate antigen 19-9 level**
  - Most sensitive and specific tumor marker for pancreatic cancer.[15]
  - Importantly, carbohydrate antigen (CA) 19-9 level is almost never elevated with small tumors (<1 cm).
  - CA 19-9 level may be abnormal due to other cancers (gastric, colorectal cancer) and with some benign conditions (cholangitis, biliary obstruction).
  - Determination of CA 19-9 levels may be useful to provide some assurance that the tumor has been resected in its entirety, to signal the presence of recurrent disease after resection, or to determine the response to adjuvant therapy.

Imaging
- **Abdominal ultrasonography**
  - May be useful in patients with jaundice to distinguish between intrahepatic and extrahepatic causes.
  - Extrahepatic obstruction from a pancreatic (or periampullary) cancer is expected to show dilated intrahepatic and extrahepatic biliary ducts.

- ○ The specificity of ultrasonography to diagnose pancreatic cancer ranges from 90% to 99%, but the sensitivity is as low as 75%.[26]
- ○ Usually, additional imaging is required when pancreatic malignancy is suspected.
- **Computed tomography**
  - ○ Triple-phase CT is an excellent tool for the preoperative staging of pancreatic cancer.
  - ○ CT provides information about the site of the lesion, including its vascular anatomy and its resectability (e.g., presence of hepatic metastases or vascular invasion).[27]
  - ○ CT can detect tumors ≥2 cm in diameter; such tumors appear as low-attenuating areas because they are poorly perfused in comparison with adjacent pancreatic tissue.[27]
  - ○ Small hepatic metastases as well as metastatic cancer in lymph nodes may not be appreciated by CT.
- **Magnetic resonance imaging**
  - ○ In patients who cannot undergo CT, magnetic resonance imaging (MRI) is a reasonable alternative for cross-sectional imaging.
  - ○ MRI does not typically provide additional information over CT.

Diagnostic Procedures
- **Endoscopic retrograde cholangiopancreatography (ERCP)**
  - ○ ERCP has a sensitivity of 95% and a specificity of 85% for the diagnosis of pancreatic cancer.[15,24]
  - ○ ERCP is performed successfully in >90% of patients and occasionally detects tumors not seen on imaging studies.[28]
  - ○ At the time of ERCP, cytology brushings from the bile duct can be obtained, which have a sensitivity between 20% and 60% in confirming the diagnosis of malignancy.[28]
  - ○ During ERCP, a stent can be placed into the obstructed common bile duct to palliate patients who are not surgical candidates.
  - ○ In addition, some surgeons and oncologists prefer stent placement in the bile duct to ensure adequate biliary drainage before initiation of chemotherapy. In these cases, endoscopists can place either a plastic or short metal stent.
  - ○ Through ERCP, hepatotoxic adverse events related to chemotherapy can be assessed, and the future risk of such events is decreased.
  - ○ Despite its utility, ERCP is not required in all patients with suspected pancreatic cancer.
  - ○ If a patient has a history typical for pancreatic cancer (e.g., pain, jaundice, weight loss) and has a mass in the head of the pancreas evident on CT, then the patient could potentially undergo surgical exploration without the need for a preoperative ERCP.
  - ○ An ERCP for drainage of the biliary tree and cytological sampling can be performed if the bilirubin is markedly elevated, nutritional status is poor, and delays in surgical intervention are anticipated.
  - ○ The only **absolute indications for an ERCP** are cholangitis, intractable pruritus, and hyperbilirubinemia that must be treated before the initiation of chemotherapy.[24,28]
- **Endoscopic ultrasonography**
  - ○ A highly sensitive tool for local and regional staging.
  - ○ EUS is complementary to cross-sectional imaging because it does not provide information about distant metastatic disease.[15]

○ EUS provides reliable information about major vascular involvement and lymph node enlargement.

○ FNA of the primary pancreatic lesion or potential lymph node metastasis can be performed during EUS (see later).

• **Fine-needle aspiration**

○ Can be performed percutaneously under CT or ultrasound guidance or can be performed endoscopically by EUS.

○ Tissue sampling should be pursued when cytologic proof of malignancy alters management—for example, as a prerequisite for chemotherapy, radiation therapy, or palliative stenting with a permanent metal stent.[29]

○ FNA is also used to establish the diagnosis when cross-sectional imaging is equivocal regarding the presence of a mass.

○ Seeding of the peritoneal cavity has been described in percutaneous sampling, but it can be avoided by employing an endoscopic approach.[29]

• **Staging laparoscopy**

○ Complements the noninvasive staging and aids the surgeon in assessing the resectability of the tumor.

○ Because of the aggressive nature of pancreatic cancer, metastatic disease at the time of presentation is common.

○ Laparoscopy can assist in identifying small or diffuse metastases (such as hepatic or peritoneal implants) that may be unrecognized in the initial diagnostic evaluation.[24]

○ A number of case series demonstrated that 10% to 40% of tumors thought to be resectable had distant or local spread that would have precluded resection.[24]

○ During laparoscopy, the abdominal cavity is inspected for frank metastases. Also, peritoneal washings are taken for cytology, peritoneal nodules or lymph nodes are sampled, and intraoperative ultrasonography of the pancreas or liver can be performed.

○ Because tumors in the pancreatic body and tail commonly metastasize to the peritoneum and liver, staging laparoscopy may be particularly useful in these patients.

TREATMENT

Surgical Management

• **Tumor resection**

○ Surgery for pancreatic cancer is performed with curative intent only if no evidence of metastatic disease is seen on preoperative imaging studies and staging laparoscopy.

○ The type of surgery performed for pancreatic cancer is dependent on the location of the tumor.

○ **Pancreaticoduodenectomy** (Whipple or pylorus-sparing Whipple resection) is typically performed for tumors involving the pancreatic head.

  ■ The classic Whipple resection involves a partial gastrectomy (antrectomy), cholecystectomy, and removal of the distal common bile duct, head of the pancreas, duodenum, proximal jejunum, and regional lymph nodes. Reconstruction requires pancreaticojejunostomy, hepaticojejunostomy, and gastrojejunostomy.[24]

○ For tumors involving the body or tail of the pancreas, distal pancreatectomy and splenectomy are performed.

○ Rarely, patients are offered a total pancreatectomy for large or multifocal tumors.

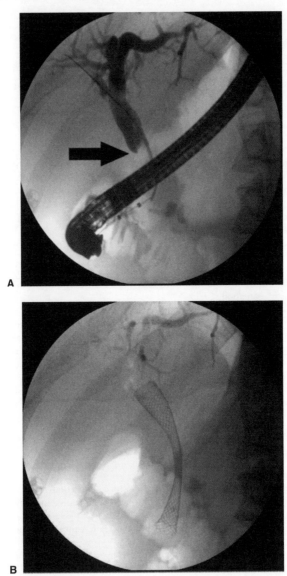

FIGURE 22-3 Endoscopic palliation of pancreatic cancer. A 69-year-old man developed jaundice, and a pancreatic mass was found that had metastasized to the liver. The decision was to administer palliative chemotherapy and place a metal biliary stent. The initial fluoroscopic cholangiogram demonstrates markedly dilated proximal and intrahepatic bile ducts with a "cutoff" (*arrow*) in the distal bile duct resulting from a malignant stricture (**A**). Fluoroscopic image demonstrates successful placement of a metallic self-expanding biliary stent across the malignant stricture (**B**).

- **Surgical palliation**
  - ○ When resection of the primary tumor is not possible, palliative procedures are performed.
  - ○ An anastomosis between the common bile duct and jejunum (choledochojejunostomy) serves to bypass the bile duct obstruction.
  - ○ Fifteen percent to 20% of these patients eventually develop duodenal obstruction, and a gastrojejunostomy is often performed during the initial surgery if a curative resection is not feasible.[15,24]

Procedures

- **Nonsurgical (endoscopic) palliation**
  - ○ Endoscopically placed metal or polyethylene **stents** are commonly used to relieve biliary obstructions.[15,24]
    - ■ Polyethylene stents need to be replaced every 3 to 4 months because of their occlusion from bacterial biofilm and precipitated debris from the bile duct.
    - ■ Metal stents may be covered or uncovered and typically cannot be removed after placement (Fig. 22-3).
    - ■ Metal stents maintain patency longer and improve both quality of life and mortality compared with plastic stents.
    - ■ Metal stents are placed with the expectation that they will remain patent for the life of the patient.
  - ○ Tumor ingrowth can result in stent occlusion, and a new stent can be placed within the old stent to relieve the recurrent biliary obstruction.
  - ○ Gastric outlet obstruction can also be palliated effectively by endoscopic placement of expandable metal stents.

Chemoradiation

- **Adjuvant and neoadjuvant treatment**
  - ○ **5-Fluorouracil,** combined **with radiation therapy,** confers a modest prolongation of survival in patients with locally advanced pancreatic cancer.[15,24]
  - ○ **Gemcitabine** has been shown to increase the quality of life in patients with advanced pancreatic cancer, but survival is only modestly improved.[15,24]
  - ○ Neoadjuvant chemotherapy is administered to some patients in the hope that downstaging of locally advanced tumors will improve resection rates. However, studies have not yet clearly demonstrated prolonged survival.

OUTCOME/PROGNOSIS

- Although surgical resection of the tumor offers the only chance for cure, patients having such "curative" resections have median survival of 18 to 20 months and a 5-year survival rate of 10%.[15]
- The overall 5-year survival rate among patients with pancreatic cancer is <5%.[15]

REFERENCES

1. Dominguez-Munoz JE, ed. *Clinical Pancreatology for Practicing Gastroenterologists and Surgeons.* Malden, MA: Blackwell; 2005.
2. Yamada T. *Textbook and Atlas of Gastroenterology [CD-ROM].* Philadelphia, PA: Lippincott Williams & Wilkins; 1999.
3. Whitcomb DC. Acute pancreatitis. *N Engl J Med.* 2006;354:2142–2150.

4. Banks PA, Freeman ML, Fass R, et al. Practice guidelines in acute pancreatitis. *Am J Gastroenterol.* 2006;101:2379–2400.

5. Forsmark CE, Baillie J; AGA Institute Clinical Practice and Economics Committee, AGA institute Governing Board. AGA Institute technical review on acute pancreatitis. *Gastroenterology.* 2007;132(5):2022–2044.

6. Grendall JH. Acute pancreatitis. *Clin Perspect Gastroenterol.* 2000;3(6):327–333.

7. Mergener K, Baillie J. Acute pancreatitis. *BMJ.* 1998;316:44–48.

8. Parenti DM, Steinberg W, Kang P. Infectious causes of acute pancreatitis. *Pancreas.* 1996;13(4):356–371.

9. Corfield AP, Williamson RCN, McMahon MJ, et al. Prediction of severity in acute pancreatitis: prospective comparison of three prognostic indices. *Lancet.* 1985;24:403–407.

10. McClave SA, Chang WK, Dhaliwal R, et al. Nutrition support in acute pancreatitis: a systematic review of the literature. *JPEN J Parenter Enteral Nutr.* 2006;30(2):143–156.

11. Yeo CJ, Bastidas JA, Lynch-Nyhan A, et al. The natural history of pancreatic pseudocysts documented by computed tomography. *Surg Gynecol Obstet.* 1990;170:411.

12. Etemad B, Whitcomb DC. Chronic pancreatitis: diagnosis, classification, and new genetic developments. *Gastroenterology.* 2001;120:682–707.

13. Steer ML, Waxman I, Freedman S. Chronic pancreatitis. *N Engl J Med.* 1995;332:1482–1490.

14. Stevens T, Conwell DL, Zuccaro G. Pathogenesis of chronic pancreatitis: an evidence-based review of past theories and recent developments. *Am J Gastroenterol.* 2004;99:2256–2270.

15. Ammann RW, Muellhaupt B. The natural history of pain in alcoholic pancreatitis. *Gastroenterology.* 1999;116(5):1132–1140.

16. Bolondi L, Li Bassi S, Gaiani S, et al. Sonography of chronic pancreatitis. *Radiol Clin North Am.* 1989;27(4):815–833.

17. Luetmer PH, Stephens DH, Ward EM. Chronic pancreatitis: reassessment with current CT. *Radiology.* 1989;171(2):353–357.

18. Axon AT, Classen M, Cotton PB, et al. Pancreatography in chronic pancreatitis: international definitions. *Gut.* 1984;25(10):1107–1112.

19. Gullo L, Ventrucci M, Tomassetti P, et al. Fecal elastase 1 determination in chronic pancreatitis. *Dig Dis Sci.* 1999;44(1):210–213.

20. Warshaw AL, Banks PA, Fernandez-del Castillo C. AGA technical review: treatment of pain in chronic pancreatitis. *Gastroenterology.* 1998;115:765–776.

21. Hidalgo M. Pancreatic cancer. *N Engl J Med.* 2010;362:1605–1617.

22. Nunes QM, Lobo DL. Pancreatic cancer. *Surgery (Oxford).* 2007;25(3):87–94.

23. Shaib YH, Davila JA, El-Serag HB. The epidemiology of pancreatic cancer in the United States: changes below the surface. *Aliment Pharmacol Ther.* 2006;24(1):87–94.

24. Lowenfels AB, Maisonneuve P, Cavallini G, et al. Pancreatitis and the risk of pancreatic cancer. *N Engl J Med.* 1993;328:1433–1437.

25. Michaud DS, Giovannucci E, Willett WC, et al. Physical activity, obesity, height, and the risk of pancreatic cancer. *JAMA.* 2001;286(8):921–929.

26. Maringhini A, Ciambra M, Raimondo M, et al. Clinical presentation and ultrasonography in the diagnosis of pancreatic cancer. *Pancreas.* 1993;8(2):146–150.

27. O'Malley ME, Boland GW, Wood BJ, et al. Adenocarcinoma of the head of the pancreas: determination of surgical unresectability with thin-section pancreatic-phase helical CT. *AJR Am J Roentgenol.* 1999;173(6):1513–1518.

28. Schofl R. Diagnostic endoscopic retrograde cholangiopancreatography. *Endoscopy.* 2001;33:147–157.

29. Dewitt J, Misra VL, Leblanc JK, et al. EUS-guided FNA of proximal biliary strictures after negative ERCP brush cytology results. *Gastrointest Endosc.* 2006;64(3):325–333.

Biliary Tract Disorders

23

Riad Azar and Andrew Reinink

Diseases of the biliary tract are frequently encountered in both primary care and specialty settings. They represent a broad spectrum of diseases, ranging from benign gallstone disease to life-threatening cholangitis and cancers. Because these disorders are widely prevalent, all physicians need to become familiar with the diagnosis and management of biliary tract disorders.

CHOLELITHIASIS AND GALLSTONE DISORDERS

GENERAL PRINCIPLES

Definition
- Cholelithiasis. The presence of concretions (gallstones) in the gallbladder or bile ducts.
- Choledocholithiasis. The presence of stones in the bile ducts, including common bile duct, common hepatic duct, right and left hepatic ducts, and intrahepatic ducts.

Classification
- Cholesterol stones
  - This is the most common type of gallstone (75% to 90%).
  - Typically formed when supersaturation of cholesterol occurs in bile.
- Brown stones
  - These form when bacteria within the biliary tree cause bilirubin to deconjugate and combine with calcium, forming the insoluble calcium bilirubinate.
- Black stones
  - These develop in conditions associated with chronic hemolysis, especially sickle cell disease and hereditary spherocytosis.
  - Black stones may also be seen in cirrhotic patients.

Epidemiology
- Overall, gallstone disease is an extremely common disorder, particularly in women and the obese.
- Prevalence ranges from 10% to 15% in 40-year-old white women to as high as 70% in female Pima Indians.[1] Although cholelithiasis is common, 80% of patients with gallstones never develop symptoms. The risk of developing biliary pain is 1% to 2% per year.

Risk Factors
- Female sex
- Multiparity

- Pregnancy
- Obesity
- Crohn's disease
- Total parenteral nutrition
- Native American race

DIAGNOSIS

Clinical Presentation

- Clinical presentation occurs when gallstones occlude the cystic duct, pass into the common bile duct, or erode through the wall of the gallbladder. Presentations of gallstone disease depend on the location of the stone in the biliary tree and include biliary pain, acute cholecystitis, choledocholithiasis, acute cholangitis, gallstone pancreatitis, and gallstone ileus (see later).
- Stones may pass from the gallbladder into the common bile duct or develop de novo in the bile ducts.

History

- Most common presentation is biliary pain.
  - Classically described as "**biliary colic,**" this consists of epigastric or right upper quadrant pain that may radiate to the right scapula or shoulder. It can be precipitated by fatty meals, which induce gallbladder contraction.
  - "Biliary colic" is a misnomer, as the pain is constant rather than colicky.
- The pain gradually increases over 30 minutes and then plateaus for 1 hour or longer before subsiding.
- Associated dyspeptic symptoms, including bloating, nausea, or vomiting, may occur.
- The interval between attacks is variable, and weeks or months may pass between episodes.
- The pain is caused by transient occlusion of the neck of the cystic duct by a gallstone.

Diagnostic Testing

Laboratories

- No laboratory abnormalities are usually noted unless a complication is present.
- Elevated levels of transaminases, alkaline phosphatase, and bilirubin can be seen with choledocholithiasis and elevations in amylase and lipase levels with pancreatitis.

Imaging

- **Ultrasonography** remains the best investigative study, with 95% sensitivity and specificity for gallbladder stones.[2]
  - The yield is highest after fasting, and stones are identified by the presence of mobile echogenic objects that produce acoustic shadowing.
  - Gallbladder sludge may also be seen as echogenic material that layers but does not produce acoustic shadowing.
- Cholelithiasis may also be identified with computed tomographic (CT) scanning, although the sensitivity is lower than that of ultrasonography.
  - CT has the additional drawbacks of radiation exposure and expense.
- Ultrasonography is the best initial study for choledocholithiasis as well. Ultrasonography is very sensitive for dilated bile ducts but less sensitive (30% to 50%) for common bile duct stones.

○ **Absence of ductal dilation does not exclude choledocholithiasis.**
○ CT scanning may also be useful but has lower sensitivity for common bile duct stones.

TREATMENT

- Gallstones are often found incidentally during evaluation for other conditions. Because 80% of patients remain asymptomatic, the consensus is that prophylactic cholecystectomy is not indicated.
  ○ Important exceptions are patients with a calcified or "porcelain" gallbladder and Native Americans with gallstones. These patients are at very high risk for gallbladder cancer, so cholecystectomy should be performed even in the absence of symptoms. Patients with chronic medical conditions that can be adversely affected by an episode of cholecystitis or pancreatitis (e.g., brittle type 1 diabetes mellitus) may benefit from elective cholecystectomy.
- For choledocholithiasis, management options include nonsurgical treatments (e.g., endoscopic papillotomy with balloon extraction, mechanical lithotripsy), and surgical approaches including cholecystectomy with laparoscopic stone removal.[3]
- Endoscopic retrograde cholangiopancreatography (ERCP) allows the diagnosis and extraction of bile duct stones.[4] In patients with high clinical suspicion for choledocholithiasis, especially in the presence of ductal dilatation on imaging and liver function test abnormalities, an ERCP should be performed even if both ultrasonography and a CT do not demonstrate choledocholithiasis.
- In patients in whom clinical suspicion is lower, a magnetic resonance cholangiopancreatography (MRCP) can be used to evaluate for choledocholithiasis. However, if an MRCP cannot be obtained, endoscopic ultrasound (EUS) has been shown to have similar sensitivity and specificity in diagnosing choledocholithiasis.[5]
- In some endoscopic suites, EUS does offer a distinct advantage in that if it is positive, a therapeutic ERCP can be performed at the same session while the patient is still under sedation.[6]
- Although improved experience with ERCP has led to improved outcomes, risks of major complications, including pancreatitis, bleeding, perforation, and sepsis, remain.
- When choledocholithiasis is encountered during laparoscopic cholecystectomy, surgeons can remove the stones through laparoscopic or open common bile duct exploration. An alternative approach is ERCP with stone extraction following cholecystectomy.

Medications
- In patients who are poor surgical candidates, oral dissolution therapy with **ursodiol** or **chenodiol** can be attempted. However, this is a slow process and rarely results in complete resolution of stones, especially stones that are larger than 5 mm.

Surgical Management
- Clinical judgment is required to determine whether gallstones are causing pain or dyspeptic symptoms.
- **Laparoscopic cholecystectomy** is the treatment of choice. The laparoscopic approach is associated with a significantly shorter hospital stay and quicker convalescence than with open cholecystectomy.

○ Complications include bile duct injuries and bile leakage from the cystic duct remnant.

- Bile peritonitis occurs when bile leaks into the peritoneal cavity leading to acute peritoneal inflammation and severe abdominal pain (bile peritonitis).

- Most bile leaks after cholecystectomy occur at the cystic duct stump or duct of Luschka. Occasionally, large collections of bile (bilomas) can form around the biliary tree, resulting in pain and leading to bacterial infections.

- Patients usually present shortly after surgery with abdominal pain. Abdominal CT scan usually reveals fluid or a biloma centered on the biliary tree. A hepatoiminodiacetic acid (HIDA) scan confirms the diagnosis by revealing spillage of radioactive tracer into the abdominal cavity.

- Large bilomas usually require percutaneous drainage, especially if they are infected.

- ERCP is often used to place biliary stents to encourage preferential flow of bile into the duodenum, which allows the leak site to heal. If bile duct stones are seen, a biliary sphincterotomy with stone extraction is usually performed before stent placement. Most leaks close within 6 weeks.

- Gallstones can also be removed through a **cholecystostomy,** but this requires multiple procedures, and the potential for gallstone recurrence remains.[7]

COMPLICATIONS

- Acute cholecystitis
- Choledocholithiasis
- Cholangitis
- Mirizzi syndrome: a stone impacted in the cystic duct or neck of the gallbladder that causes external compression of the common bile duct
- Gallstone pancreatitis
  ○ Gallstone pancreatitis is discussed in detail in Chapter 22.
- **Gallstone ileus**
  ○ This consists of mechanical intestinal obstruction resulting from the passage of a large gallstone into the bowel lumen.[8]
  ○ The process starts with a gallstone eroding through the gallbladder wall into the small intestine. The stone can then cause obstruction, usually at the terminal ileum. Patients present with acute partial small bowel obstruction.
  ○ Gallstone ileus is responsible for 1% to 4% of all cases of intestinal obstruction and develops in 0.3% to 3% of all cholelithiasis patients. It is seen more commonly in the elderly (eighth decade) and in women, leading to high mortality (7.1% to 18%) from frequent comorbidities.
  ○ The diagnosis is suggested by the findings of air in the biliary tree with dilated loops of bowel and air fluid levels on an x-ray study, with or without an ectopic gallstone.
  ○ Abdominal ultrasonography is useful in detecting biliary stones, and barium upper gastrointestinal series x-ray study may be needed to detect a duodenal-biliary fistula.
  ○ Treatment is surgical enterotomy with removal of the stones (enterolithotomy). In addition, cholecystectomy with surgical closure of the duodenal fistula may be performed. However, this procedure is associated with high

morbidity and mortality and should be pursued only in patients in excellent general health.
- ○ Rare large stones cause most cases of gallstone ileus and therefore recurrent obstruction is uncommon.

ACUTE CHOLECYSTITIS

General Principles

Definition
- Acute **calculous cholecystitis** consists of inflammation or hemorrhagic necrosis, with variable infection, ulceration, and neutrophilic infiltration of the gallbladder wall, usually resulting from impaction of a stone in the cystic duct.
- In contrast, **acalculous cholecystitis** is an acute inflammatory disease of the gallbladder not associated with gallstones but associated with bile stasis in the gallbladder due to impaired gallbladder motility from ischemia, usually in the setting of significant comorbid illnesses.

Epidemiology
- Acute cholecystitis develops in 20% of symptomatic biliary colic patients per year.[9]

Etiology
- Cystic duct occlusion results in bile stasis, gallbladder wall edema, gallbladder distention, inflammatory exudate, and bacterial infection.

Diagnosis

Clinical Presentation
- Patients typically present with steady upper abdominal pain that lasts hours, with associated nausea, vomiting, and fever.
- The presentation may be more subtle in the elderly.
- If bacteremic, patients may present with high fever, rigors, and severe abdominal tenderness.
- Examination often reveals right upper quadrant tenderness or a positive Murphy's sign, consisting of pain with palpation of the right upper quadrant during inspiration with subsequent inhibition of inspiration. **Murphy's sign** can also be elicited during ultrasonography, when pressure is applied directly on the gallbladder with the ultrasound probe.

Diagnostic Testing
Laboratories
- Most patients have a modest leukocytosis and normal or only slightly increased transaminases and bilirubin.
- Significantly elevated transaminases or bilirubin should raise suspicion of common bile duct stone.

Imaging
- Patients with suspected acute cholecystitis should undergo **ultrasonography.** Important findings include gallstones, sonographic Murphy's sign, gallbladder wall thickening, and pericholecystic fluid.
- If the diagnosis remains in doubt, cholescintigraphy (HIDA, *para*-isopropyl iminodiacetic acid, or diisopropyl iminodiacetic acid scan) should be performed.

Radiolabeled iminodiacetic acid derivatives are administered, which are rapidly extracted by the liver and then excreted into bile. A normal study shows radioactivity in the gallbladder, common bile duct, and small intestine within 60 minutes. In acute cholecystitis, there is delayed filling of the gallbladder because of cystic duct obstruction.

Treatment

- Patients with acute cholecystitis are made **NPO** and are given **intravenous fluids** and **broad-spectrum antibiotics** to treat secondary infection.
- **Nasogastric suction** is performed if the abdomen is distended or if the patient is vomiting.
- Prompt **surgical consultation** should be obtained. **Definitive management is laparoscopic or open cholecystectomy.**
- Most clinicians recommend waiting 24 to 48 hours until the patient has clinically stabilized, but surgery should be performed more urgently if the condition deteriorates.
- If possible, cholecystectomy should be performed during the initial hospitalization, as delaying the procedure to a subsequent return visit has been shown to increase costs with no clinical benefit.[10,11]
- Patients who are poor surgical candidates should have percutaneous cholecystostomy or transpapillary endoscopic drainage of the gallbladder.

Complications

- Complications of acute cholecystitis include gallbladder perforation, emphysematous cholecystitis caused by gas-forming bacteria, and gallstone ileus.

ACUTE CHOLANGITIS

GENERAL PRINCIPLES

Definition

- Acute cholangitis consists of inflammation of the bile duct, typically from bacterial infection complicating an obstructed duct.[12]

Etiology

- **Choledocholithiasis** causes most cases of cholangitis, although patients with biliary neoplasms or inflammatory biliary strictures from primary sclerosing cholangitis (PSC) can develop cholangitis, especially if they have undergone prior biliary interventions (e.g., ERCP).
- Gallstones can cause cholangitis even after a cholecystectomy, as stones are retained in the common bile duct with some frequency, and can be present for years after cholecystectomy before causing any problems. These retained stones can be identified during a cholecystectomy through intraoperative cholangiography.
- Most common pathogens are enterobacteria (68%), enterococci (14%), bacteroides (10%), and clostridium species (7%).

Risk Factors

- Choledocholithiasis
- Instrumentation of the biliary tract

DIAGNOSIS

Clinical Presentation

- Approximately 70% of patients present with all three components of Charcot's triad: pain, jaundice, and fever.
- If suppurative cholangitis develops, patients will additionally present with mental status changes and hypotension (Reynold's pentad).
- Leukocytosis and markedly increased bilirubin and alkaline phosphatase are usually present.
- Blood cultures are frequently positive if gram-negative bacteria are the cause of the infection, especially in cases of suppurative cholangitis.
- The most common organisms isolated are gram-negative rods such as *Escherichia coli,* enterococci, and anaerobes, particularly in the elderly.

Diagnostic Testing

- The diagnosis must be made quickly, as patients are at risk of developing severe sepsis.

Imaging

- **Ultrasonography or abdominal CT** should be performed, looking for ductal dilatation or common bile duct stones.
- A negative study finding, however, does not rule out cholangitis, because the common duct may not be dilated early in the course of disease and common duct stones may be missed.

Diagnostic Procedures

- **ERCP must be performed emergently** in suspected cases of cholangitis, especially if the patient is clinically deteriorating.[13] Therefore, the ERCP team should be notified immediately in any case of suspected acute cholangitis.
- ERCP identifies common duct stones or strictures and allows therapeutic interventions, such as sphincterotomy, biliary drainage, stone extraction, and biliary stent placement.
- If ERCP is unsuccessful or cannot be performed, percutaneous transhepatic cholangiography (PTC) or surgical decompression should be pursued.
- Both of these procedures, however, have higher mortality and morbidity rates than ERCP.

TREATMENT

- ERCP provides for drainage of the biliary tree and may resolve obstruction from choledocholithiasis. Furthermore, stents can be placed to keep bile flowing, especially when unsurmountable obstructions (e.g., neoplasms) are encountered.

Medications

- **Broad-spectrum antibiotics** and **aggressive fluid resuscitation** should be immediately started if cholangitis is suspected.
  - Typically, ureidopenicillins, carbapenems, or the combination of third/fourth-generation cephalosporins + metronidazole are the empiric antibiotics of choice.
  - If penicillin-allergic metronidazole with either aztreonam or ciprofloxacin can be used.

- Antibiotics are usually given for a total of 7 to 10 days, but they can be stopped earlier if good biliary drainage is established.
- For patients who have not undergone cholecystectomy, resolution of cholangitis should lead to prompt laparoscopic cholecystectomy.

GALLBLADDER CARCINOMA

GENERAL PRINCIPLES

Definition
- This consists of neoplasia involving the gallbladder, typically adenocarcinoma.

Epidemiology
- Gallbladder cancer represents the most common biliary tract malignancy.[14]
- This is predominantly seen in elderly women. It is the most common gastrointestinal malignancy in Native Americans.
- Up to 80% have a history of gallstones, and there is a higher incidence of gallstones with longer duration of p53 or K-ras mutations.
- Approximately 90% of patients are diagnosed after the neoplasm has spread beyond the gallbladder.
- Patients who have a calcified or "porcelain" gallbladder are at very high risk of gallbladder cancer and should undergo cholecystectomy even if asymptomatic.

DIAGNOSIS

Clinical Presentation
- Patients typically present with **prolonged abdominal pain,** which may be difficult to differentiate from biliary pain, or acute cholecystitis.
- Other common symptoms include nausea, vomiting, weight loss, and jaundice.

Differential Diagnosis
- Biliary pain
- Acute cholecystitis

Diagnostic Testing
Laboratories
- Carcinoembryonic antigen and carbohydrate antigen 19-9 (CA19-9) are both often elevated.
- Increases in serum bilirubin and alkaline phosphatase generally indicate the presence of advanced disease.

Imaging
- **Ultrasonography** often detects masses within the gallbladder lumen or irregular gallbladder wall thickening. A normal ultrasonography does not rule out gallbladder cancer, however.
- CT scanning demonstrates masses and gallbladder thickening and provides additional evidence for extent of disease.

Diagnostic Procedures
- Fine-needle aspiration during EUS has also been used to evaluate peripancreatic and periportal lymphadenopathy.[15]

- ERCP or percutaneous transhepatic cholangiography is indicated in patients with evidence of biliary obstruction.
- Histologic diagnosis for tumors that appear unresectable can be accomplished with percutaneous biopsy or ERCP.
- If resection is planned, preoperative tissue diagnosis is unnecessary.

TREATMENT

- Most patients present with advanced unresectable disease.
- The overall 5-year survival rate is <5%, but patients with advanced cancer have a median survival of only 45 to 127 days.

Surgical Management

- Patients whose cancers are staged between I and III have potentially resectable tumors.
- Depending on the extent of spread, surgery may be as simple as cholecystectomy or require extensive hepatic, pancreatic, and duodenal resection.

Palliative Management

- Patients with unresectable disease may be given **chemotherapy** with agents such as 5-fluorouracil, adriamycin, gemcitabine, and nitroureases, but results are not encouraging.
- Most patients with unresectable disease will need palliative treatments, such as **endoscopic stent placement** or **percutaneous biliary drainage.**

PRIMARY SCLEROSING CHOLANGITIS

GENERAL PRINCIPLES

Definition

- PSC consists of inflammation of the intrahepatic and extrahepatic bile ducts, from an autoimmune or idiopathic mechanism.[16] The disease is discussed here from a biliary obstruction point of view, see Chapter 19 for further details.
- Insidious in onset, PSC typically begins with fatigue, jaundice, and cholestasis and progresses irreversibly to end-stage liver disease (ESLD).[17]

Epidemiology

- Seventy-five percent of patients are male.
- The average age at diagnosis is 40 years, although the disease can often be diagnosed in childhood.

Etiology

- The etiology of PSC is unknown.
- Animal and *in vitro* models have identified infections, autoimmunity, cytokines, and bile acid transporter or ion channel abnormalities as underlying causes for PSC.

Pathophysiology

- Both intrahepatic and extrahepatic bile ducts are involved with strictures.
- The disease process is usually diffuse, with obliterative fibrosis distributed throughout the biliary system.

- Tight strictures predispose the patient to intermittent obstruction of biliary flow with subsequent bacterial cholangitis. Obstruction of biliary flow causes reflux of bile into the hepatocytes.

Risk Factors

- Up to 70% of PSC occurs in the setting of **inflammatory bowel disease** (IBD), with **ulcerative colitis** accounting for 90% of those cases.
- No relationship exists between the duration and severity of IBD and the development of PSC.
- Although colectomy is curative for colonic disease in ulcerative colitis, it does not eliminate the risk of PSC.

Associated Conditions

- **Metabolic bone disease,** most commonly osteoporosis, occurs frequently in PSC for unclear reasons.
- Patients with PSC have a 10% to 30% chance of developing **cholangiocarcinoma,** which is often very difficult to diagnose in the setting of PSC.
- Despite knowing that patients with PSC are at high risk for cholangiocarcinoma, no effective way has been found to screen for cholangiocarcinoma.
- Patients with PSC with concomitant IBD also have an increased risk of **colon cancer,** but preliminary reports suggest that this risk may be decreased with the use of ursodeoxycholic acid.

DIAGNOSIS

Clinical Presentation

- The onset of disease is often insidious, with the gradual onset of fatigue, pruritus, and jaundice.
- **Pruritus** can be particularly severe in PSC and can be difficult to manage.
- The exact mechanism remains unknown but may involve the accumulation of pruritogenic substances secondary to decreased bile excretion or increased opioidergic tone.
- If advanced liver disease has already developed, some patients present with variceal bleeding, encephalopathy, or ascites.
- Steatorrhea and malabsorption of fat-soluble vitamins may develop late in disease because of decreased secretion of bile acids.

Diagnostic Testing
Laboratories

- Approximately 25% of patients are diagnosed from abnormal laboratory tests before symptoms have developed.
- Most have significantly elevated alkaline phosphatase, γ-glutamyltransferase, and bilirubin.
- The transaminases are elevated to a lesser degree.
- In addition, many patients will have positive antinuclear antibodies and antineutrophil cytoplasmic antibodies (p-ANCA) levels, suggesting that PSC is immune mediated.
- Patients with IBD who present with **elevated alkaline phosphatase** levels should have an aggressive evaluation to look for PSC.

Imaging
- Definitive diagnosis is made by imaging of the biliary tree with either **ERCP or PTC**. MRCP is increasingly being used as a noninvasive option.
- The classic finding is multifocal stricturing of the intrahepatic and extrahepatic bile ducts with intervening normal or dilated segments. This is often described as a **"string of beads" appearance.**
- Secondary causes of strictures, including trauma, ischemia, tumors, and certain infections (cytomegalovirus, *Cryptosporidium*), need to be excluded.
- A minority of patients who do not have the classic cholangiographic findings demonstrate small duct cholangitis on liver biopsy.

TREATMENT

- Various medical therapies, such as immunosuppressants, corticosteroids, and antibiotics, have not been proved successful in slowing progression of disease, although **ursodeoxycholic acid** improves biochemical abnormalities.
- Management is therefore primarily supportive until ESLD develops, at which point liver transplantation is offered.
- **Indications for transplantation** include refractory ascites, recurrent bacterial cholangitis, encephalopathy, and variceal bleeding.
- The survival rate 10 years after transplantation is ~79%, although patients with PSC have a higher retransplantation rate than all other patients with ESLD caused by recurrent disease.

Medications
- **Pruritus:** Symptoms often respond to bile acid-binding resins, such as **cholestyramine** at a dose of 4 g PO BID to QID.[18]
- Other medical options include colestipol, ursodiol, rifampicin, odansetron, and immunosuppressants.
- Antihistamines seem to have no effect on pruritus beyond possible sedation effects.[19]
- Nonpharmacologic therapies that have shown promise include photodynamic therapy and, in extreme cases, liver transplantation.
- Other supportive therapies, such as emollients, lotions, or cold compressives, have not proved efficacious in PSC.

COMPLICATIONS

- **Dominant stricture.** Approximately 20% of patients develop a dominant stricture.
  - Cholangiography demonstrates the dominant stricture, and balloon dilatation with stent placement can be performed.
  - It is often very difficult to differentiate a dominant stricture from cholangiocarcinoma.
  - Tumor markers, such as CA19-9, carcinoembryonic antigen, and cytologic brushings, may be of some value in identifying patients with cholangiocarcinoma.
  - A recently developed technology called "spyglass" allows direct visualization of the bile duct during ERCP through fiber optics.
  - Direct biopsy of the strictures can also be obtained, potentially improving the detection of early cholangiocarcinomas.

- **Cholangiocarcinoma**[20]
- **Bacterial cholangitis.** Bacterial cholangitis is more frequent in patients who have had manipulation of the biliary tract or have developed a dominant stricture.
  - Cholelithiasis or choledocholithiasis can also contribute to the development of bacterial cholangitis.
  - Patients typically present with fever and worsening jaundice, and they often have recurrent episodes.
  - After empiric antibiotics are started, treatment is directed at relieving the obstruction, usually endoscopically.
  - ERCP allows dilation of large strictures, biliary decompression, and removal of stones.
  - Prospective studies have not shown any benefit in placing endoprostheses across strictures.
  - Furthermore, stent occlusion and cholangitis frequently occur with stent placement.
  - Long-term prophylactic antibiotics have not been shown to have any benefit in preventing cholangitis.

OUTCOME/PROGNOSIS

- PSC follows a slowly progressive course, with a median survival of ~10 years from diagnosis.

CHOLANGIOCARCINOMA

GENERAL PRINCIPLES

Definition
- This consists of neoplasia developing within the bile ducts.

Epidemiology
- A relatively rare tumor—reported incidence of 8 per million in the United States.[21]
- Seen primarily in middle-aged men.

Etiology
- Unknown

Pathophysiology
- Chronic biliary inflammation is thought to contribute to cancer formation.

Associated Conditions
- The strongest association is with PSC.
- Also seen with chronic liver disease, ulcerative colitis, parasitic biliary disease, choledochal cysts, hepatitis C, and smoking.

DIAGNOSIS

Clinical Presentation
- Patients typically present with anorexia, weight loss, acholic stool, abdominal pain, pruritus, and jaundice when the tumor causes significant obstruction.

- A **Klatskin tumor** is a bile duct cancer with involvement of the hilum of the right and left hepatic ducts.
- Some bile duct tumors spread diffusely throughout the liver, making it difficult to distinguish from PSC.
- Most tumors are locally invasive and do not metastasize.
- Prognosis is grim, with rare patient survival of >1 year.

Diagnostic Testing

Laboratories

- Most patients have **elevated alkaline phosphatase and bilirubin** levels.
- **Elevations in CA19-9** levels are the most sensitive and specific tumor marker in cholangiocarcinoma, but this marker is also elevated many times in concomitant bacterial cholangitis.

Imaging

- **Ultrasonography and abdominal CT** scan are useful in identifying intrahepatic or extrahepatic ductal dilation, but the primary tumors are often difficult to visualize.
- Magnetic resonance imaging (MRI) or MRCP may be more sensitive in identifying the primary tumor.

Diagnostic Procedures

- **ERCP or PTC** provides direct imaging of the biliary system and can define the extent of tumor spread.
- During ERCP, tissue diagnosis can be made using bile cytology, cytologic brushings, or cholangioscopic biopsies.
- Biopsies obtained through percutaneous or transluminal means are not recommended because of the danger of tumor seeding.
- Regional lymph node sampling can also be done during EUS in early-stage disease to evaluate for surgical resectability or liver transplantation.
- EUS can also be used to obtain a fine-needle aspirate for cytology in patients with unsuccessful ERCP or those who have had negative brush cytology results.
- The histologic diagnosis of cholangiocarcinoma may be challenging, because many tumors are well differentiated and occur in the setting of PSC.

TREATMENT

- Surgical resection represents the only option for long-term survival.
- Chemotherapy and radiation therapy are uniformly ineffective in prolonging survival.

Surgical Management

- Distal extrahepatic and intrahepatic tumors are more likely to be resectable than proximal extrahepatic tumors.
- A high recurrence rate is seen for patients after resection, and adjuvant chemoradiation has not been shown to improve survival.
- Liver transplantation combined with neoadjuvant chemoradiation has led to increased survival rates in patients with locally unresectable cancer with otherwise normal hepatic and biliary function and patients with a history of PSC.

Palliative Management

- Patients who have unresectable tumors are usually offered **ERCP with stent placement** versus **percutaneous biliary drainage**.

- This has replaced palliative biliary-enteric anastomosis in most centers.
- Recent preliminary reports of other palliative treatments (e.g., photodynamic therapy) have been encouraging, but more studies are needed.

OUTCOME/PROGNOSIS

- Median survival for resectable tumors is 3 years but only 1 year if unresectable.
- Death usually results from recurrent biliary sepsis or liver abscess formation.

REFERENCES

1. Diehl AK. Epidemiology and natural history of gallstone disease. *Gastroenterol Clin North Am.* 1991;20:1–19.
2. Bortoff GA, Chen MY, Ott DJ, et al. Gallbladder stones: imaging and intervention. *Radiographics.* 2000;20(3):751–766.
3. Hungness ES, Soper NJ. Management of common bile duct stones. *J Gastrointest Surg.* 2006; 10(4):612–619.
4. Fogel EL, McHenry L, Sherman S, et al. Therapeutic biliary endoscopy. *Endoscopy.* 2005; 37(2):139–145.
5. Verma D, Kapadia A, Eisen GM, et al. EUS vs. MRCP for detection of choledocholithiasis. *Gastrointest Endosc.* 2006;64(2):248–254.
6. Petrov MS, Savides TJ. Systematic review of endoscopic ultrasonography versus endoscopic retrograde cholangiopancreatography for suspected choledocholithiasis. *Br J Surg.* 2009; 96(9):967–974.
7. Rogers S, Cello J, Horn J, et al. Prospective randomized trial of LC+LCBDE vs ERCP/S+LC for common bile duct stone disease. *Arch Surg.* 2010;145(1):28–33.
8. Webb L, Ott M, Gunter O. Once bitten, twice incised: recurrent gallstone ileus. *Am J Surg.* 2010;200:e72–e74.
9. Strasberg SM. Acute calculous cholecystitis. *N Engl J Med.* 2008;358:2804–2811.
10. Gurusamy K, Samraj K, Gluud C, et al. Meta-analysis of randomized controlled trials on the safety and effectiveness of early versus delayed laparoscopic cholecystectomy for acute cholecystitis. *Br J Surg.* 2010;97:2.
11. Wilson E, Gurusamy K, Gluud C, et al. A cost utility and value of information analysis of early *versus* delayed laparoscopic cholecystectomy for acute cholecystitis. *Br J Surg.* 2010; 97:210–219.
12. Qureshi WA. Approach to the patient who has suspected acute bacterial cholangitis. *Gastroenterol Clin North Am.* 2006;35(2):409–423.
13. Lai ECS, Mok FPT, Tan ESY. Endoscopic biliary drainage for severe acute cholangitis. *N Engl J Med.* 1992;326:1582–1586.
14. Jones RS. Carcinoma of the gallbladder. *Surg Clin North Am.* 1990;70:1419–1428.
15. Chang KJ. State of the art lecture: endoscopic ultrasound (EUS) and FNA in pancreatico-biliary tumors. *Endoscopy.* 2006;38(suppl 1):S56–S60.
16. LaRusso N, Shneider B, Black D, et al. Primary sclerosing cholangitis: summary of a workshop. *Hepatology.* 2006;44(3):746–764.
17. Lee YM, Kaplan MM. Primary sclerosing cholangitis. *N Engl J Med.* 1995;332:924–937.
18. Mela M, Mancuso A, Burroughs AK. Review article: pruritus in cholestatic and other diseases. *Aliment Pharmacol Ther.* 2003;17(7):857–870.
19. Holtmeier J, Leuschner U. Medical treatment of primary biliary cirrhosis and primary sclerosing cholangitis. *Digestion.* 2001;64(3):137–150.
20. Rosen CB, Nagorney DM, Wiesner RH. Cholangiocarcinoma complicating primary sclerosing cholangitis. *Ann Surg.* 1991;213:21–25.
21. Malhi H, Gores GJ. Cholangiocarcinoma: modern advances in understanding a deadly old disease. *J Hepatol.* 2006;45(6):856–867.

Genetic Testing in Gastrointestinal Diseases

Elizabeth Blaney and Chien-Huan Chen

- Many gastrointestinal diseases have known causative mutations and testing is available for clinical use (Table 24-1).
- Identification of familial cancer syndromes provides the opportunity for early detection and prevention. A familial form of cancer is suspected in the following setting:[1]
  - Early age of diagnosis
  - Synchronous or metachronous tumors
  - Multiple primary tumor types
  - Family history of the same cancer type in one or more first-degree relatives
  - High rate of cancer occurrence in a family
  - Associated congenital anomalies or known phenotypic syndromes
- Genetic counseling should be offered to all patients before testing due to potential psychological impact and possibility of insurance or employment discrimination in the event of a positive test result.
- In addition to determining risk for heritable diseases, genetic testing is also used to determine polymorphisms that can guide pharmacotherapy.

HEREDITARY DIFFUSE GASTRIC CANCER

GENERAL PRINCIPLES

Genetics

- Hereditary diffuse gastric cancer (HDGC) is an **autosomal dominant** inherited form of diffuse type gastric cancer.
- HDGC is associated with germ line truncating **mutations in the gene E-cadherin (CDH1)**, resulting in defective intercellular adhesion.
- Lifetime cumulative risk for advanced gastric cancer is 40% to 70% in men and 60% to 80% in women, with 38 years as the average age of onset.[2]
- Women with HDGC are also at high risk for lobular breast cancer (60% by age 80), so enhanced breast cancer screening is recommended.
- CDH1 gene mutation is suspected in the following settings:
  - Diffuse gastric cancer at age <50
  - Any gastric cancer at age <40
  - Multiple cases in on family
  - Suggestive pathology on biopsy—in situ signet ring cells or pagetoid spread of signet ring cells adjacent to diffuse type gastric cancer

DIAGNOSIS

Genetic Testing

- Genetic testing is commercially available and consists of direct gene sequencing of peripheral blood to identify a specific mutation in an affected individual.

TABLE 24-1 SUMMARY OF GENETICS AND GASTROINTESTINAL DISEASES

Disease	Inheritance	Gene	Test	Indication for Testing	Follow-up of Test Result
HDGC	Autosomal dominant	CDH1	Gene sequence analysis on blood sample	Diffuse gastric cancer at age <50, family history, characteristic pathology on tumor specimen	If mutation identified, at-risk family members screened with mutation-specific assay
PJS	Autosomal dominant	LKB1, STK11	Gene sequence analysis on blood sample	PJS phenotype	If mutation identified, at-risk family members screened
Celiac disease	HLA associated	HLA DQ2, DQ8	HLA typing	Exclude celiac disease in patients already on gluten free diet	Rules out celiac disease in absence of DQ2 or DQ8
Lynch syndrome or HNPCC	Autosomal dominant	MMR genes— MLH1, MSH2, MSH6, PMS2	IHC of tumor or polypectomy specimen to determine loss of expression of MMR genes MSI testing of tumor or polypectomy specimen	Patients with suspected Lynch syndrome undergoing resection of tumors or polyps	Once IHC determines which gene is likely mutated or MSI-H is found in the tumor, gene sequencing and mutational analysis is performed; at-risk family members may then be screened
FAP	Autosomal dominant	APC	Gene sequence analysis on blood sample	Patient with polyposis phenotype	If mutation is identified, at-risk family members screened

Disease	Inheritance	Gene	Method	Indication	Comment
MUTYH-associated polyposis	Autosomal recessive	MUTYH	Gene sequence analysis on blood sample	Patients with polyposis but lacking APC mutation or apparent autosomal recessive inheritance	If mutation is identified, at-risk family members screened
IBD	Genetic polymorphisms in pharmacokinetics	TPMT	TPMT genotype by gene sequence analysis of blood sample; TPMT phenotype by enzyme activity RBC assay	Prior to the start of thiopurine-based treatment for IBD	Patients with homozygous mutant alleles are not candidates for thiopurine therapy; Those with low enzyme activity require decreased drug dosage
HH	Complex genetics with variable penetrance	HFE—C282Y, H63D	HFE gene mutation testing on blood sample	Patients with clinical iron-overload state	First-degree relatives of patients with symptomatic HH may be screened
Hereditary pancreatitis	Autosomal dominant; Autosomal recessive	PRSS1 CFTR, SPINK1	Gene sequence analysis on blood sample	Patients with unexplained pancreatitis as child, unexplained recurrent acute or chronic pancreatitis as adult, suggestive family history	Identifies the etiology of pancreatitis

FAP, familial adenomatous polyposis; HDGC, hereditary diffuse gastric cancer; HH, hereditary hemochromatosis; HNPCC, hereditary nonpolyposis colon cancer; IBD, inflammatory bowel disease; IHC, immunohistochemistry; MMR, mismatch repair; MSI, microsatellite instability; MSI-H, high level of microsatellite instability; MUTYH, mutY homolog; PJS, Peutz–Jeghers syndrome.

Subsequently mutation-specific assays may be performed on at-risk family members. Mutations are identified in 25% to 50% of families.

TREATMENT

- There are no reliable screening tests for carriers of germ line mutation of CDH1 to allow early diagnosis of diffuse gastric cancer, as endoscopic visualization fails to identify early-stage disease and random biopsies may miss focal advanced lesions.
- **Prophylactic total gastrectomy** is often recommended in early twenties or 5 years earlier than the youngest family member who developed gastric cancer.
- Women in HDGC families are at high risks of developing lobular breast cancer, and are recommended for **enhanced breast cancer screening**.

PEUTZ–JEGHERS SYNDROME

GENERAL PRINCIPLES

Genetics

- Peutz–Jeghers syndrome (PJS) is an **autosomal dominant** disease of multiple hamartomatous polyps in the gastrointestinal tract associated with mucocutaneous pigmentation.
- The genetic defect is in a gene encoding a **serine threonine kinase (LKB1 or STK11)**, which is proposed to function as a tumor suppressor.

DIAGNOSIS

Clinical Manifestations

- Patients with PJS manifest **melanin spots,** appearing as blue-gray to brown lesions on the lips and perioral region (94%), hands (74%), buccal mucosa (66%), and feet (62%). Pigmentations appear in infancy and regress after puberty, with exception of buccal lesions.
- **Hamartomatous polyps** are most commonly in small intestine, but can also be found in stomach, colon, and rectum. They are unique in that they contain a proliferation of smooth muscle extending into the lamina propria in a tree-like fashion with normal overlying mucosa.
  ○ Polyps may lead to obstruction, intussusception, infarction, and bleeding.
- Patients with PJS are at **increased risk for malignancy of the gastrointestinal tract,** most commonly colon cancer, followed by pancreas, stomach, and small bowel.
- Women are at increased risk for **gynecological cancers** such as breast, ovary, and cervical cancers.
- Young men are at increased risk for **sertoli cell testicular tumors.**

Genetic Testing

- Genetic testing on blood samples is commercially available through several laboratories and LKB1 mutations can be identified in about 80% of families with PJS.[3]
- Genetic testing is **offered starting at age 8,** as up to 30% to 40% of patients may start to develop complications such as bowel obstruction by age 10.

TREATMENT

- **Regular surveillance** of affected individuals aims to detect cancers of the breast, colon, pancreas, stomach, small bowel, ovaries, uterus, cervix, and testicles.
  - ○ Upper endoscopy, colonoscopy, small bowel video capsule endoscopy every 2 to 3 years starting age 8.[4]
  - ○ Endoscopic ultrasound, CT and/or CA 19–9 every 1 or 2 years starting age 25 to screen for pancreatic cancer.
  - ○ Women require pelvic examination with Papanicolaou smear, mammography, breast MRI, transvaginal ultrasound, and CA-125 starting age 25.
  - ○ Men require testicular exams.
- Screening and clinical examination for at-risk first-degree relatives should start at birth.

LYNCH SYNDROME

GENERAL PRINCIPLES

Genetics

- Lynch syndrome or **hereditary nonpolyposis colon cancer (HNPCC)** is an **autosomal dominant** disorder, representing the most common familial colorectal cancer (CRC) syndrome. It also accounts for 2% to 6% of all CRC.
- Up to 75% of patients with Lynch syndrome develop CRC by age 65, with average age of cancer diagnosis being 45 years.[5]
- Lynch syndrome is also associated with extracolonic cancers, including endometrial, ovarian, stomach, small bowel, pancreatic, hepatobiliary, renal pelvis, and ureter cancers.
- Lynch syndrome is the result of **dysfunction in DNA mismatch repair (MMR) enzymes.** Germ line mutations of MLH1 or MSH2 account for 90% of Lynch syndrome cases. MSH6 and PMS2 are additional clinically relevant MMR genes.
- MMR gene mutations lead to accumulation of abnormalities in microsatellites of growth regulatory genes, leaving cells vulnerable to accumulating mutations that promote development of cancer.

DIAGNOSIS

Clinical Presentation

- It is important to identify individuals with Lynch syndrome, which lacks an easy to identify phenotype, as surveillance decreases the incidence of CRC and associated death.
- Diagnosis is based on criteria in Amsterdam I and Amsterdam II as well as Bethesda guidelines (Table 24-2).

Genetic Testing

- Direct sequencing of MMR gene to look for germ line mutation is expensive and may lead to discovery of variants of uncertain significance.[6]
- When Lynch syndrome is suspected, **immunohistochemistry (IHC) testing** on tumor or polypectomy specimen is performed to identify loss of expression of MLH1, MSH2, MSH6, or PMS2.

TABLE 24-2   DIAGNOSTIC CRITERIA FOR LYNCH SYNDROME

Amsterdam I criteria

At least three relatives with histologically verified CRC

1. One is a first-degree relative of the other two
2. At least two successive generations affected
3. At least one of the relatives was diagnosed with CRC at age <50
4. FAP is excluded

Amsterdam II criteria

At least three relatives with an HNPCC-associated cancer (CRC, endometrial, stomach, ovary, ureter/renal pelvis, brain, small bowel, hepatobiliary tract, and sebaceous tumors of skin)

1. One is a first-degree relative of other two
2. At least two successive generations affected
3. At least one HNPCC-associated cancer diagnosed at age <50
4. FAP is excluded

Bethesda guidelines

1. CRC diagnosed in a patient aged <50
2. Presence of synchronous or metachronous CRC or other HNPCC-associated cancers, regardless of age
3. CRC with MSI-high histology in a patient aged <60
4. CRC or HNPCC-associated tumor diagnosed at age <50 in at least one first-degree relative
5. CRC or HNPCC-associated tumor diagnosed at any age in two first- or second-degree relatives

CRC, colorectal cancer; FAP, familial adenomatous polyposis; HNPCC, hereditary nonpolyposis colon cancer; MSI, microsatellite instability.

- **Microsatellite instability (MSI)** is another useful test to identify patients with Lynch syndrome. It is measured by PCR of tumor tissue.
  - Greater than 90% of HNPCC-associated tumors have high level of microsatellite instability (MSI-H), whereas sporadic CRC usually have low level of MSI. Therefore, MSI-H should prompt further testing for Lynch syndrome.
  - Up to 15% of sporadic CRC can have MSI-H, which is associated with epigenetic inactivation of MLH1 by methylation or BRAF mutation.
  - Therefore, MLH1 hypermethylation or BRAF mutation can exclude Lynch syndrome in MSI-H tumors.
- **IHC and MSI analysis** have similar sensitivity and prove complementary to maximize the sensitivity in identifying Lynch syndrome. Choice of testing may depend on the expertise of the pathology department.
- Once IHC has determined which gene is most likely to be mutated, or MSI-H is found in the tumor suggesting possible MMR mutation, germ line mutational analysis is performed on the proband by gene sequencing and deletion analysis. Positive test confirms the diagnosis, but in some families a specific mutation is not identified.

TREATMENT

- **Enhanced cancer surveillance** is recommended for those who carry MMR gene mutation or if there is a strong suspicion for Lynch syndrome based on family history or testing for IHC or MSI.
  - **Annual colonoscopy** starting at age 20 to 25 or 10 years prior to the earliest age of colon cancer diagnosis in the family.
  - **Upper endoscopy** every 1 to 2 years can be considered beginning at age 30 to 35 to screen for gastric cancer.
  - Screening for small bowel tumors with **capsule endoscopy** has been suggested.
  - Annual screening for endometrial and ovarian cancer starting at age 30 to 35, or 10 years prior to the earliest age of first diagnosis of these cancers in the family.
  - Annual urinalysis and cytological examination beginning at age 25 to 35.
- Total colectomy or subtotal colectomy with continued surveillance of remaining rectum is recommended for those who develop CRC or advanced adenomas, as there is high incidence of synchronous or metachronous cancers.
- Primary prophylactic surgery is generally not recommended.

FAMILIAL ADENOMATOUS POLYPOSIS

GENERAL PRINCIPLES

Genetics

- Familial adenomatous polyposis (FAP) is an **autosomal dominant** disease characterized by 100 or more colorectal adenomas.
- Risk of colon cancer in classic FAP approaches 100% by age 35 to 40.[7]
- It is the most common inherited polyposis syndrome, with prevalence of 1 of 5000 to 7500.
- Patients with FAP usually develop symptoms after puberty, and polyposis is diagnosed by an average age of 36, with death from cancer at age 42.
  - CRC develops 10 to 15 years from the onset of polyposis.
- The genetic basis for disease is germ line **loss of function in APC gene** on chromosome 5q21–q22, which leads to cellular resistance to apoptosis and chromosomal instability, predisposing the cell to tumorigenesis.
  - More than 800 mutations in the APC gene have been associated with FAP, with almost all mutations resulting in protein truncation.
  - One-third of patients have no family history of the disease, many representing sporadic germ line mutations.
- **Attenuated familial adenomatous polyposis (AFAP)** is a variant of FAP in which patients have fewer polyps (>20 for diagnosis), later onset of polyp development and cancer, and infrequent rectal involvement, with 75% of tumors occurring in the proximal colon. Adenomas are often flat rather than polyploid.
  - Although it is also due to APC gene mutation, it may not be detected by available testing.
- Mutations in base excision repair gene mutY homolog (MUTYH) leads to recessive inheritance of a variant form of FAP called **MUTYH-associated polyposis.**

○ Testing is available for MUTYH mutations in those with polyposis but lacking APC mutation and those with apparent autosomal recessive pattern inheritance.

DIAGNOSIS

Genetic Testing

• Commercial blood tests are available for APC mutations, although they do not detect all mutations that cause FAP.
• APC gene sequencing should be performed on an affected family member with polyposis phenotype to determine if a mutation is found.
  ○ If mutation is present, other at-risk family members may be screened for the same mutation.
  ○ Genetic screening for children should start at age 10 to 12.

TREATMENT

Screening and Management

• Gene carriers, at-risk family members who did not undergo genetic testing, or whose genetic testing is uninformative should be offered annual screening starting age 10 to 12.
• Classic FAP may be screened with sigmoidoscopy or colonoscopy, whereas AFAP requires colonoscopy given predominance of right-sided tumors.
• Colectomy should be performed when polyposis is diagnosed. The preferred procedure is total proctocolectomy with ileoanal anastomosis. Because adenomas or cancers can still arise from the ileal pouch, continued annual surveillance of the ileal pouch, rectal cuff and anastomosis by endoscopy is required.

Management of Extracolonic Tumors Associated with FAP

• Patients with FAP are also at risk for duodenal ampullary carcinoma, follicular and papillary thyroid cancer, childhood hepatoblastoma, gastric carcinomas, and CNS tumors (mostly medulloblastomas).
• Gastric polyps occur in 30% to 50% of cases, but most are non-neoplastic, characterized by hyperplasia of fundic glands without epithelial dysplasia.
• The lifetime risk of duodenal adenoma approaches 100%, and duodenal and ampullary adenocarcinoma has become the leading cause of death in FAP patients who have undergone prophylactic colectomy.
  ○ The second and third portion of the duodenum and especially the periampullary region are the most commonly affected areas. Polyps may cause biliary obstruction.
  ○ Surveillance for duodenal polyps should include baseline examination with both forward and side-viewing upper endoscopy at the time of colectomy or early in the third decade of life, with repeat screening in 3 to 5 years.
  ○ Patients with a history of duodenal polyps should undergo surveillance endoscopy on the basis of the Spigelman stage of duodenal polyps (Table 24-3).[8]
  ○ Surveillance can be performed every 2 to 3 years for stage I and II, and every 6 to 12 months for stage III and IV.

TABLE 24-3	SPIGELMAN STAGE OF DUODENAL POLYPS		
Score	1	2	3
No. of polyps	1–4	5–20	>20
Size (mm)	1–4	5–10	>10
Histologic type	Tubular	Tubulovillous	Villous
Dysplasia	Mild	Moderate	Severe

- Stage I: score 1–4
- Stage II: score 5–6
- Stage III: score 7–8
- Stage IV: score 9–12

SPECIAL CONSIDERATIONS

Gardner's Syndrome

- Gardner's syndrome includes the same genetic lesions (APC gene) and gastrointestinal manifestations as FAP and is distinguished by **prominence of extraintestinal lesions** including desmoid tumors, sebaceous or epidermoid cysts, lipomas, osteomas (particularly of the mandible), supernumerary teeth, gastric polyps, and juvenile nasopharyngeal angiofibromas.
- More than 90% of patients with Gardner's syndrome have **congenital hypertrophy of the retinal pigmented epithelium (CHRPE).** Consisting of pigmented ocular fundic lesions, CHRPE is present in only 5% of controls; therefore, this examination finding is highly suggestive of gene carriage of adenomatous polyposis, especially when present bilaterally in patients with a positive family history.
- **Desmoid tumors or diffuse mesenteric fibromatosis** is found in 4% to 20% of FAP patients and can lead to intestinal obstruction or constriction of the mesenteric vasculature or uterus.
- Desmoid tumors frequently develop in areas of previous surgical procedures such as colectomy or ceasarian section. Desmoid tumors can prove a lethal complication, ranking second behind metastatic disease in patients with FAP. There is no proven treatment or prevention strategy.

Turcot's Syndrome

- Turcot's syndrome refers to the **association between brain tumors and FAP or HNPCC.** There is no directly established mechanism for the development of brain tumors with the mutations that lead to colorectal cancer.
  - Mutations to APC tend to be associated with medulloblastomas.
  - Mutations in mismatch repair genes are typically associated with glioblastoma.

HEREDITARY HEMOCHROMATOSIS

GENERAL PRINCIPLES

Genetics

- Hereditary hemochromatosis (HH) is an inherited **disorder of increased intestinal iron absorption resulting in systemic iron overload.**

- HH is due to mutations in the HFE gene on chromosome 6 or rarely other genes (hemojuvelin, hepcidin, ferrportin, transferring receptor-2).
- Fifty percent to 100% of patients with HH are homozygous for C282Y among patients of European ancestry.[9]
- Although 3 of 1000 people are homozygous for C282Y, there is variable disease penetrance.
- Patients may also be homozygous for the H63D mutation, heterozygous for C282Y or H63D or compound heterozygotes.
  - Of the patients with phenotypic HH, 5% to 11% are compound heterozygotes, with overall decreased iron overload compared with C282Y homozygotes.
  - Approximately 1.5% of patients with HFE gene defects are homozygotes for H63D, but it is unclear if this leads to significant iron overload.
  - Three percent to 10% of patients with phenotypic HH are heterozygotes for either C282Y or H63D, with the development of iron overload likely explained by the presence of additional mutations.

DIAGNOSIS

Genetic Testing

- Early detection of disease can allow treatment, preventing the late consequences of iron overload including cirrhosis, hepatocellular carcinoma, diabetes mellitus, and cardiomyopathy.
- Testing for HFE gene mutation should be performed on patients with a clinical iron overload state, that is, transferrin saturation >45% and/or elevated ferritin.
- First-degree relatives of patients with symptomatic HH benefit from screening, which includes transferrin saturation, ferritin, and HFE gene mutation.
- Optimal timing of screening is between 18 and 30 years of age, when hemochromatosis is evident by iron tests, but prior to onset of end-organ damage.
- Many patients with HFE gene mutations may not develop organ damage or require treatment, but should be monitored with yearly examination and iron studies.

HEREDITARY PANCREATITIS

GENERAL PRINCIPLES

- Hereditary pancreatitis typically presents as acute pancreatitis in childhood or early adolescence, chronic pancreatitis in late adolescence or early adulthood, and patients are at risk for pancreatic cancer later in life.
- Autosomal dominant hereditary pancreatitis is usually caused by mutations in the serine protease 1 gene (PRSS1) on chromosome 7q35, which encodes cationic trypsin.[10] One-third of patients with PRSS1-associated hereditary pancreatitis develop pancreatic insufficiency and/or diabetes mellitus.
- Autosomal recessive pancreatitis is most commonly associated with cystic fibrosis (CFTR gene mutation).
- Mutations in the serine protease inhibitor Kazal type 1 gene (SPINK1) also result in autosomal recessive or complex genetic pattern of inherited pancreatitis.
- Both CFTR and SPINK1 code for molecules that protect the pancreas from active trypsin.

- Genetic testing can be performed on those with a suggestive family history, unexplained pancreatitis in a child, or unexplained recurrent acute or chronic pancreatitis in older patients.

OTHER USES OF GENETIC TESTING

INFLAMMATORY BOWEL DISEASE AND TPMT

General Principles
- Azathiaprine (AZA) and 6-mercaptopurine (6-MP) are successfully used in patients with inflammatory bowel disease for inducing and maintaining remission, and as steroid sparing agents.
- AZA is metabolized to 6-MP, which is then metabolized to 6-thioguanine (6-TG) and 6-methylmercaptopurine (6-MMP) through the enzyme thiopurine methyltransferase (TPMT). 6-TG and 6-MMP are related to the bone marrow and liver toxicities, respectively.
- TPMT enzyme activity is a major determining factor of 6-MP metabolism and its toxicity.

Genetic Polymorphisms of TPMT
- Approximately 89% of population has wild-type TPMT genotype, which is associated with normal TPMT enzyme activity. Eleven percent of population is heterozygous for TPMT and has intermediate TPMT enzyme activity. About 0.3% of population is homozygous for TPMT mutant alleles, and has almost no TPMT enzyme activity, which leads to high 6-TG levels and bone marrow toxicity in patients taking AZA or 6-MP.
- Testing for genetic polymorphisms to determine the TPMT genotype before initiating therapy with thiopurines can identify patients with low or absent TPMT activity.
  - Patients with homozygous mutant alleles are not candidates for therapy with AZA or 6-MP.
- TPMT genotypes correlate with enzyme activity or phenotype, which may be determined directly by RBC assay. Testing of TPMT enzyme activity can be confounded by recent blood transfusion or concomitant medications. Empiric dosing of thiopurines may be initiated on the basis of TPMT enzyme activity level, such that the lower the enzyme activity, the lower the dose of AZA or 6-MP. For example, patients with intermediate TPMT enzyme activity may be dosed with AZA 1.0 to 1.5 mg/kg/day rather than 2.0 to 2.5 mg/kg/day.
- It is important to note that regardless of TPMT genotype or phenotype, monitoring of blood cell counts and liver function tests are still required, as normal TPMT screening testing does not preclude development of adverse drug reactions.

Thiopurine Metabolite Monitoring
- Metabolite monitoring is also useful in guiding therapy.[11]
  - 6-TG levels between 230 and 400 may correlate with clinical response to AZA or 6-MP, whereas levels >400 may correlate with bone marrow suppression.
  - 6-MMP levels >5700 may correlate with liver toxicity.

- Determining metabolite levels can also help distinguish patients who are non-compliant from those who are underdosed, resistant to treatment, or refractory to therapy with thiopurines.

CELIAC DISEASE

General Principles

- Celiac disease is characterized by a chronic inflammatory response to gluten in small bowel mucosa in genetically susceptible individuals. See Chapter 14 for further details.
- In the United States, the prevalence is approximately 1%.

Genetics

- Celiac disease is associated with HLA DQ2 and DQ8, which are necessary but not sufficient to produce the celiac phenotype.

Diagnosis

Genetic Testing

- HLA typing, a commercially available blood test, can be useful in the diagnosis of celiac disease when patients are already on a gluten-free diet without a confirmed diagnosis. The absence of HLA DQ2 or DQ8 essentially rules out celiac disease.[12]

REFERENCES

1. Gallagher DJ, Smith JD, Offit K, et al. Diagnosing hereditary colorectal cancer. *Clin Colorectal Cancer.* 2010;9:205–211.
2. Fitzgerald RC, Hardwick R, Huntsman D, et al. Hereditary diffuse gastric cancer: updated consensus guidelines for clinical management and directions for future research. *J Med Genet.* 2010;47:436–444.
3. van Lier MG, Wagner A, Mathus-Vliegen EM, et al. High cancer risk in Peutz-Jeghers syndrome: a systematic review and surveillance recommendations. *Am J Gastroenterol.* 2010;105:1258–1264; author reply 65.
4. Beggs AD, Latchford AR, Vasen HF, et al. Peutz-Jeghers syndrome: a systematic review and recommendations for management. *Gut.* 2010;59:975–986.
5. Jasperson KW, Tuohy TM, Neklason DW, et al. Hereditary and familial colon cancer. *Gastroenterology.* 2010;138:2044–2058.
6. Pino MS, Chung DC. Application of molecular diagnostics for the detection of Lynch syndrome. *Expert Rev Mol Diagn.* 2010;10:651–665.
7. Galiatsatos P, Foulkes WD. Familial adenomatous polyposis. *Am J Gastroenterol.* 2006; 101:385–398.
8. Brosens LA, Keller JJ, Offerhaus GJ, et al. Prevention and management of duodenal polyps in familial adenomatous polyposis. *Gut.* 2005;54:1034–1043.
9. Neghina AM, Anghel A. Hemochromatosis genotypes and risk of iron overload–a meta-analysis. *Ann Epidemiol.* 2011;21:1–14.
10. Rosendahl J, Bodeker H, Mossner J, et al. Hereditary chronic pancreatitis. *Orphanet J Rare Dis.* 2007;2:1.
11. Teml A, Schaeffeler E, Herrlinger KR, et al. Thiopurine treatment in inflammatory bowel disease: clinical pharmacology and implication of pharmacogenetically guided dosing. *Clin Pharmacokinet.* 2007;46:187–208.
12. American Gastroenterological Association medical position statement: Celiac Sprue. *Gastroenterology.* 2001;120:1522–1525.

Gastrointestinal Procedures

25

Sachin Wani and Daniel Mullady

- The ability to perform endoscopic procedures has radically changed the practice of gastroenterology.
- Endoscopy allows for direct visual inspection, tissue sampling, and minimally invasive therapeutic intervention. An endoscopic procedure is worth performing if the benefit for the patient exceeds the risks by a sufficiently wide margin.
- Preparation for endoscopy involves addressing important issues specific to each patient, such as assessing contraindications and relative contraindications, medication allergies, patient medications, and possible interactions with medicines used for sedation. In addition, the presence of coagulopathy, comorbid factors, and conditions potentially requiring antibiotic prophylaxis must be considered. Furthermore, each patient, or a designated guardian, should understand the benefits and risks associated with the procedure, and informed consent must be obtained before the procedure is initiated.
- General indications for endoscopic procedures are listed in Table 25-1.

UPPER GASTROINTESTINAL ENDOSCOPY

GENERAL PRINCIPLES

- Esophagogastroduodenoscopy (EGD) allows high-resolution visual inspection of the upper gastrointestinal (GI) tract from the esophagus to the second or third portion of the duodenum.

DIAGNOSIS

- EGD is performed for various indications, such as
  - **diagnosis** and **management** of abdominal pain or upper GI bleeding;
  - **screening** and diagnosis of esophageal or gastric malignancies;
  - **surveillance** of premalignant conditions such as Barrett's esophagus;
  - application of endoscopic **eradication therapies** for management of Barrett's esophagus–associated dysplasia and early esophageal adenocarcinoma; and
  - **palliation** of dysphagia resulting from both malignant and benign causes.

Procedure

- At most institutions, examinations are performed using **topical anesthetics** applied to the oropharynx in combination with **intravenous (IV) conscious sedation.**
- **Monitored anesthesia** care can be used with assistance from an anesthesiologist when conscious sedation is anticipated to be unsuccessful.
- The only patient preparation required is to **avoid oral intake for ≥6 hours before the procedure.**

TABLE 25-1	GENERAL INDICATIONS FOR ENDOSCOPIC PROCEDURES

Gastrointestinal endoscopy is generally indicated:

If a change in management is probable based on results of endoscopy

After an empiric trial of therapy for a suspected benign digestive disorder has been unsuccessful

As the initial method of evaluation as an alternative to radiographic studies

When a primary therapeutic procedure is contemplated

Gastrointestinal endoscopy is generally not indicated:

When the results are not expected to contribute to a management choice

For periodic follow-up of healed benign disease unless surveillance of a premalignant condition is warranted

Gastrointestinal endoscopy is generally contraindicated:

When the risks to patient health or life are judged to outweigh the most favorable benefits of the procedure

When adequate patient cooperation or consent cannot be obtained

When a perforated viscus is known or suspected

TREATMENT

- Various instruments may be passed through the therapeutic channel of the endoscope for use in tissue biopsy, medication delivery, cauterization, clip application, enteral stenting, and application of endoscopic eradication therapies.

COMPLICATIONS

- Endoscopy has a small risk of complications, overall estimated to occur in 0.1% having the procedure.[1,2]
  - Significant **bleeding** has been reported in 0.025% to 0.15%.
  - **Perforation** has been reported in 0.02% to 0.2%.
  - **Cardiorespiratory complications,** mostly attributed to premedication or sedation, can occur in 0.05% to 0.73% of patients.
- The risk of **mortality** as a result of upper endoscopy has been estimated to range from 0.005% to 0.04%.

COLONOSCOPY

GENERAL PRINCIPLES

- Colonoscopy is performed to examine the colonic and terminal ileal mucosa.

DIAGNOSIS

- Colonoscopy is performed for various indications, including
  - **evaluation** and **treatment** of overt lower GI bleeding;
  - **evaluation** of iron-deficiency anemia;
  - **screening** and **surveillance** of colorectal cancer and polyps;

○ **diagnosis** and cancer surveillance in inflammatory bowel disease;
○ **palliative treatment of** stenosing or bleeding neoplasms; and
○ **evaluation** of clinically significant diarrhea of unexplained origin.

Procedure

* As with EGD, colonoscopy almost always involves the use of **IV conscious sedation** or **monitored anesthesia.**
* **Colon preparation** is required before the procedure. This usually involves a lavage or purgative method used on the day or evening before the patient's colonoscopy.
  ○ **Polyethylene glycol preparations** are preferred (GoLYTELY or MiraLax) to phospho-soda–based preparations which may lead to electrolyte derangements and renal failure.

TREATMENT

* Various instruments may be passed through the therapeutic channel of the endoscope for use in tissue biopsy, cauterization or fulguration of tissue, polypectomy, and colonic stent placement.

COMPLICATIONS

* Colonoscopy has a small risk of complications,[1,2] estimated to occur in 0.1% to 1.9% of patients having the procedure.
  ○ Significant **bleeding** can be seen in up to 1.9% of patients. The rate of bleeding complications seen with therapeutic colonoscopy is roughly double than that seen with diagnostic colonoscopy.
  ○ **Perforation** can occur in up to 0.4% of patients. Surgical consultation should be obtained in the event of suspected perforation; however, if possible, attempts to close the defect with hemoclips should be made.
  ○ **Cardiorespiratory complications,** which are also a concern, are mostly attributed to the sedation used during the procedure.
* **Mortality** has been reported in up to 0.06% of patients.

FLEXIBLE SIGMOIDOSCOPY

GENERAL PRINCIPLES

* Flexible sigmoidoscopy involves a shorter examination compared with colonoscopy and is used to examine the distal colon up to the splenic flexure.

DIAGNOSIS

* Flexible sigmoidoscopy is generally used for evaluation of
  ○ suspected distal colonic disease when colonoscopy is not indicated;
  ○ anastomotic recurrence in rectosigmoid carcinoma; and
  ○ exclusion of infection or immune-mediated processes (e.g., graft-versus-host disease) in certain patient subsets, including those with inflammatory bowel disease or following bone marrow transplantation.

Procedure

- This examination is usually performed **without sedation,** which adds the advantages of decreased cost; fewer complications associated with sedation; and decreased lost work time for the patient.
- This procedure also eliminates the need for a complete colon preparation. Two enemas given a few hours before the procedure are usually adequate preparation.

TREATMENT

- As above for colonoscopy.

COMPLICATIONS

- Complications of flexible sigmoidoscopy are similar to those listed above under colonoscopy.
- The overall risk of perforation during flexible sigmoidoscopy is low (0.01%).

SMALL BOWEL ENTEROSCOPY

GENERAL PRINCIPLES

- Since standard upper GI endoscopy is limited to the proximal duodenum, longer endoscopes are needed to examine the upper GI tract beyond the ligament of Treitz.
  - Two types of enteroscopes developed for this purpose are the **push enteroscope** and the **single- or double-balloon enteroscope.**[3] Instead of a dedicated push enteroscope, a small caliber colonoscope (pediatric colonoscope) can also be used for push enteroscopy.
  - **Sonde enteroscopy,** a procedure involving a long, thin endoscope advanced by small bowel peristalsis, is no longer in use.
  - **Capsule enteroscopy** is currently being used in many settings as a means to visualize segments of the bowel previously inaccessible to endoscopy.

DIAGNOSIS

- Small bowel enteroscopy is performed **for evaluation of obscure (occult or overt) GI bleeding.**
- It is also indicated for **diagnosis and treatment of small bowel polyps and masses.**

Procedure

- **Push enteroscopes** are 160 to 240 cm in length and can be used for therapeutic intervention. They allow for controlled insertion and withdrawal.
  - Push enteroscopy is traditionally used after a negative upper endoscopy and colonoscopy.
  - The yield of push enteroscopy in this setting is approximately 60%.

- **Balloon enteroscopy** utilizes single or double inflatable balloons on the end of the endoscope and an accompanying overtube to grip the intestinal wall and allow deep cannulation of the small bowel.
  - Both transoral and transanal approaches can be used and often the entire length of the small bowel can be examined when both approaches are used in combination.
  - This form of enteroscopy allows biopsy or treatment of lesions noted beyond the reach of push enteroscopes and is replacing intraoperative enteroscopy in some centers.
- **Capsule enteroscopy** visualizes segments of the bowel previously inaccessible to endoscopy.
  - The patient swallows a capsule that contains a camera, light source, battery, and radio transmitter.
  - As the capsule traverses the GI tract, it takes pictures and transmits these images to a receiver that the patient wears on the belt. The capsule takes 8 hours of images, usually sufficient time to traverse the ileocecal valve.
  - The images are then loaded onto a computer where they can be viewed in a movie format at up to 25 frames per second.
  - The current indications for capsule endoscopy include evaluation of obscure GI bleeding and persistent occult GI bleeding.
  - The major contraindication is the presence of intestinal strictures which can obstruct passage of the capsule.[4,5]

TREATMENT

- While capsule endoscopy is only a diagnostic procedure, small bowel enteroscopy using push enteroscopes and single/double balloon enteroscopes not only provides diagnosis but also allows tissue acquisition, resection of polyps, and ablation of vascular lesions.

COMPLICATIONS

- These are similar to that seen with endoscopic procedures described above.
- The **main complication associated with capsule endoscopy is capsule retention,** rates of which are dependent on the indication of the procedure. Capsule retention frequently occurs in the area of pathology in the small bowel.
  - Intestinal obstruction from a retained capsule is a rare complication, frequently requiring surgical intervention when it occurs.

ENDOSCOPIC RETROGRADE CHOLANGIOPANCREATOGRAPHY

GENERAL PRINCIPLES

- Endoscopic retrograde cholangiopancreatography (ERCP) is performed using a specially designed endoscope that involves a side-viewing imaging system.
- This system allows direct visualization of the major and minor papillae and facilitates insertion of devices into the desired duct.

DIAGNOSIS

- With the advent of improved cross-sectional imaging technology with computed tomography (CT) and magnetic resonance cholangiopancreatography, the role of diagnostic ERCP had diminished considerably.
- ERCP is used predominantly for the evaluation and management of
  - choledocholithiasis, especially in the presence of biliary obstruction or cholangitis;
  - benign and malignant biliary strictures;
  - bile leak;
  - suspected sphincter of Oddi dysfunction, frequently combined with sphincter manometry;
  - pancreatic duct leak;
  - complications of acute and chronic pancreatitis such as pancreatic duct disruption, strictures, and stones; and
  - resection of ampullary adenomas.

Procedure

- An ERCP can be used effectively in **detecting and treating choledocholithiasis.** **Sphincterotomy** may be performed at the time of stone removal to reduce the chance of recurrent choledocholithiasis.
- ERCP may also be used therapeutically to **dilate benign and malignant strictures** in the biliary tree with or without subsequent stent placement.
- **Brushings for cytology** may also be obtained during ERCP to assist in the diagnosis of cholangiocarcinoma and pancreatic neoplasms.
- **Palliation of jaundice** in patients with pancreatic and biliary malignancies can be achieved by placement of self-expanding metallic stents.

TREATMENT

- Various devices can be passed through the working channel of the duodenoscope to achieve access and cannulation of the common bile duct and pancreatic duct, sphincterotomy, balloon dilation, tissue biopsies and brushings, biliary and pancreatic stenting, stone extraction, and biliary/pancreatic manometry.

COMPLICATIONS

- The ERCP procedure is associated with **all the risks of upper endoscopy.**[6]
  - Approximately 5% to 7% of patients develop **postprocedural pancreatitis.** This is usually mild and self-limited; however, in a small percentage of cases, this can be life threatening.
  - The incidence is higher in patients with suspected sphincter of Oddi dysfunction.

ENDOSCOPIC ULTRASONOGRAPHY

GENERAL PRINCIPLES

- Endoscopic ultrasound (EUS) allows for high-resolution imaging of the luminal GI tract combining endoscopic visualization and high-frequency ultrasound. It uses higher frequencies than transabdominal ultrasound and provides resolution of the GI tract wall into distinct layers that correlate closely with histology.

DIAGNOSIS

- EUS has become widely accepted as an effective modality in evaluating lesions in the GI tract, mediastinum, and other organs such as the left adrenal gland and the liver.[7]
- **EUS-guided fine-needle aspiration (FNA)** provides clinically important diagnostic and prognostic information including cytologic confirmation of the presence (or absence) of malignancy and metastasis to secondary sites.
- The **most common indications of EUS-guided FNA** include evaluation of
  - ○ pancreatic masses;
  - ○ mediastinal and intra-abdominal lymphadenopathy;
  - ○ liver masses;
  - ○ left adrenal masses; and
  - ○ GI submucosal lesions.
- EUS-guided FNA has supplanted CT-guided biopsy and ERCP in the diagnosis of pancreatic cancer.
- EUS is the most sensitive imaging study for the diagnosis of chronic pancreatitis and choledocholithiasis.
- EUS is also an adjunctive tool in the evaluation of patients with fecal incontinence to assess for internal and external anal sphincter defects.

Procedure

- EUS is performed using a specially designed endoscope that involves a side-viewing imaging system.
  - ○ The endoscope is passed to different areas in the upper and lower GI tract allowing for targeted inspection of areas of interest.
  - ○ The FNA needle can be passed through the working channel of the endoscope to perform FNA of solid lesions or aspiration of fluid from pancreatic cysts.

COMPLICATIONS

- EUS is associated with **all the risks associated with upper endoscopy** including those associated with sedation.
- **Bacteremia** is a rare occurrence after EUS-guided FNA, with an incidence of approximately 0.4% to 1%.
- There is a small risk of **pancreatitis** (1% to 2%) associated with EUS-guided FNA of pancreatic masses.
- **Bleeding and bile peritonitis** as complications of EUS-guided FNA are rare and described anecdotally in the literature.

LIVER BIOPSY

GENERAL PRINCIPLES

- Liver biopsy can be achieved by two different techniques:
  - ○ **Percutaneous liver biopsy,** performed at the bedside, sometimes with ultrasound guidance; rarely, it is performed under computed tomographic guidance.
  - ○ **Transjugular liver biopsy** under fluoroscopic guidance.

DIAGNOSIS

- **Common indications** for liver biopsy include evaluation of abnormal liver chemistries, assessment of degree of inflammation and fibrosis in chronic liver disease (e.g., hepatitis C), and diagnosis of liver masses.[8]

Procedure

- Bedside percutaneous liver biopsy is commonly performed by gastroenterologists or hepatologists.
  - The patient is placed supine with the right arm behind the head.
  - With ultrasound guidance or percussion, an appropriate biopsy location is chosen in the right lateral chest wall, usually near the eighth intercostal space.
  - The area is prepared and draped in sterile fashion, and lidocaine is used to infiltrate the skin, subcutaneous fat, intercostal muscles, and liver capsule.
  - A small incision is made, and the liver biopsy needle is advanced to the liver capsule.
  - With the patient held in full expiration, the biopsy needle is advanced into the liver parenchyma, and a core of tissue is obtained.
  - The patient is then observed closely for at least 4 hours for complications.
  - **Contraindications to percutaneous liver biopsy** include severe coagulopathy, thrombocytopenia, or ascites.[8]
- If percutaneous liver biopsy cannot be safely performed or if portal pressure measurements are needed, transjugular liver biopsy under radiologic guidance may be performed.
- Directed biopsy with ultrasound or CT guidance may be necessary for sampling of liver masses.

COMPLICATIONS

- Complications of liver biopsy are rare but can be severe.
  - The most common complication is **pain at the biopsy site or in the right shoulder.**
  - Less common complications are **bleeding, pneumothorax, gallbladder perforation, inadvertent kidney biopsy, or death.**
  - Most complications are apparent within the first 4 to 6 hours, but they can occur up to 48 hours after biopsy.

PERCUTANEOUS ENDOSCOPIC GASTROSTOMY/JEJUNOSTOMY

GENERAL PRINCIPLES

- Percutaneous endoscopic gastrostomy/jejunostomy (PEG/PEJ) and jejunal extension through PEG (PEG-J) tubes are indicated in patients requiring long-term nutritional support.

DIAGNOSIS

- **Common indications** include oropharyngeal dysphagia secondary to neurologic conditions, oropharyngeal and laryngeal cancer, esophageal cancer, and head and facial trauma.[9]

Procedure

- Enteral feeding through a gastrostomy or jejunostomy has several advantages over parenteral nutrition such as lower risks of infection, preservation of gut integrity, and costs.
- Percutaneous enterostomies should not be performed in individuals with rapidly progressive diseases with a short life expectancy or when oral feeds are expected to resume within 30 days.
- Other contraindications include coagulopathy, pharyngeal or esophageal obstruction, inability to achieve apposition of stomach with the abdominal wall, lack of adequate gastric transillumination due to prior gastric surgery, ascites, hepatomegaly, and obesity and bowel obstruction.
- The two common techniques of PEG and PEJ include the "pull" and "push" technique.
- PEJ is a modification of PEG and more difficult to perform.
- Feeding via the PEG/PEJ is typically initiated the next day or 24 hours post-procedure.

COMPLICATIONS

- Complications include wound infections, bleeding, perforation, ileus, injury to internal organs, tumor seeding, buried bumper syndrome, and death.
- Antibiotic prophylaxis is recommended to reduce the risk of peristomal wound infection.

SPECIAL CONSIDERATIONS

Conscious Sedation

- Conscious sedation provides adequate analgesia and sedation for most GI procedures while allowing the patient to cooperate with verbal commands.
- Conscious sedation for endoscopic procedures usually involves a **benzodiazepine** (i.e., midazolam) **and an opiate** (i.e., meperidine or fentanyl).
- In patients not adequately sedated with this combination, addition of other IV agents such as promethazine or diphenhydramine can be considered.
- **Propofol** is an ultrashort-acting sedative, and its use **requires the presence of an anesthesiologist** for both the administration of the drug and airway control. Using propofol results in deep, not conscious, sedation.[10]
- The American Society of Anesthesiologists (ASA) assessment (categories I to V) is useful in evaluating the sedation risk for a patient.
  - ASA category I represents the lowest risk.
  - Advanced age, obesity, pregnancy, sleep apnea, a history of substance abuse, or severe cardiac, respiratory, hepatic, renal, or central nervous system disease places patients at higher risk for sedation.
  - Anesthesia assistance should be considered for patients with ASA class III and above, for those who have had adverse reaction or inadequate response to moderate sedation, for patients who take opiates chronically, and for lengthy or complex endoscopic procedures.
  - The ASA guidelines state that patients should fast a minimum of 2 hours after consumption of clear liquids and 6 hours after consuming light meals before the administration of sedation.

- The most common sedation complications include airway obstruction and respiratory depression, oversedation, hypoxia, and hypotension. Patients are monitored during the procedure using continuous pulse oximetry, heart monitoring, intermittent blood pressure recordings, and in some situations, end-tidal CO_2. These parameters are supplemental to vigilant clinical observation of the patient.

Antibiotic Prophylaxis for Endoscopy

- Mucosal trauma during GI endoscopy can result in bacterial translocation of microbial flora into the bloodstream. Bacteremia as a result of this carries a risk of localization of infection in remote tissues (e.g., infective endocarditis). Endoscopy can also contaminate a sterile space or tissue by an endoscopic accessory or by contrast injection.
- **Bacterial endocarditis** is a potentially life-threatening infection.
  - Approximately 4% of patients develop bacteremia associated with endoscopy, but this varies depending on the specific procedure performed.
  - Although infective endocarditis is a potentially life-threatening infection, this has rarely been reported post-GI endoscopy. There are no data demonstrating a causal link between endoscopic procedures and infective endocarditis.
  - Similarly, there are no data that demonstrate that antibiotic prophylaxis before endoscopic procedures protects against infective endocarditis.
  - The guidelines for antibiotic prophylaxis for GI endoscopy were recently updated by the American Society for Gastrointestinal Endoscopy and have been highlighted in Table 25-2.[11] These recommendations are in accordance with the recommendations of the American Heart Association.
  - Antibiotic prophylaxis solely to prevent infective endocarditis is no longer recommended before endoscopic procedures.
- Antibiotic prophylaxis should be administered in patients undergoing ERCP for biliary obstruction in whom complete drainage may not be achieved (hilar stricture and primary sclerosing cholangitis) and in patients with communicating pancreatic cysts or pseudocysts and prior to transpapillary or transmural drainage of pseudocysts. Antibiotic prophylaxis is routinely recommended prior to EUS-guided FNA of cystic lesions along the GI tract.
- Antibiotics should be administered in all patients prior to placement of PEG/PEJ tube and in all cirrhotic patients admitted with GI bleeding.

Anticoagulation and Antiplatelet Agents

- Patients on chronic anticoagulation (warfarin, heparin, and low-molecular-weight heparin), antiplatelet agents [aspirin, non-steroidal anti-inflammatory drugs (NSAIDs), thienopyridines (clopidogrel)], and glycoprotein IIb/IIIa receptor inhibitors requiring GI procedures pose a challenging problem.
- Ideally, the **platelet count should be >50,000 and INR should be <1.5 prior to endoscopic procedures.**
- The three issues that should be considered include
  - risk of bleeding from antithrombotic therapy;
  - risk of bleeding from an endoscopic intervention in the setting of antithrombotic medication use; and
  - risk of thromboembolic event from interruption of antithrombotic therapy.

| TABLE 25-2 | AMERICAN SOCIETY FOR GASTROINTESTINAL ENDOSCOPY RECOMMENDATIONS FOR ANTIBIOTIC PROPHYLAXIS |

Antibiotic recommended:

Patients with bile duct obstruction in absence of cholangitis undergoing ERCP with anticipated incomplete drainage (e.g., hilar strictures, PSC)

Sterile pancreatic fluid collection (e.g., pseudocyst, necrosis) which communicates with the pancreatic duct undergoing ERCP and sterile pancreatic fluid collection undergoing transmural drainage

Cystic lesions along GI tract undergoing EUS-guided FNA

Acute GI bleeding in the cirrhotic patient

Endoscopic feeding tube placement

Antibiotic optional:

Solid lesion along lower GI tract undergoing EUS-guided FNA

Antibiotic not recommended:

Prior to any endoscopic procedure regardless of cardiac condition to prevent infective endocarditis

Bile duct obstruction in the absence of cholangitis undergoing ERCP with complete drainage

Solid lesion along upper GI tract undergoing EUS-guided FNA

Prior to any endoscopic procedure to prevent graft and device infection in patients with synthetic vascular graft and other nonvalvular cardiovascular devices

Prior to any endoscopic procedure to prevent septic arthritis in patients with prosthetic joints

---

ERCP, endoscopic retrograde cholangiopancreatography; EUS-guided FNA, endoscopic ultrasound-guided fine-needle aspiration; GI, gastrointestinal; PSC, primary sclerosing cholangitis.

- Management of antithrombotic agents is **based on the risk of the GI procedure** (low vs. high risk), **indication for use of antithrombotic agent** (low vs. high risk for thromboembolic event), and **indication of procedure** (elective vs. emergent).
  - **Low risk GI procedures** include all diagnostic procedures including ERCP without sphincterotomy and EUS without FNA.
  - **High-risk procedures** include polypectomy, sphincterotomy, stricture dilation, PEG, and EUS-guided FNA.
- The guidelines for management of anticoagulation and antiplatelet therapy for GI endoscopy were recently updated by the American Society for Gastrointestinal Endoscopy.[12] The salient recommendations from this guideline are as follows:
  - **Aspirin and/or NSAIDs** may be continued for all endoscopic procedures. If discontinued prior to high-risk procedures, they should be held for 5 to 7 days prior to the procedure.
  - Patients with a **recently placed vascular stent or acute coronary syndrome** should have elective procedures deferred until administration of antithrombotic therapy for minimum recommended duration has been completed. Any changes to the antithrombotic regimen should be based on consultation with the patient's cardiologist.
  - Patients on **clopidogrel or ticlopidine** alone or in combination with aspirin should be on aspirin during the periendoscopic period. If these medications

need to be held, patients need to be off clopidogrel or ticlopidine for 7 to 10 days prior to endoscopy.

○ While anticoagulation can be held in patients with low risk of thromboembolic events (e.g., lone atrial fibrillation, bioprosthetic valve, deep vein thrombosis), **patients at high risk** (e.g., atrial fibrillation associated with comorbid conditions, coronary stent within 1 year, acute coronary syndrome, mechanical mitral valve) should be **bridged with low-molecular-weight heparin or unfractionated heparin.**

○ **Warfarin** should be held for 3 to 5 days, **low-molecular-weight heparin** for 12 to 24 hours, and **unfractionated heparin** for 4 to 6 hours prior to the procedure.

○ Consensus regarding **resumption of anticoagulant therapy** after endoscopic intervention is lacking and should be based on procedure details and indications for anticoagulation.

○ For patients with **acute bleeding who require endoscopic therapy,** antiplatelet and anticoagulants should be held until hemostasis is achieved and attempts should be made to correct any coagulopathy using a combination of fresh-frozen plasma, vitamin K, and platelets.

REFERENCES

1. Froehlich F, Gonvers JJ, Vader JP, et al. Appropriateness of gastrointestinal endoscopy: risk of complications. *Endoscopy.* 1999;31(8):684–686.
2. Kavic S, Basson M. Complications of endoscopy. *Am J Surg.* 2001;181:319–332.
3. May A, Färber M, Aschmoneit I, et al. Prospective multicenter trial comparing push-and-pull enteroscopy with the single- and double-balloon techniques in patients with small-bowel disorders. *Am J Gastroenterol.* 2010;105(3):575–581.
4. ASGE Standards of Practice Committee, Fisher L, Lee Krinsky M, Anderson MA, et al. The role of endoscopy in the management of obscure GI bleeding. *Gastrointest Endosc.* 2010;72(3):471–479.
5. Laine L, Sahota A, Shah A. Does capsule endoscopy improve outcomes in obscure gastrointestinal bleeding? Randomized trial versus dedicated small bowel radiography. *Gastroenterology.* 2010;138(5):1673–1680.
6. Dumonceau JM, Andriulli A, Deviere J, et al. European Society of Gastrointestinal Endoscopy. European Society of Gastrointestinal Endoscopy (ESGE) Guideline: prophylaxis of post-ERCP pancreatitis. *Endoscopy.* 2010;42(6):503–515.
7. Hawes RH. The evolution of endoscopic ultrasound: improved imaging, higher accuracy for fine needle aspiration and the reality of endoscopic ultrasound-guided interventions. *Curr Opin Gastroenterol.* 2010;26(5):436–444.
8. Rockey DC, Caldwell SH, Goodman ZD, et al; American Association for the Study of Liver Diseases. Liver biopsy. *Hepatology.* 2009;49(3):1017–1044.
9. ASGE Technology Committee, Kwon RS, Banerjee S, Desilets D, et al. Enteral nutrition access devices. *Gastrointest Endosc.* 2010;72(2):236–248.
10. Cohen LB, Ladas SD, Vargo JJ, et al. Sedation in digestive endoscopy: the Athens international position statements. *Aliment Pharmacol Ther.* 2010;32(3):425–442.
11. ASGE Standards of Practice Committee, Banerjee S, Shen B, Baron TH, et al. Antibiotic prophylaxis for GI endoscopy. *Gastrointest Endosc.* 2008;67(6):791–798.
12. ASGE Standards of Practice Committee, Anderson MA, Ben-Menachem T, Gan SI, et al. Management of antithrombotic agents for endoscopic procedures. *Gastrointest Endosc.* 2009;70(6):1060–1070.

Index

Page numbers followed by *f* refer to figures; page numbers followed by *t* refer to tables.